theclinics.com

HEART FAILURE CLINICS

Function Follows Form

GUEST EDITORS
Jagat Narula, MD, PhD
Gerald D. Buckberg, MD
Bijoy K. Khandheria, MBBS

July 2008 • Volume 4 • Number 3

SAUNDERS

An Imprint of Elsevier, Inc.
PHILADELPHIA LONDON TORONTO MONTREAL SYDNEY TOKYO

W.B. SAUNDERS COMPANY
A Division of Elsevier Inc.

1600 John F. Kennedy Boulevard. • Suite 1800 • Philadelphia, Pennsylvania 19103-2899

http://www.theclinics.com

HEART FAILURE CLINICS
July 2008
Editor: Barbara Cohen-Kligerman

Volume 4, Number 3
ISSN 1551-7136
ISBN-13: 978-1-4160-5782-6
ISBN-10: 1-4160-5782-X

Heart Failure Clinics (ISSN 1551-7136) is published quarterly by Elsevier Inc., 360 Park Avenue South, New York, NY 10010-1710. Months of publication are January, April, July, and October. Business and editorial offices: 1600 John F. Kennedy Boulevard, Suite 1800, Phliadelphia, PA 19103-2899. Customer service office: 6277 Sea Harbor Drive, Orlando, FL 32887-4800. Pending periodicals postage paid at New York, NY and additional mailing offices. Subscription prices are USD 179 per year for US individuals, USD 286 per year for US institutions, USD 62 per year for US students and residents, USD 215 per year for Canadian individuals, USD 321 per year for Canadian institutions, USD 215 per year for international individuals, USD 321 per year for international institutions and USD 74 per year for foreign students/residents. To receive student and resident rate, orders must be accompanied by name of affiliated institution, date of term, and the *signature* of program/residency coordinator on institution letterhead. Orders will be billed at individual rate until proof of status is received. Foreign air speed delivery is included in all *Clinics* subscription prices. All prices are subject to change without notice. POSTMASTER: Send address changes to *Heart Failure Clinics*, Elsevier Journals Customer Service, 6277 Sea Harbor Drive, Orlando, FL 32887-4800. **Customer Service: 1-800-654-2452 (US). From outside of the US, call (+1) 407-563-6020. Fax: 1-407-363-9661. E-mail: JournalCustomerService-usa@elsevier.com.**

Heart Failure Clinics is covered in *Index Medicus*.

Printed in the United States of America.

Cover artwork courtesy of Umberto M. Jezek.

CONSULTING EDITORS

RAGAVENDRA R. BALIGA, MD, MBA, Director, Section of Cardiovascular Medicine, University Hospital East; and Clinical Professor of Internal Medicine, The Ohio State University, Columbus, Ohio

JAMES B. YOUNG, MD, Chairman and Professor, Department of Medicine, Lerner College of Medicine; and George and Linda Kaufman Chair, Cleveland Clinic Foundation, Case Western Reserve University; Cleveland, Ohio

GUEST EDITORS

JAGAT NARULA, MD, PhD, Professor of Medicine; Chief, Division of Cardiology; and Associate Dean, University of California Irvine College of Medicine, Orange, California

GERALD D. BUCKBERG, MD, Distinguished Professor of Surgery, David Geffen School of Medicine, University of California Los Angeles, Los Angeles, California

BIJOY K. KHANDHERIA, MBBS, Professor of Medicine and Chair, Division of Cardiovascular Diseases, Mayo Clinic, Scottsdale, Arizona

CONTRIBUTORS

ROBERT H. ANDERSON, MD, Professor of Medicine, Cardiac Unit of Child Health, Pediatrics Cardiac Morphology, National Heart and Lung Institute, Imperial College, London, United Kingdom

CONSTANTINE L. ATHANASULEAS, MD, Professor of Surgery, Division of Cardiothoracic Surgery, University of Alabama Birmingham, Birmingham, Alabama

NICHOLAS AYACHE, PhD, Professor, Institut National de Recherche en Informatique et en Automatique, Asclepios Project, Sophia Antipolis, France

MANEL BALLESTER, MD, Faculty of Medicine, University of Lleida, Barcelona, Spain

MAREK BELOHLAVEK, MD, PhD, Professor of Medicine and Biomedical Engineering, Division of Cardiovascular Diseases, Mayo Clinic, Scottsdale, Arizona

FLORENCE BILLET, MSc, PhD Candidate, Institut National de Recherche en Informatique et en Automatique, Asclepios Project, Sophia Antipolis, France

GERALD D. BUCKBERG, MD, Distinguished Professor of Surgery, David Geffen School of Medicine, University of California Los Angeles, Los Angeles, California

ROBERT BURKE, MD, Peter J. Grant Fellow in Echocardiography, Division of Cardiovascular Diseases, Mayo Clinic, Scottsdale, Arizona

FRANCESC CARRERAS, MD, Hospital de la Santa Creu i Sant Pau, Barcelona, Spain

PHANI CHINCHAPATNAM, PhD, Research Fellow, Centre for Medical Image Computing, University College London, London, United Kingdom

CECIL COGHLAN, MD, Professor of Medicine, University of Alabama at Birmingham, Birmingham, Alabama

SABINE DÄBRITZ, MD, Professor of Medicine, Department of Grown-Up Congenital Heart Disease, University Hospital Münster, EMAH-Zentrum, Münster, Germany

BART W.L. de BOECK, MD, Department of Cardiology, University Medical Centre, Utrecht, the Netherlands

HERVÉ DELINGETTE, PhD, Professor, Institut National de Recherche en Informatique et en Automatique, Asclepios Project, Sophia Antipolis, France

ANA FERREIRA, MD, Hospital Royo Villanova, Zaragoza, Spain

MORTEZA GHARIB, PhD, Professor, Option in Bioengineering; and Hans W. Liepmann Professor of Aeronautics, Graduate Aeronautical Laboratories, California Institute of Technology, Pasadena, California

ANNA GROSBERG, PhD, Post-Doctoral Scholar, Option in Bioengineering, California Institute of Technology, Pasadena, California

JULIEN I.E. HOFFMAN, MD, Professor of Pediatrics (Emeritus) and Senior Member, Cardiovascular Research Institute, University of California, San Francisco, California

ARSHAD JAHANGIR, MD, Associate Professor of Medicine, Division of Cardiovascular Diseases, Mayo Clinic, Rochester, Minnesota

ROY C.P. KERCKHOFFS, PhD, Assistant Project Scientist, Department of Bioengineering, The Whitaker Institute for Biomedical Engineering, University of California San Diego, La Jolla, California

BIJOY K. KHANDHERIA, MBBS, Professor of Medicine and Chair, Division of Cardiovascular Diseases, Mayo Clinic, Scottsdale, Arizona

PAUL P. LUNKENHEIMER, MD, Professor of Physiology and Pathophysiology, Experimental Thoraco-vascular Surgery, University of Münster, Münster, Germany

JOS G. MAESSEN, MD, PhD, Department of Cardiothoracic Surgery, Cardiovascular Research Institute Maastricth, Maastricht, the Netherlands

AMAN MAHAJAN, MD, PhD, Associate Professor, Cardiac Anesthesiology, David Geffen School of Medicine, University of California Los Angeles, Los Angeles, California

TOMMASO MANSI, MSc, PhD Candidate, Institut National de Recherche en Informatique et en Automatique, Asclepios Project, Sophia Antipolis, France

ANDREW D. McCULLOCH, PhD, Professor and Chair, Department of Bioengineering, The Whitaker Institute for Biomedical Engineering, University of California San Diego, La Jolla, California

TIM McQUINN, MD, Associate Professor, Department of Cell Biology and Anatomy; and Associate Professor of Pediatric Cardiology, Medical University of South Carolina, Charleston, South Carolina

LAWRENCE J. MULLIGAN, PhD, Senior Principal Scientist, Therapy Delivery Systems/Leads Research, Medtronic Inc., Mounds View, Minnesota

SANJIV M. NARAYAN, MD, FACC, Director of Cardiac Electrophysiology, Veterans Affairs Medical Center, University of California, San Diego, California

JAGAT NARULA, MD, PhD, Professor of Medicine; Chief, Division of Cardiology; and Associate Dean, University of California Irvine College of Medicine, Orange, California

PETER NIEDERER, MD, Professor of Biomedical Engineering, Institute of Biomedical Engineering, ETH and University of Zurich, Zurich, Switzerland

JEFFREY H. OMENS, PhD, Professor, Department of Medicine; and Department of Bioengineering, University of California San Diego, La Jolla, California

JEAN-MARC PEYRAT, MSc, PhD Candidate, Institut National de Recherche en Informatique et en Automatique, Asclepios Project, Sophia Antipolis, France

FRITZ W. PRINZEN, PhD, Department of Physiology, Cardiovascular Research Institute Maastricth, Maastricht, the Netherlands

LEONARD M. RADEMAKERS, MD, Department of Cardiothoracic Surgery, Cardiovascular Research Institute Maastricht, Maastricht, the Netherlands

REZA RAZAVI, MD, Professor, Division of Imaging Sciences, King's College London, The Rayne Institute, St. Thomas Hospital, London, United Kingdom

KLAUS REDMANN, MD, Senior Scientist, Experimental Thoraco-vascular Surgery, University of Münster, Münster, Germany

KAWAL RHODE, PhD, Lecturer, Division of Imaging Sciences, King's College London, The Rayne Institute, St. Thomas Hospital, London, United Kingdom

KAI ROTHAUS, MD, Senior Scientist, Institut für Informatik, University of Münster, Münster, Germany

SALEH SALEH, MD, Clinical Associate Professor of Medicine, David Geffen School of Medicine, University of California Los Angeles, Los Angeles, California

PETER SCHMID, MD, Senior Scientist, Institute of Biomedical Engineering, ETH and University of Zurich, Zurich, Switzerland

DAVID SEDMERA, MD, PhD, Lab Head, Institute of Animal Physiology and Genetics, Laboratory of Cardiovascular Morphogenesis; and Associate Professor, Institute of Anatomy, First Faculty of Medicine, Charles University, Prague, Czech Republic

PARTHO P. SENGUPTA, MBBS, MD, DM, Assistant Professor of Medicine, Division of Cardiovascular Diseases, Mayo Clinic, Scottsdale, Arizona

MAXIME SERMESANT, PhD, Research Scientist and Lecturer, Institut National de Recherche en Informatique et en Automatique, Asclepios Project, Sophia Antipolis, France; Division of Imaging Sciences, King's College London, The Rayne Institute, St. Thomas Hospital, London, United Kingdom

MORTEN SMERUP, MD, PhD, Senior Scientist, Department of Cardiothoracic and Vascular Surgery, University Hospital, Århus, Denmark

JÖRG STYPMANN, MD, Senior Scientist, Medizinische Klinik und Poliklinik C—Kardiologie und Angiologie, University of Münster, Münster, Germany

FERNANDO TONDATO, MD, Division of Cardiovascular Diseases, Mayo Clinic, Scottsdale, Arizona

CONTENTS

FORTHCOMING ISSUES

October 2008

Renal Disease in Heart Failure
George Bakris, MD, *Guest Editor*

January 2009

Hemodynamic Monitoring in the Diagnosis and Management of Heart Failure
Ragavendra R. Baliga, MD, MBA,
and William T. Abraham, MD, *Guest Editors*

April 2009

Management of Heart Failure in the Emergency Department
W. Frank Peacock, MD,
and James F. Neuenschwander II, MD, FACEP,
Guest Editors

RECENT ISSUES

April 2008

The Role of Statins in Heart Failure
Gregg C. Fonarow, MD, *Guest Editor*

January 2008

Diastolic Dysfunction and Heart Failure
Manni A. Vannan, MBBS,
and Bertram Pitt, MD, *Guest Editors*

October 2007

Heart Failure in the Elderly
Wilbert S. Aronow, MD, *Guest Editor*

ELSEVIER
SAUNDERS

Heart Failure Clin 4 (2008) xiii–xix

HEART
FAILURE
CLINICS

Editorial

The Concertina Pump

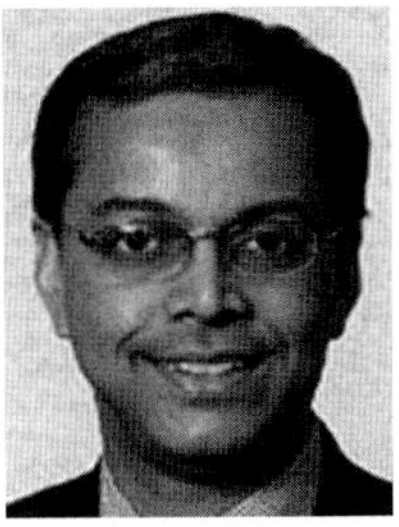

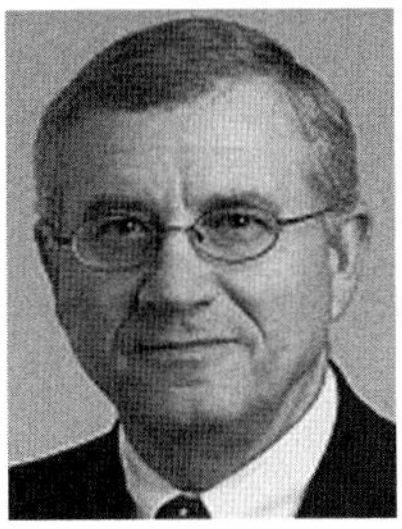

Ragavendra R. Baliga, MD, MBA James B. Young, MD
Consulting Editors

> When I first gave my mind to vivisection, as a means of discovering the motions and uses of the heart, and sought to discover these from actual inspection, and not from the writings of others, I found the task so truly arduous, so full of difficulties, that I was almost tempted to think, with Fracastorius, that the motion of the heart was only to be comprehended by God.
>
> —William Harvey, *Exercitatio Anatomica de Motu Cordis et Sanguinis in Animalibus*, 1628, as quoted by E.H. Starling in his Linacre Lecture on the Law of the Heart, 1918.

In the second century AD, Galen proposed that there were two distinct types of blood: "nutritive blood" that was made by the liver and carried through veins to the organs where it was consumed, and "vital blood" that was made by the heart and then flowed through arteries to carry the "vital spirits." Galen also proposed that the heart served not to pump blood but to suck it in from the veins. Galen taught that blood flowed through the septum of the heart from one ventricle to the other through a system of tiny pores. He was unaware that the blood left each ventricle through arteries.

Galen's teachings remained unchallenged until 1628, when William Harvey proposed that there is more to "blood flowing in and blood flowing out." In his book, *Exercitatio Anatomica de Motu Cordis et Sanguinis in Animalibus* (On the Movement of the Heart and Blood in Animals), Harvey proposed that "blood flows in and blood is pumped out" by the heart. It is hard to imagine the notions going through Galen's mind and Harvey's mind when they looked at static anatomy and tried to determine the function of the heart, let alone the anatomy and the pathophysiology. Nonetheless, they set the stage for more remarkable iconoclastic views of heart pump muscle function. More recently, Robinson, Factor, and Sonnenblick combined both Galen and Harveys' observations and concepts to propose that the heart is a "suction pump" [1], wherein the "blood is sucked in and then blood is pumped out" by the heart.

In this editorial, we would like to bring to your attention to another iconoclastic emerging concept that suggests, in addition to having the properties of a suction pump, the heart functions as a sort of twisting bellows pump that is similar to the accordion or concertina air drivers (Fig. 1). What beautiful music can, indeed, be made by this pump.

The accordion or the bellows pump acts by the positive displacement principle, generating both suction and compression with expanding cavity volume on the suction side and a decreasing cavity

1551-7136/08/$ - see front matter
doi:10.1016/j.hfc.2008.04.003

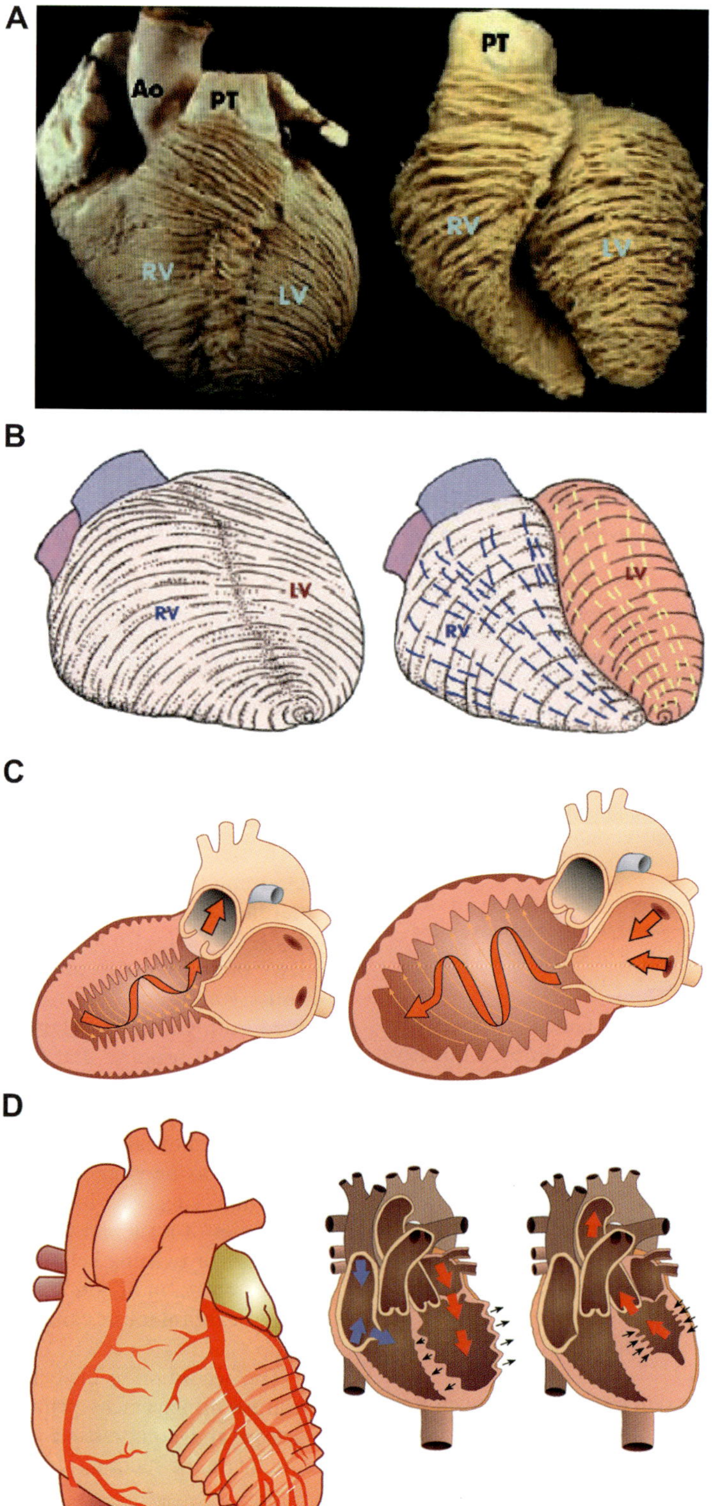
A
Ao
PT
RV
LV
PT
RV
LV
B
RV
LV
RV
LV
C
D

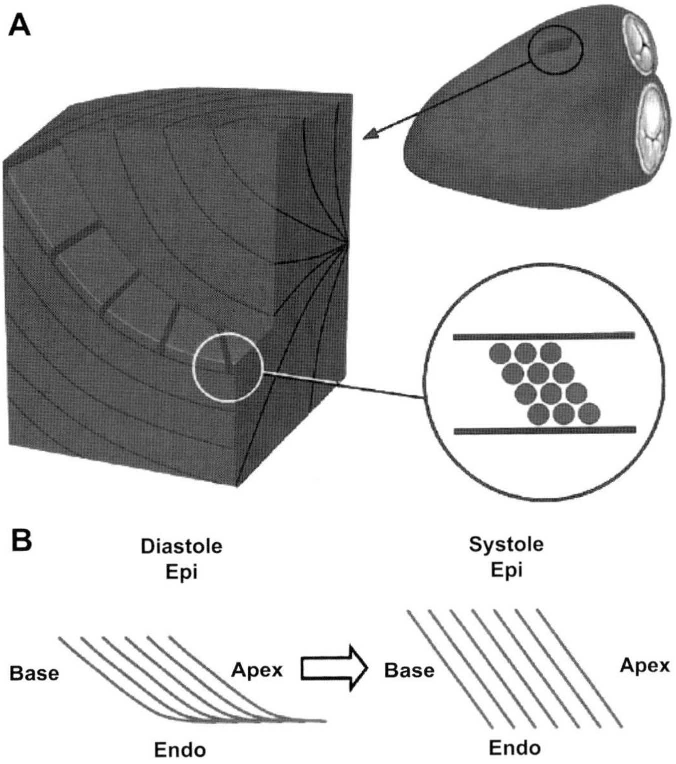

Fig. 2. (*A*) Myocardial fiber and sheet orientation within a block of muscle excised from the anterior wall of the left ventricle. Myocytes lie in planes parallel to the long axis of the heart. Within these planes, myocyte orientation is circumferential at the mid-wall, but rotates clockwise (when viewed from the outside) to form a 60 degree left-handed helix in the epicardium (Epi) and counterclockwise to a +60 degree right-handed helix in the endocardium (Endo). Myocytes are organized into sheets 4 cells thick that are stacked like shingles. (*B*) Myocardial sheet movement during cardiac cycle. During systole, due to rearrangement of myocytes, sheets are becoming more perpendicular toward the endocardium, thus helping to transform a 14 percent decrease in myocyte length to 40 percent thickening of the left ventricular wall. (*From* Thomas JD, Popovic ZB. Assessment of left ventricular function by cardiac ultrasound. J Am Coll Cardiol 2006;48(10):2012–25; with permission.)

volume on the discharge side. Liquid flows into the pumps as the cavity on the suction side expands and the liquid flows out of the discharge as the cavity collapses. The volume is constant, given each cycle of operation, and alternating positive and negative pressure is developed. The bellows pump is used to generate whirlpools. The accordion properties of the left ventricle, therefore, could also explain the suction effect of the embryonic and adult heart [1–3]. The accordion, or the "squeezebox" in common parlance, is able to generate the maximum intensity of sound energy when

Fig. 1. (*A, B*) Muscular architecture demonstrating the feasibility of the concertina or bellows mechanism The upper panels are sequential dissections by Professor Damian Sanchez-Quintana, University of Extremadura, Spain. (*A*) A normal heart viewed from the front shows the circumferential to oblique arrangement of the myofibers in the subepicardium. (*B*) Myofibers lying deeper than the subepicardium retain the circumferential arrangement in the right ventricle but change from oblique to circumferential in the left ventricle. The lower panels depict, in simplistic fashion, the subepicardial myofibers (*left panel*) and the deeper myofibers (*right panel*) in the ventricles of the normal heart. (*C, D*) Artist's rendition of the concertina pump. Ao, aorta; CS, coronary sinus; ICV, inferior caval vein; LA, left atrium; LV, left ventricle; PT, pulmonary trunk; RA, right atrium; RV, right ventricle. (*Parts A and B from* Ho SY, Nihoyannopoulos P. Anatomy, echocardiography, and normal right ventricular dimensions. Heart 2006;92(Suppl 1):i2–13; with permission; and *Parts C and D courtesy of* Dennis Mathias, Ohio State University Cardiovascular Division, Columbus, OH.)

it is most expanded before the musician compresses it to generate the sound. Similarly, one can visualize the heart being able to generate the highest cardiac output when it contracts from a maximally relaxed state. The converse is possibly true that when the heart is not maximally relaxed, it is more likely to generate a lesser cardiac output, which may result in symptoms of heart failure when it is not commensurate with the requirements of the body. We would like to propose that the heart functions as a gyrating accordion or concertina.

The walls of the ventricles itself undergo pleating, like an accordion in animal models [4], and, more recently, myocardial disarray in the form of clefts or fissures has been described in humans [5]. In a sheep model of myocardial wall thickening of the left ventricle, one group of investigators found that laminar deformation, when combined with lateral transmural distribution of alternating families of myocardial sheets, created an accordion-like wall thickening mechanism [4]. The mechanism by which myocyte contraction is translated into this pattern of sheet deformation is not completely understood, but one mechanism postulated is that the extracellular collagen matrix provides a coupling between the fiber and the sheets.

Myocardial fiber orientation varies from approximately -60 degrees at the epicardium to 60 degrees at the endocardium in several species (Fig. 2). The directions of fiber and cleavage planes were inferred indirectly from three orthogonal views until recently [6]. Using methods developed by JC Criscione to measure directly sheet orientations across the left ventricle (LV) wall, Ashikaga and colleagues [7] found a relatively uniform transmural distribution of negative myocardial sheet angles (β) in the anterior wall of the canine heart. The same group, studying the anterolateral region of the ovine heart, found a hitherto unknown alternating transmural angular distribution of two separate sheet families. The presence of these families allowed a new interpretation of myocardial mechanics that suggested accordion- or concertina-like properties of the heart. Radial thickening of the ventricular wall during systole is an important contributor to normal LV function because of its role in increasing stroke volume [8,9] and its sensitivity to hypoperfusion of the myocardium [10]. LeGrice and colleagues [11] suggested that (a) sliding of adjacent myocardial sheets along their cleavage planes due to inter-laminar transverse shear played a major role in systolic wall thickening in the subendocardium, and (b) the magnitude of ventricular wall thickening due to shearing of the laminae is dependent on the initial cleavage plane orientation and myocardial sheets have opposite signs of transverse shear when oriented perpendicular to each other. In fact, most systolic wall thickening could be accounted for by laminar thinning or thickening and extension, together with interlaminar transverse shear. Harrington and colleagues' transmural myocardial sheet characterization provides additional information into these models of wall thickening [4]. In Fig. 3, they show how combining their

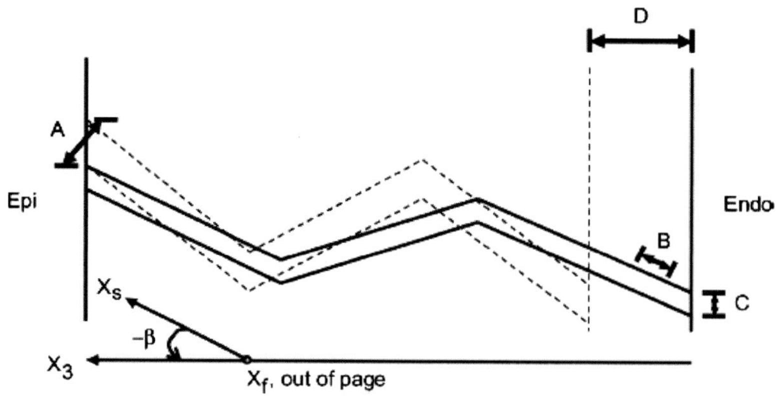

Fig. 3. Two-dimensional representation of the plane, which, in reality, twists through the wall, as the sheets are perpendicular to the helically progressing fibers across the wall. (*Solid and dashed lines*) Lateral myolaminar sheets in systole and diastole, respectively. With alternating sheet families through the wall, wall thickening (D) may be due to laminar transverse shear (A), laminar extension (B), and laminar thinning (C) of each population. (*From* Harrington KB, Rodriguez F, Cheng A, et al. Direct measurement of transmural laminar architecture in the anterolateral wall of the ovine left ventricle: new implications for wall thickening mechanics. Am J Physiol Heart Circ Physiol 2005;288(3):H1324–30; with permission.)

A

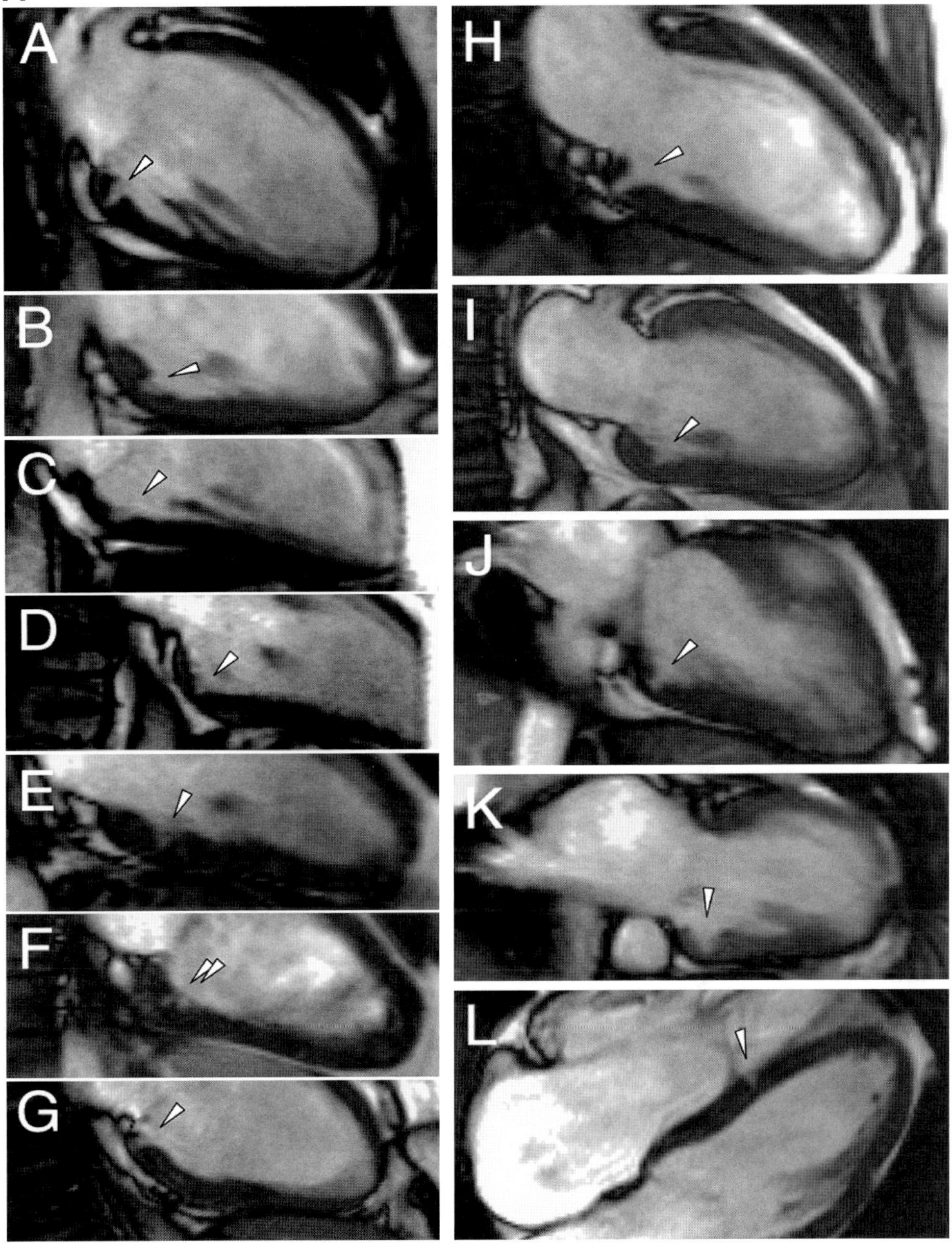

Fig. 4. (*A*) Clefts seen in 7 volunteers and 5 patients. (A to G) Vertical long-axis cine images in all 7 of the 120 healthy volunteers studied who had clefts (*arrowheads*) visible in diastole in the basal inferior wall. (H to K) Comparable appearances in patients who had (H) hypertrophic cardiomyopathy, (I) systemic hypertension, (J) repaired tetralogy of Fallot, and (K) relieved pulmonary stenosis. (L) Arrowhead pointing to a cleft from the right ventricular side in the interventricular septum of a patient who had repaired tetralogy of Fallot, located adjacent to the insertions of right ventricular trabecular bands. (*B*) Clefts viewed in specifically aligned orthogonal planes short-axis (A, B), oblique long-axis (C, D), and tangential (E, F) diastolic images of a male patient with suspected hypertrophic cardiomyopathy. The left ventricular mass index of 93 g/m^2 was just within normal limits. In A, C, and E, the arrowheads point to an anteroseptal cleft, which was shown in other views to penetrate to a very small muscular ventricular septal defect in early systole, occluding later in systole. In B, D, and F, the arrowheads point to an inferoseptal cleft. Dotted lines and arrows indicate the relative orientations of slices. Note that both clefts were located adjacent to the insertion of the right ventricle into the left ventricle (A, B). (*From* Johansson B, Maceira AM, Babu-Narayan S, et al. Clefts can be seen in the basal inferior wall of the left ventricle and the interventricular septum in healthy volunteers as well as patients by cardiovascular magnetic resonance. J Am Coll Cardiol 2007;50(13):1294–5; with permission.)

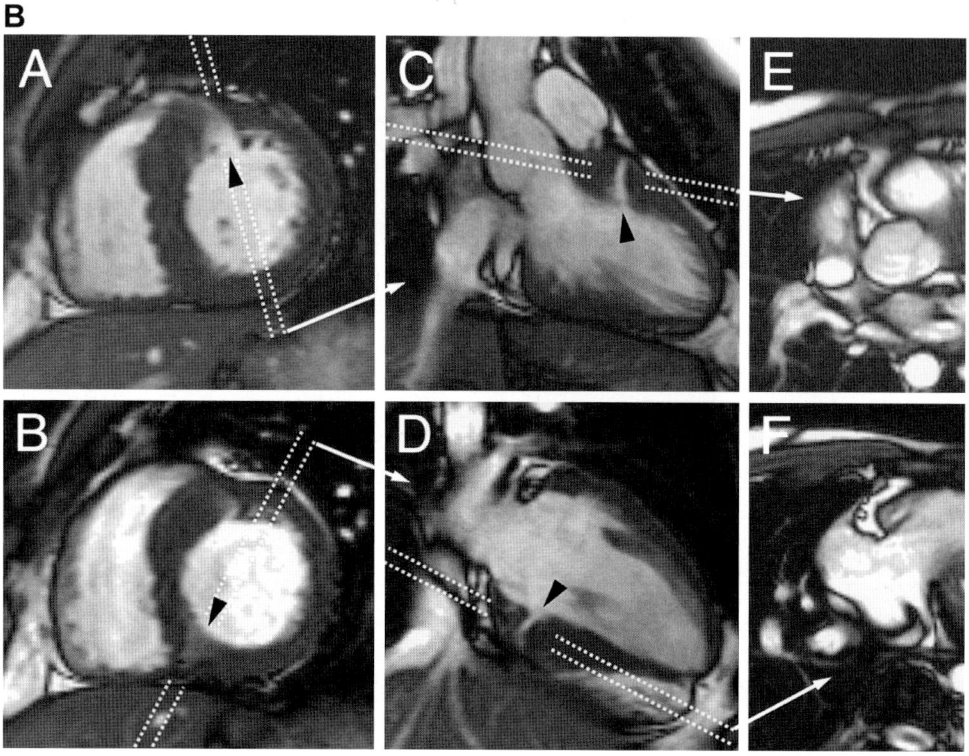

Fig. 4 (*continued*)

lateral transmural distribution of alternating families of myocardial sheets with a two-dimensional representation of how previously described mechanisms of laminar deformation creates an accordion-like thickening of the ventricular wall. In fact, the accordion configuration reported by them may facilitate wall thickening by way of laminar shear in the cylindrical ventricle. They argued that indeed, if only one population of sheets were present throughout the wall from epicardium to endocardium, thickening due to laminar shear could happen only if the endocardium moved parallel to the epicardium as much as they move away from each other (ie, thickening and shearlike translocation would). They also suggested that alternating shear displacement within the wall is allowed by the accordion laminar distribution such that minimal shear displacement of the epicardium occurs relative to the endocardium. In this mechanism proposed by Harrington and colleagues, the shear deformation can be similar throughout the myocardial wall, but the direction of sheet sliding alternates. Similarly, the basal anterior region has the reverse accordion distribution. In addition to the concertina effect, the heart undergoes torsion before completing systole—the "gyrating" accordion. It is likely that as the heart stiffens in left ventricular hypertrophy, the accordion mechanism is less forceful, resulting in diastolic dysfunction. Perhaps a better understanding of this will prompt newer and more innovative approaches to the prevention of diastolic dysfunction.

Magnetic resonance steady-state free-precession (SSFP) cine imaging of the heart is capable of presenting excellent contrast between the blood and the myocardium with outstanding in-plane resolution of interstitial spaces (or thin structures), as long as their boundaries extend parallel to the elongated voxels, orthogonal to the plane of acquisition [5,12]. This increased resolution has allowed another group of investigators [5] to describe clefts in the wall of the left ventricle and the interventricular septum in some healthy volunteers (Fig. 4A,B). These intramyocardial fissures or clefts suggest that the myocardium is capable of disarray. Better resolution of imaging techniques may allow visualization of accordion-like wall thickening and clefts in human left ventricles proposed in this editorial. Further investigation of myocardial sheet mechanics in the human heart with particular attention to transmural microstructure and wall thickening mechanism may be the key to understanding normal left ventricular systole and diastole. This characterization of myocardial architecture is also important because the degradation of collagen in myocardial disease states has been described to alter baseline fiber architecture [13, 14] and therefore contribute to the understanding of ventricular function and dysfunction [15].

In our proposed model, where the heart functions like a gyrating accordion (like the motion of twisting a washcloth) with the torsion of the LV and contraction of the bellows sucking blood from the atrium and generate, the vortices more recently described in the contracting left ventricle assume new meaning and particular importance, while allowing us to focus on different medical and surgical therapies to correct harmful cardiac remodeling. In this exciting issue on myocardial mechanics edited by Drs. Jagat Narula, Geoffrey Buckberg, and Bijoy Khandheria, there are more provocative (and controversial) articles on myocardial mechanics. We hope that this hypothesis-generating editorial, and all of the articles in this issue, will stimulate further research in this area.

We would like to close this editorial, as we began, with the words of William Harvey: "All we know is still infinitely less than all that remains unknown."

Ragavendra R. Baliga, MD, MBA
The Ohio State University
Columbus, OH, USA

E-mail address: Ragavendra.Baliga@osumc.edu

James B. Young, MD
Division of Medicine
Lerner College of Medicine
Cleveland Clinic
Cleveland, OH, USA

E-mail address: YOUNGJ@ccf.org

References

[1] Robinson TF, Factor SM, Sonnenblick EH. The heart as a suction pump. Sci Am 1986;254(6):84–91.
[2] Buckberg GD, Castellá M, Gharib M, et al. Active myocyte shortening during the 'isovolumetric relaxation' phase of diastole is responsible for ventricular suction; 'systolic ventricular filling'. Eur J Cardiothorac Surg 2006;29(Suppl 1):S98–106.
[3] Forouhar AS, Liebling M, Hickerson A, et al. The embryonic vertebrate heart tube is a dynamic suction pump. Science 2006;312(5774):751–3.
[4] Harrington KB, Rodriguez F, Cheng A, et al. Direct measurement of transmural laminar architecture in the anterolateral wall of the ovine left ventricle: new implications for wall thickening mechanics. Am J Physiol Heart Circ Physiol 2005;288(3): H1324–30.
[5] Johansson B, Maceira AM, Babu-Narayan S, et al. Clefts can be seen in the basal inferior wall of the left ventricle and the interventricular septum in healthy volunteers as well as patients by cardiovascular magnetic resonance. J Am Coll Cardiol 2007;50(13): 1294–5.
[6] Costa KD, Takayama Y, McCulloch AD, et al. Laminar fiber architecture and three-dimensional systolic mechanics in canine ventricular myocardium. Am J Physiol 1999;276(2 Pt 2):H595–607.
[7] Ashikaga H, Criscione JC, Omens JH, et al. Transmural left ventricular mechanics underlying torsional recoil during relaxation. Am J Physiol Heart Circ Physiol 2004;286(2):H640–7.
[8] Dumesnil JG, Shoucri RM. Quantitative relationships between left ventricular ejection and wall thickening and geometry. J Appl Physiol 1991;70(1): 48–54.
[9] Gould KL, Kennedy JW, Frimer M, et al. Analysis of wall dynamics and directional components of left ventricular contraction in man. Am J Cardiol 1976; 38(3):322–31.
[10] Gallagher KP, Gerren RA, Stirling MC, et al. The distribution of functional impairment across the lateral border of acutely ischemic myocardium. Circ Res 1986;58(4):570–83.
[11] LeGrice IJ, Takayama Y, Covell JW. Transverse shear along myocardial cleavage planes provides a mechanism for normal systolic wall thickening. Circ Res 1995;77(1):182–93.
[12] Maceira AM, Prasad SK, Khan M, et al. Normalized left ventricular systolic and diastolic function by steady state free precession cardiovascular magnetic resonance. J Cardiovasc Magn Reson 2006; 8(3):417–26.
[13] Weis SM, Emery JL, Becker KD, et al. Myocardial mechanics and collagen structure in the osteogenesis imperfecta murine (oim). Circ Res 2000;87(8): 663–9.
[14] Chen J, Song SK, Liu W, et al. Remodeling of cardiac fiber structure after infarction in rats quantified with diffusion tensor MRI. Am J Physiol Heart Circ Physiol 2003;285(3):H946–54.
[15] Weber KT, Sun Y, Tyagi SC, et al. Collagen network of the myocardium: function, structural remodeling and regulatory mechanisms. J Mol Cell Cardiol 1994;26(3):279–92.
[16] Thomas JD, Popovic ZB. Assessment of left ventricular function by cardiac ultrasound. J Am Coll Cardiol 2006;48(10):2012–25.

ELSEVIER
SAUNDERS

Heart Failure Clin 4 (2008) xxi–xxii

HEART
FAILURE
CLINICS

Preface

It Is Not Just a Squeezebox!

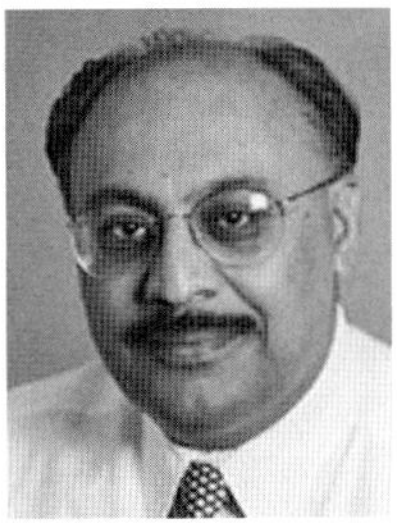

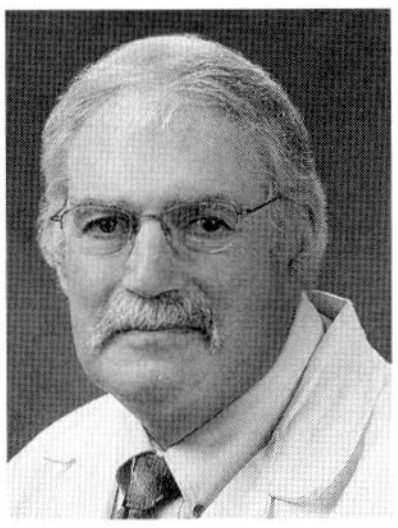

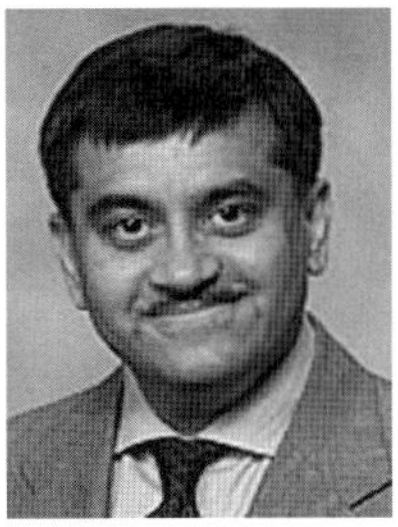

Jagat Narula, MD, PhD   Gerald D. Buckberg, MD   Bijoy K. Khandheria, MBBS
Guest Editors

The heart has always been perceived as a squeezebox, with blood flowing in and out of cardiac chambers and supporting the metabolic demands of the body. This simplistic explanation of pump function has prevailed for centuries. Sporadic strokes of discontent with this philosophy, coupled with unorthodox descriptions, have often made ripples that became lost in the ocean of data focusing upon ejection fraction and myocardial contractility.

The heart has been perceived as a squeezebox since the era of Leonardo da Vinci [1], who painted the left ventricle wall with uniform thickness. Centuries later, Wiggers [2] proposed the left ventricle as a pressure chamber whereby aortic and left ventricular pressures were presumed to be identical during all of systole; peak flow followed the peak pressure, as intraventricular pressure rose faster than the movement of fluid. Noble [3] contradicted this notion by making simultaneous pressure measurements in the left ventricle and the aortic root. His studies revealed higher left ventricular pressure during the first half of systole and higher aortic pressure in the second half of systole, which created a paradoxical observation that the blood flow from the left ventricle could continue to enter into the aorta against the positive pressure gradient. Noble [3] proposed that this type of pressure pattern would result from a flow momentum, yet this idea was overshadowed by the prevailing theories of cardiac ejection and pressure propulsion.

A fundamental problem in understanding cardiac function may relate to overdependence on comprehending the heart's action based upon variables deduced from pressure curves. If pressure is defined as force per unit area, then the force of moving blood and the momentum of flow may become the primary variable, and pressure may reflect a secondary variable that is derived from the average force of the moving blood. In any momentum system, pressure becomes a variable that is quantified only at boundary layers where the velocity is impeded. During transfer of momentum between the heart muscle and blood, the muscle must somehow sense the rheologic sequence of the blood and then respond to it with an impulse that is consistent with rheologic efficiency. Although blood has inertia as it enters the cardiac chambers, streams intermingle without chaos. During the ejection phase into the aorta, blood is propelled in the opposite direction with immaculate synchrony. During this interval, chaos and turbulence may be a graveyard for

1551-7136/08/$ - see front matter
doi:10.1016/j.hfc.2008.05.001

erythrocytes, but stagnation may perpetuate thrombosis. Consequently, flow swirls emerge spontaneously to prevent hemodynamic stasis.

Numerous questions arise. How does this muscular organ work so meticulously? How does it maintain such an organized pattern for eight or more decades without a breather? What is the nature of such an energy-efficient performance that does not exhaust itself, an action that differs from the limited endurance of skeletal muscle? How is traffic regulated through the ventricular cavities? What maintains the smooth and harmonious opening and closing of valves? How do valvular oars facilitate flow through the cardiac chambers? The ingenuity of myocardial fiber architecture, the peculiarity of looping of the cardiac tube, and biochemical heterogeneity of muscle fibers have been proposed to explain the most exquisite pump that the nature has engineered.

This issue of *Heart Failure Clinics*, entitled "Function Follows Form," involves our effort to offer you the intricacies of this unique pump. To accomplish this task, we have been fortunate to receive contributions from established investigators. This issue is divided into four parts: embryologic evolution of the myocardium, myocardial architecture, clinical correlates of the morphology, and applications of this knowledge to clinical management of the afflictions of the myocardium. The organizational pattern aims to develop presentations that are of equal interest to basic scientists and clinicians. We hope that our issue will generate cross-talk and simultaneously convince the readers that we are not dealing with just another squeezebox! The heart is an example of evolution at its best!

Jagat Narula, MD, PhD
University of California
Irvine, CA, USA

E-mail address: Narula@uci.edu

Gerald D. Buckberg, MD
University of California
Los Angeles, CA, USA

E-mail address: gbuckberg@mednet.ucla.edu

Bijoy K. Khandheria, MBBS
Mayo Clinic
Scottsdale, AZ, USA

E-mail address: Khandheria@mayo.edu

References

[1] Holmes KC. Muscle contraction. Novartis Found Symp 1998;213:76–89 [discussion 89–92].

[2] Wiggers CJ. Some significant advances in cardiac physiology during the nineteenth century. Bull Hist Med 1960;34:1–15.

[3] Noble MI. The contribution of blood momentum to left ventricular ejection in dog. Circulation Res 1968;26:663–70.

ELSEVIER
SAUNDERS

Heart Failure Clin 4 (2008) 235–245

HEART
FAILURE
CLINICS

Embryogenesis of the Heart Muscle

David Sedmera, MD, PhD[a,b,*], Tim McQuinn, MD[c]

[a]*Institute of Animal Physiology and Genetics, Prague, Czech Republic*
[b]*Charles University, Prague, Czech Republic*
[c]*Medical University of South Carolina, Charleston, SC, USA*

This article focuses on the development of two distinct components of the myocardium: the so-called "working myocardium," which encompasses the bulk of the cardiac mass, and the specialized network of pacemaking and conduction myocardium, known as the cardiac conduction system. Of course, the heart contains other critical tissues, including serous and fibrous covering (epicardium), fibrous tissue derivatives (valves and cardiac skeleton), blood supply (coronary arteries and cardiac veins), and an endocardial lining. Each of these tissues is important for proper heart function, and the developmental story of each is the subject of much ongoing research. For those interested in an overview of these dynamic subfields and for an introduction to these topics, the reader is referred to a recent dedicated handbook, ML Kirby's *Cardiac development* [1].

Before one can consider the working myocardium and cardiac conduction system populations in detail, the events that lead to the formation of at least the tubular heart from the precardiac mesoderm have to be addressed, and current knowledge of genes involved in myocardial differentiation needs to be summarized.

This research was supported by the National Institutes of Health grant RR16434, MSMT VZ 206100-3, AS CR AVOZ50450515, and the Purkinje Fellowship of the Academy of Sciences of the Czech Republic. This work was conducted in part in a facility constructed with support from the National Institutes of Health, Grant Number C06 RR018823 from the Extramural Research Facilities Program of the National Center for Research Resources.

* Corresponding author. Laboratory of Cardiovascular Morphogenesis, Institute of Animal Physiology and Genetics, Videnska 1083, 142 20 Prague 4 - Krc, Czech Republic.

E-mail address: sedmera@iapg.cas.cz (D. Sedmera).

Early stages of heart formation

The heart takes its origin from paired cardiac mesodermal primordia that fuse in the midline to create a primitive tubular heart [2]. Soon after initiation of a heartbeat, the cardiac tube undergoes a process of looping, which leads to creation of the first grossly visible asymmetry in the embryo. The looped heart then enters a period of chamber formation, with five compartments identifiable by morphologic as well as molecular criteria. Following the blood flow, the first segment is the sinus venosus. The sinus venosus functions as a blood reservoir and pacemaker of the heart, which correlates with its more robust expression of genes necessary for spontaneous action potential generation [3]. Morphologically and histologically, the sinus venosus is characterized by thin walls, small cell size, and scarce intracellular myofibrils. Next come the yet unseparated atrial chambers, with faster impulse propagation, absence of cardiac jelly, and no trabeculae (although they develop the pectinate muscles later on). The third segment is the atrioventricular channel. Atrioventricular channel myocardium is noted for a strongly circular myofiber alignment, as well as a lining of cardiac jelly; it also exhibits a slow conduction velocity. This gives it the role of delay generator for conduction between the atrial and ventricular myocardium (similar to the function of the atrioventricular node in the mature heart). The cardiac jelly is molded into atrioventricular cushions, which participate later on in chamber septation and formation

1551-7136/08/$ - see front matter
doi:10.1016/j.hfc.2008.02.007

of the atrioventricular valves. Next come the ventricles, which are distinguished by development of an extensive trabecular network on the luminal side, fast impulse propagation, and most rapid differentiation of myocytes with respect to their contractility, channels, and energy metabolism.

Most of the remaining discussion will focus on development of the ventricular myocardium, because the ventricles are the main pumping chambers of the heart, and cardiac failure is essentially failure of the ventricles. The last myocardial segment in the tubular heart is the conotruncus, or the outflow tract. Similar to the atrioventricular canal, the conotruncus myocardium also has the characteristic of the earlier primitive tube [4]: that is, slow conduction [5,6] and prevailing circular myocyte alignment. Derived from the secondary heart field, it is a transitory structure that undergoes extensive remodeling to give rise to important structures in the mature heart. The outflow cushions take part in division of the cardiac outlet into an aortic and pulmonary component, and their distal parts form the semilunar valves. The conotruncus myocardium mostly disappears through apoptosis [7], with the exception of the portion forming the pulmonary infundibulum.

Box 1. Genes involved in differentiation of myocardial lineage

Transcription factors (targets)
GATA
Nkx
Myocardin
MEF
Tbx
SRF

Stimulation
Activin
TGFbeta
Wnt (non-canonical)
BMP
FGF
Shh

Inhibition
Wnt (canonical)
Notch
Noggin

Data from Kirby ML. Cardiac development. New York: Oxford University Press; 2007.

Molecular determination of cardiac lineage

The cardiomyocytes differentiate from horseshoe-shaped mesodermal primordia (Box 1). In vitro studies have shown that there are more of these cells capable of forming cardiac myocytes than what actually occurs in vivo [8], pointing to a combination of positive and negative regulators of cardiomyogenic differentiation. A list of currently identified genes participating in commitment to, as well as restriction of this program, derived from a recent reference [1], is provided for overview (see Box 1).

Structure and function of the tubular heart

Although already diversified functionally [9], there is minimal variation in structure along the early cardiac tube (Fig. 1, Video 1). In sections, the tube is composed of a one or two cells-thick myocardial mantle, an acellular cardiac jelly, and the endocardium. The first morphologic sign of regional myocardial diversification can be perceived in more pronounced circumferential arrangement of actin and fibronectin [10] in the inner layer. Regional differences in myofibrillar patterns become more obvious at the looping stage of the rat heart [11,12]. Whether this regional asymmetry is responsible for the process of looping or its direction needs yet to be established.

The tubular heart (see Fig. 1) differs in its mode of contraction from the mature one, or even a preseptation trabeculated heart, which is similar to the adult in, for example, observing the Frank-Starling law [13,14]. Ventricular contraction in the tube heart is fundamentally asymmetric, a factor not often considered in biomechanical models of the tube heart [15,16]. The fact that the opposite endocardial surfaces contract to fully occlude the cardiac lumen in a contractile wave from the atrioventricular canal to the muscularized outflow tract has implications for determination of cardiac function at these

Video 1. Video recording (25 fps) of tubular heart action. Ventral view of a Stage 12 chick embryo in modified New culture. Best viewed as a loop. Available in the online version of this article at: http://www.heartfailure.theclinics.com.

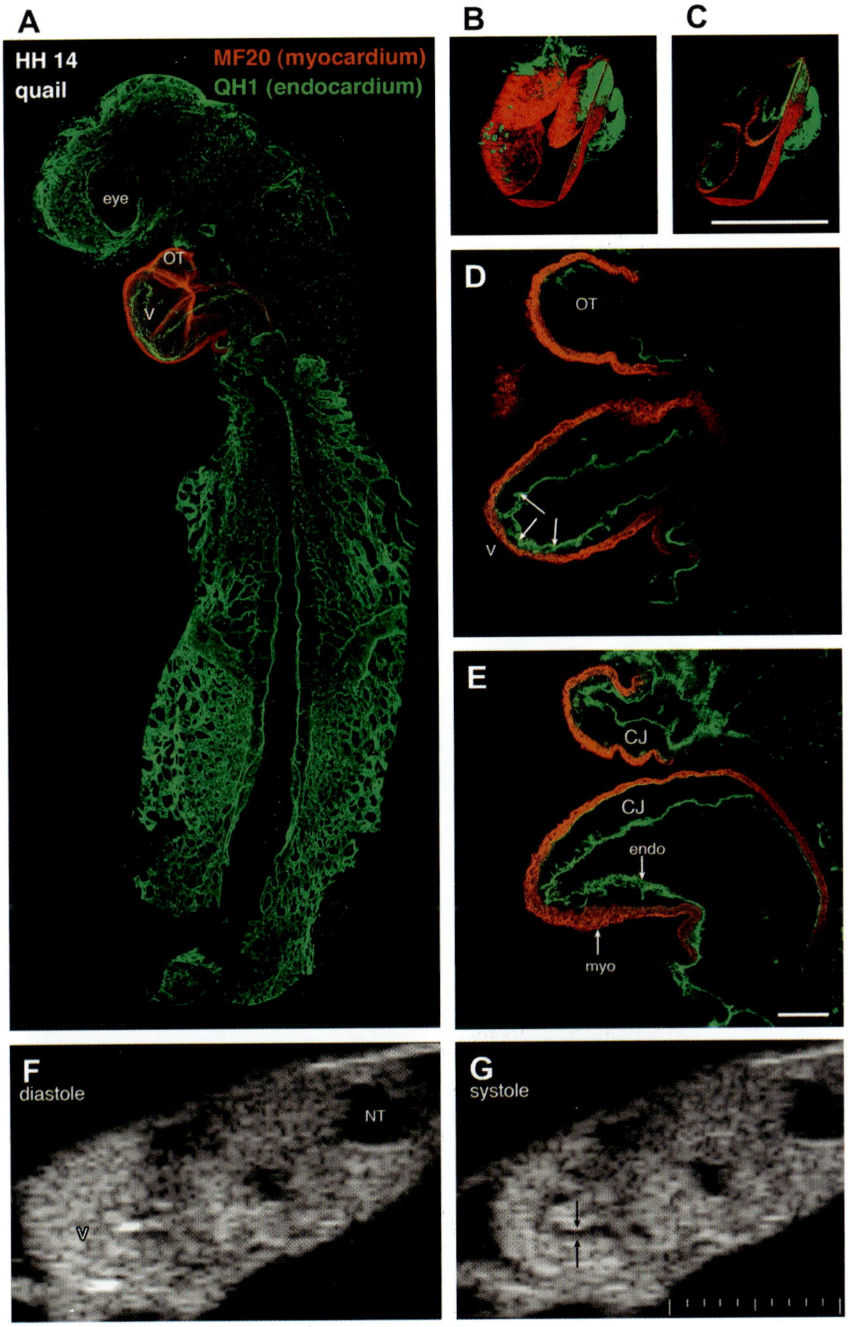

Fig. 1. Structure of a tubular heart. (*A–E*) Whole mount immunostaining for myocardial marker myosin heavy chain (*red*) and endothelial QH1 marker (*green*) shows beautifully the shape of the heart (S-loop). Individual confocal sections (*D, E*) show the diminished amount of cardiac jelly in the ventricular apex, resulting in close contact between these two layers. Endocardial ruffles (*arrowheads*) show the site of prospective trabecular formation. Three-dimensional reconstructions (*B, C*) show the whole heart and an oblique section illustrating the variable extent of the cardiac jelly. Scale bars are 500 μm (*B, C*) and 100 μm (*D, E*). Echocardiographic views (*F, G*) show the heart loop in two different phases of cardiac cycle. Note the echo-free acellular layer of cardiac jelly (*arrows*) along the inner curvature during systole. CJ, cardiac jelly; endo, endocardium; myo, myocardium; NT, neural tube; OT, outflow tract; V, ventricle. Scale bar 100-μm smallest division.

stages. There is no residual nonejected systolic volume under normal conditions until the ventricular cardiac jelly regresses and cardiac ventricular outgrowth ("ballooning") begins [4]. The ejection phase of contraction in the early tube heart therefore has little in common with ventricular systole in the septating and septated heart with their apex-to-base electromechanical activity. Because there is complete occlusion of the lumen at each point along the early tube heart (see Video 1), there is no back flow, and perhaps no dependence on valves as the whole tube acts as an impedance pump [15,17]. The relevance of measurements of global systolic performance based on calculations of fractional shortening, ejection fraction, and end-systolic volume measurements for measurement of cardiac function during these stages of development is not clear.

Development of myocardial trabeculation

The development of myocardial architecture of the ventricular wall passes through several distinct steps (Fig. 2, Video 2). At first, in the tubular heart, the myocardium has an epithelial character with just two layers of cells. The second step is the formation of sheet-like myocardial protrusions into the lumen, so-called "trabeculations" (see Fig. 2). The next step is compaction of the basal portions of these trabeculations, which correlates with the establishment of the coronary vascular system derived from the epicardium. The final stage is the development of multilayered spiral system.

It is possible, only after looping, to discern changes in the luminal appearance of the different components of the tube (see Fig. 1), with trabeculations first becoming evident along the inner

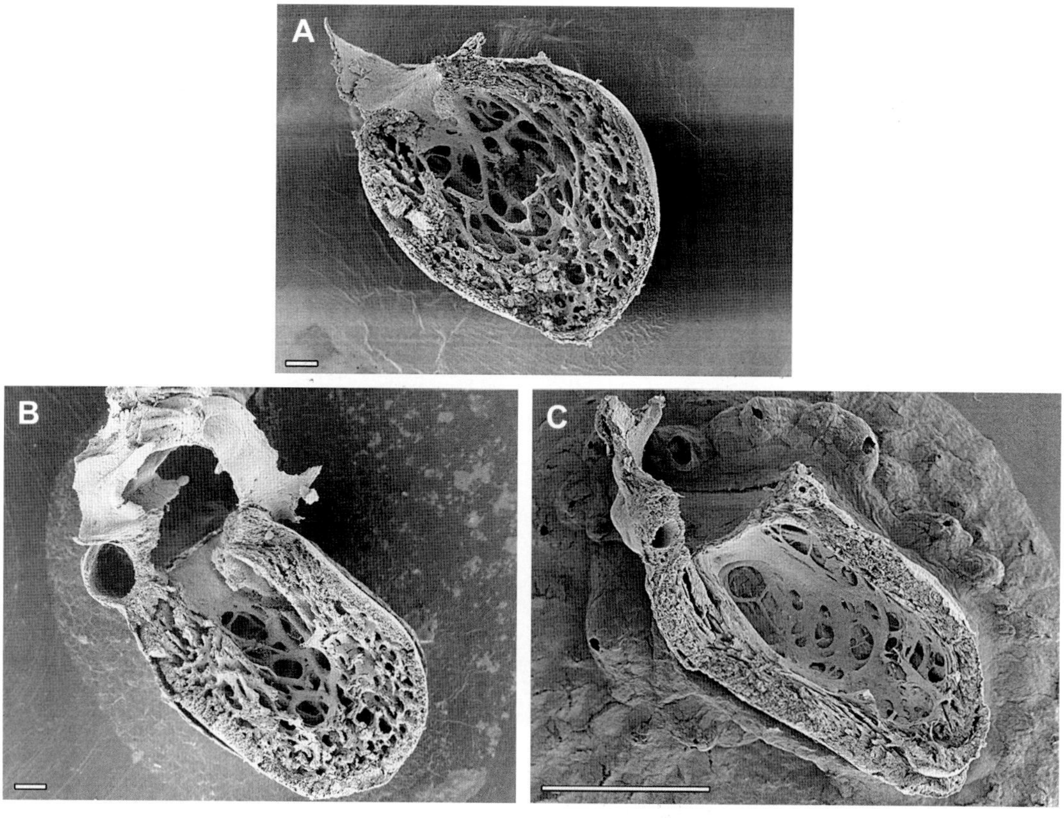

Fig. 2. Time course of ventricular compaction in the human left ventricle. Note increasing proportion and thickness of the outer compact layer. (*A*) Numerous fine trabeculae are present at 6 weeks. (*B*) The trabeculae start to compact at their basal portion, contributing to added thickness of the compact layer at 12 weeks when ventricular septation is completed. (*C*) The compact layer forms the bulk of the myocardial mass after completion of compaction in the early fetal period. Scale bars 100 microns (*A, B*), 1 mm (*C*). (*A and C from* Sedmera D, Pexieder T, Vuillemin M, et al. Developmental patterning of the myocardium. Anat Rec 2000;258:319; with permission.)

Video 2. Ultrasound recording of preseptation trabeculated heart. Four-chamber view of a Stage 24 heart shows the reciprocating contraction of atria (*center*) and septating ventricle (*right*), as well as flowing blood in the branchial arch arteries (*left*) and paired dorsal aortae (*far left, in cross section*). Recorded at 30 fps, smallest division on scale bar 100 μm. Available in the online version of this article at: http://www.heartfailure.theclinics.com.

myocardial layers near the maximum or greater curvature of the looped primitive ventricle [19,20]. This happens in the chick embryo at stage 16/17, in a mouse at 10 days of gestation, a rat at 11 days, and in human beings at the end of the first month of gestation (Carnegie stage 12, the embryo is approximately 4-mm long [21]). The pattern of early trabecular ridges in the ventricular apex runs dorsoventrally (circumferential to the heart tube) and appears similar in different species [18]. At this early stage, the tube itself still contracts in a fashion most consistent with an impedance pump [22]. Maximal stresses and the most highly differentiated cells are concentrated in the myocardial layers adjacent to the lumen, where they may serve to stimulate early trabecular formation [23]. The spacing of such trabecular sheets may depend upon material properties [24,25] of the ventricular wall that result in buckling to relieve tension in response to compression along its longitudinal axis, similar to a long thick carpet pushed from both ends. The early trabeculations effectively increase the surface to volume ratio, enabling the myocardial mass to increase before establishment of a coronary circulation, and may also serve to compartmentalize blood flow as separate ventricular streams before septation [26].

After buckling, the distribution of stresses is no longer uniform, which favors growth of the trabeculations toward the center of the ventricle (see Fig. 2). The trabeculae become transformed into fenestrated trabecular sheets with no free ends; this is conceptually and topologically different from villi in the intestine [27]. Patterns of trabeculations specific for the morphologically left, as opposed to the right, ventricles become apparent at the beginning of ventricular septation [28,29].

The exact patterns of trabeculations in the adult heart show appreciable variability between individuals, and, similar to fingerprints, they seem to be unique for each individual heart. The arrangement of the moderator band, which contains the right bundle branch, and the anatomy of the medial papillary muscle complex of the mitral valve are more uniform, but by no means constant [30].

Atrial myoachitecture

Compared with the ventricle, the atrial myoarchitecture has received much less attention, except as a substrate for propagation of atrial arrhythmias [31,32]. The pectinate muscles appear in the future atrial appendages after the beginning of the atrial septation. A preferential conduction pathway appears during development within the roof of the atria, transmitting the impulse rapidly from the right-sided sinoatrial node to the left atrium. The morphologic substrate of this pathway—the bundle of Bachman—is apparent from embryonic day 6 in the chick onward, and is a prominent ridge of pectinate muscles continuous with the terminal crest [33]. Similar activation patterns are apparent in the embryonic rat and mouse (D. Sedmera, unpublished data, 2003–2005). Further acceleration of impulse propagation (relative to interposed atrial myocardium) is noted along the ridges formed by the forming pectinate muscles, which branch from the terminal crest toward the atrioventricular sulcus. Thus, the pectinate muscles seem to serve a dual role: to strengthen the rather thin atrial wall akin to the struts of an umbrella and act as a morphologic substrate of the preferential conduction pathways, which appear to exist to assure synchronous atrial activation and contraction rather than rapid impulse conduction between the sinoatrial and atrioventricular nodes.

Myocardial (non)compaction

Marked developmental modifications, significant in terms of both structure and function, occur in the compact myocardium (see Fig. 2; Fig. 3). In early embryonic stages in birds and mammals [35], and also in hearts of lower vertebrates (summarized in Ref. [36]), almost the entire thickness of the ventricular wall is made up of a trabecular layer, with little or no coronary vascular supply.

The initial thickening of the compact layer is based on cell proliferation [37]. Subsequent thickening occurs because of compaction of trabeculations, this process coinciding with invasion by the

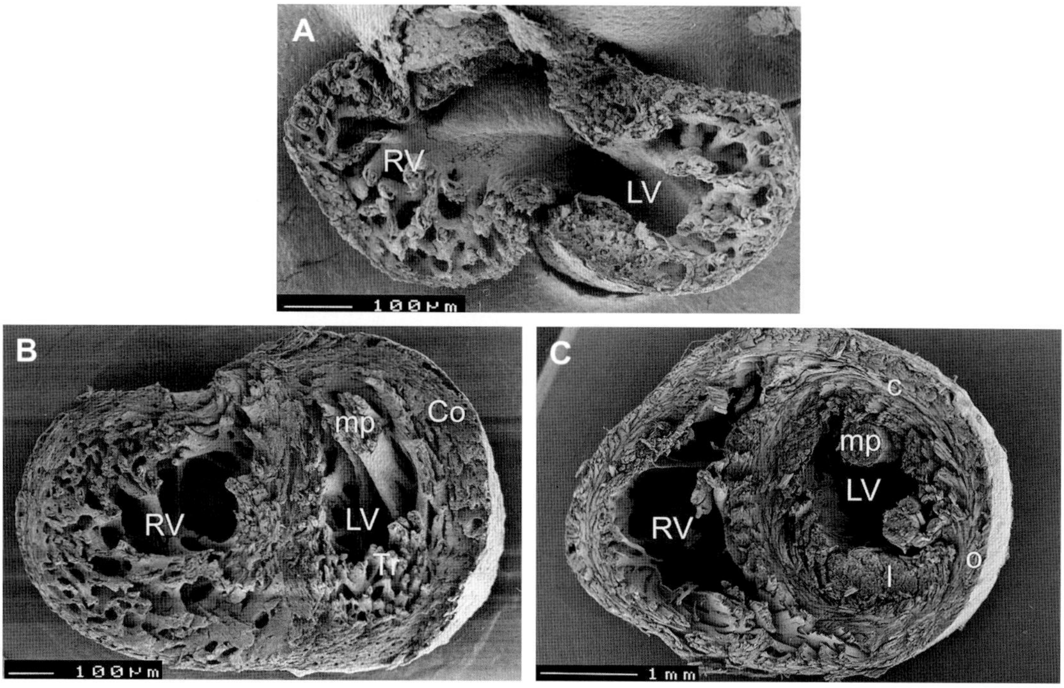

Fig. 3. Development of spiral architecture in the compact layer. (*A*) Pre-compaction stage (E13.5 embryonic mouse heart in transverse section), showing thin, avascular compact layer with circumferential arrangement of myocytes. (*B*) After compaction, vascularized compact layer at E15.5 shows spiral arrangement in both compact myocardium (Co) and trabeculae (Tr). (*C*) In the adult mouse heart, the typical three-layered structure with inner predominantly longitudinal (l), middle circular (c), and outer oblique (o) orientation can be seen in the left ventricle (although recent quantitative studies show that the change in orientation occurs in continuum [34]). Ventricular midportion slabs, viewed from the apex toward the outflow. The first two specimens were prepared by late Dr. Si Minh Pham at University of Lausanne. LV, left ventricle; mp, papillary muscles; RV, right ventricle.

developing coronary vasculature (discussed further in the following section) from the epicardium [38,39]. Compaction is more pronounced in the left ventricle [18], and substantial further growth and compaction occur through the postnatal development [40] with increasing systemic pressure.

The process of trabecular compaction is fairly rapid (in a chick, between embryonic day [E]7 to 10; in a mouse, between E13 and E14; in a human being between 10 and 12 weeks [18]). From E16 in the mouse and the fourth month of gestation in a human being, the compact layer forms the bulk of the ventricular myocardium (see Figs. 2 and 3). Noncompaction of the myocardium presents serious functional consequences for the heart. Several mouse null mutants, such as RXRalpha knockout, present with a complete lack of compaction, which results in lethality around E14 (reviewed in [18]), stressing the importance of the compact myocardium for contractile performance in later fetal stages. In human beings, ventricular noncompaction is usually localized. Although it can occur as an isolated entity, it can be associated with heart failure and sudden cardiac death [41]. Even if only a minor proportion of the ventricular wall is affected, ventricular contractile dynamics may be perturbed [42]. This condition is diagnosed today by ultrasound and is classified as a distinct cardiomyopathy, and several genetic etiologies are recognized [43–46]. There is mounting evidence that the epicardium and the epicardially-derived cells play a crucial role in the development of the compact layer of the ventricular myocardial walls. Not only is the "thin compact myocardium syndrome" observed in several mouse models with perturbed epicardial development, such as in the vascular cell adhesion molecule-1 knockout [47], but experimental studies in avian embryos in which epicardial development is perturbed also show inhibition of ventricular compaction [48]. The exact molecular mechanisms responsible for the regulation of ventricular myocardial differentiation, growth, and trabecular compaction are currently poorly understood, although retinoid signaling from the epicardium to the myocardium appears to be crucial [49]. More research into this area can bring more clues to the molecular etiology of this condition in human beings.

The progressive thickening of the compact myocardium is accompanied by an improved level of its organization. In 1672 Malpighi had observed that "spiral muscle fibers were successively wrapped" around both ventricles of the chick from the fifth day of incubation onwards. This results in development of a three-layered spiral system of myocardial fibers [50,51]. Development of the spiraling alignment of the fibers (see Fig. 3) likely reflects the twisting pattern of contraction and can be experimentally accelerated by increased workload [52].

Remodeling of the blood supply

Once the size and metabolic activity of an animal exceed the limits of oxygen diffusion, a circulatory system needs to be established. This is true also for the heart, both phylogenetically and ontogenetically. The primitive pulsatile vessels or even sophisticated hearts of more complex invertebrates, such as large marine crustaceans or mollusks, are devoid of coronary vascularization.

If an increase in myocardial mass is necessary, the heart muscle is organized into a spongy network of trabeculae. This arrangement of myocardium is found in larger invertebrates (crabs, oysters), and some lower vertebrates, typically cold-blooded, relatively sedentary animals with low blood pressure, notably certain fish [53,54] and amphibian species, such as Xenopus [36], that have a ventricle devoid of coronary arteries.

The origin of the coronary vessels, including the capillaries, was for a long period controversial. Recent studies using retroviral targeting [55] and chick-quail chimeras [56] clearly showed the extracardiac origin of the angioblasts, which form the primitive vascular bed that will become the coronary vasculature, and in that way supplant older concepts of participation of the trabecular endocardium in the definitive coronary bed, or the sprouting of coronary arteries from the aorta. Indeed, connection to the aorta is the final stage of development (reviewed in [57]). The stimulus for the angioblast invasion is probably local tissue hypoxia [58,59], most pronounced in the outermost subepicardial layers. The mediators are fibroblast and vascular endothelial growth factors. Interestingly, the process of vascularization itself does not seem to be dependent on ventricular loading, as demonstrated by studies of Rongish and colleagues [60]. They used the avascular rat embryonic heart transplanted into anterior eye chamber to study the relationship of the various components of the extracellular matrix to coronary vascularization, and found that angioblast invasion occurred even in the absence of any functional loading.

Unlike most organs in the vertebrate body, the heart has to function continuously from very early stages of its development to support the embryo's increasing demands. Consequently, the coronaryless stages are recapitulated in the ontogenesis of the higher vertebrates, and the lacunar system of the trabeculated heart was recognized more than a century ago [61,62] as a way to increase the surface-to-volume ratio to facilitate the exchange of nutrients and oxygen. The external, coronary blood supply becomes necessary when increasing circulatory demands cannot be met by the trabeculated heart, and increased thickness of the compact layer precludes its adequate nutrition and oxygenation by diffusion from the ventricular lumen.

Development of pacemaking and conduction system

The intrinsic rhythm of the adult heart is determined within the tissues of the cardiac pacemaker: the sinoatrial (SA) node. The SA node is situated at the inflow portion of the heart, at the border of the superior caval vein and the right atrium. Following initiation of a cardiac action potential within the node, the activation wave is propagated through the atrial myocardium, eventually converging into the atrioventricular (AV) node. As its name suggests, the AV node is found at the junction of the atria and ventricles, and functions as a delay generator in the propagation of activation. Following the exit from the AV node, activation rapidly propagates along the His bundle and its branches, finally activating the ventricles via a ramified network of Purkinje fibers. Together, this rapid-conduction system of His-Purkinje tissues forms the last of the main elements of the cardiac conduction system (CCS).

The main components of the CCS show remarkable evolutionary conservation. The development of a mature CCS function during embryogenesis follows significant phases of cardiac morphogenesis [63]. Initially, the impulse propagates in a slow and apparently isotropic fashion from the sinus venosus, the most caudal portion of the tubular heart, toward the cranially located primitive outflow tract [9]. While the apparent speed of impulse propagation gradually increases (based on total activation time inferred from isochronal epicardial maps), the sequence of ventricular activation as the heart loops still follows the flow of blood. Eventually, the immature base-to-apex sequence of ventricular activation undergoes an apparent reversal, altering to a mature apex-to-base pattern [64–66], which is a hallmark of the His-Purkinje system function.

The cascade of events resulting in the differential gene expression that distinguishes CCS from the working myocardium is becoming unveiled [67,68]. Molecular determinants of the SA node have been recently described [3], and consist of a combination of transcription factors Nkx2.5, Tbx3, and Pitx2c. Nkx2.5 in the atrial myocardium suppresses the expression of pacemaker channel gene Hcn4 and T-box transcription factor Tbx3, restricting their expression domain to the forming of Nkx2.5-negative sinoatrial node and sinus horns and defining a gene expression boundary between the atrium and SA node. Tbx3 in turn suppresses the chamber differentiation program, providing an additional mechanism of reinforcing the nodal identity. Deficiency in Tbx3 results in an expansion of the atrial gene expression program into the nodal area and a partial loss of nodal gene expression, whereas its overexpression reciprocally suppresses the atrial program and induces a pacemaking phenotype [69]. Pitx2c is a laterality determination gene that suppresses the program for SA node formation on the left side, resulting in the normal right-sided position of the node.

Determination of the AV node is linked to formation of the AV canal in the developing heart, or rather, differentiation of the atrial and ventricular chambers from the "primitive" myocardium of the cardiac tube [4]. A combination of T-box transcription factors Tbx2 and Tbx5 signaling is involved [70], with Tbx5 being the determinant of the AV canal as well as the ventricular conduction system. Tbx2 is induced by BMP2 expression, and repressed by Hesr1 expressed in the atrial and Hesr2 in the ventricular myocardium [71]. Nkx2.5 signaling is critical not only for the early stages of cardiogenesis [72], but is up-regulated during the later stages of the ventricular conduction system formation, namely differentiation of the Purkinje fibers in the chick [73]. In mammals, it is required for normal formation of the AV node and bundle branches [74].

In the chick, endothelin was identified as a secreted factor capable of turning on CCS markers in embryonic cardiomyocytes in vivo [75], and further studies suggest that it is also involved in turning on the Purkinje fiber-specific program in vivo [76]. There is some evidence that it is also involved in CCS induction in mammals (reviewed in [68]), but further research is needed to confirm this hypothesis.

In summary, myocardium is derived from precardiac mesoderm, and its formation is subject of positive and negative regulation by a number of genes. After formation of a tubular heart with a mode of contraction distinct from subsequent stages, initial increase in ventricular mass during the period of chamber formation is achieved by development of trabeculations, a hallmark of sponge-like hearts. Similar structures (pectinate muscles) develop later on in the atria. Trabecular compaction coincides with deployment of coronary circulation, and results in formation of ventricular chambers with significant, vascularized compact layers and clearly delineated lumen, which are capable of superior performance (pressure generation, ejection fraction) than the avascular, spongy ventricles. The contraction of the developing heart is orchestrated by its pacemaking and conduction system, which develops and changes parallel to heart morphogenesis. While the molecular determination of the sinoatrial node and atrioventricular was recently unraveled, the pathways implicated in induction and patterning of ventricular His-Purkinje system are still subject to research.

References

[1] Kirby ML. Cardiac development. New York: Oxford University Press; 2007.

[2] Yutzey KE, Bader D. Diversification of cardiomyogenic cell lineages during early heart development. Circ Res 1995;77:216–9.

[3] Mommersteeg MT, Hoogaars WM, Prall OW, et al. Molecular Pathway for the Localized Formation of the Sinoatrial Node. Circ Res 2007;100:354–62.

[4] Moorman AF, Christoffels VM. Cardiac chamber formation: development, genes, and evolution. Physiol Rev 2003;83:1223–67.

[5] de Jong F, Opthof T, Wilde AA, et al. Persisting zones of slow impulse conduction in developing chicken hearts. Circ Res 1992;71:240–50.

[6] Sedmera D, Reckova M, DeAlmeida A, et al. Spatiotemporal pattern of commitment to slowed proliferation in the embryonic mouse heart indicates

progressive differentiation of the cardiac conduction system. Anat Rec A Discov Mol Cell Evol Biol 2003; 274:773–7.
[7] Schaefer KS, Doughman YQ, Fisher SA, et al. Dynamic patterns of apoptosis in the developing chicken heart. Dev Dyn 2004;229:489–99.
[8] Eisenberg LM, Eisenberg CA. An in vitro analysis of myocardial potential indicates that phenotypic plasticity is an innate property of early embryonic tissue. Stem Cells Dev 2004;13:614–24.
[9] Kamino K. Optical approaches to ontogeny of electrical activity and related functional organization during early heart development. Physiol Rev 1991;71:53–91.
[10] Shiraishi I, Takamatsu T, Fujita S. Three-dimensional observation with a confocal scanning laser microscope of fibronectin immunolabeling during cardiac looping in the chick embryo. Anat Embryol (Berl) 1995;191:183–9.
[11] Price RL, Chintanowonges C, Shiraishi I, et al. Local and regional variations in myofibrillar patterns in looping rat hearts. Anat Rec 1996;245:83–93.
[12] Wenink AC, Knaapen MW, Vrolijk BC, et al. Development of myocardial fiber organization in the rat heart. Anat Embryol (Berl) 1996;193:559–67.
[13] Clark EB, Hu N, Dummett JL, et al. Ventricular function and morphology in chick embryo from stages 18 to 29. Am J Phys 1986;250:H407–13.
[14] Hu N, Clark EB. Hemodynamics of the stage 12 to stage 29 chick embryo. Circ Res 1989;65:1665–70.
[15] Forouhar AS, Liebling M, Hickerson A, et al. The embryonic vertebrate heart tube is a dynamic suction pump. Science 2006;312:751–3.
[16] Taber LA. Biomechanics of cardiovascular development. Annu Rev Biomed Eng 2001;3:1–25.
[17] McQuinn TC, Bratoeva M, Dealmeida A, et al. High-frequency ultrasonographic imaging of avian cardiovascular development. Dev Dyn 2007;236: 3503–13.
[18] Sedmera D, Pexieder T, Vuillemin M, et al. Developmental patterning of the myocardium. Anat Rec 2000;258:319–37.
[19] Ben-Shachar G, Arcilla RA, Lucas RV, et al. Ventricular trabeculations in the chick embryo heart and their contribution to ventricular and muscular septal development. Circ Res 1985;57:759–66.
[20] Challice CE, Viragh S. The embryonic development of the mammalian heart. In: Challice CE, Viragh S, editors. Ultrastructure of the mammalian heart. New York: Academic Press; 1973. p. 91–126.
[21] Mall FP. On the development of the human heart. Am J Anat 1912;13:249–98.
[22] Butcher JT, McQuinn TC, Sedmera D, et al. Transitions in early embryonic atrioventricular valvular function correspond with changes in cushion biomechanics that are predictable by tissue composition. Circ Res 2007;100:1503–11.
[23] Thompson RP, Reckova M, DeAlmeida A, et al. The oldest, toughest cells in the heart. In: Chadwick DJ, Goode J, editors. Development of the cardiac conduction system, vol. 250. Chichester (England): Wiley; 2003. p. 157–76.
[24] Miller CE, Wong CL. Trabeculated embryonic myocardium shows rapid stress relaxation and non-quasi-linear viscoelastic behavior. J Biomech 2000;33:615–22.
[25] Miller CE, Wong CL, Sedmera D. Pressure overload alters stress-strain properties of the developing chick heart. Am J Physiol Heart Circ Physiol 2003;285: H1849–56.
[26] Van Mierop LHS, Kutsche LM. Comparative anatomy and embryology of the ventricles and arterial pole of the vertebrate heart. In: Nora Kutsche JJ, Takao A , editors. Congenital heart disease: causes and processes. New York: Futura Publishing; 1984. p. 459–79.
[27] Sedmera D, Thomas PS. Trabeculation in the embryonic heart [letter]. Bioessays 1996;18:607.
[28] Wenink AC. Quantitative morphology of the embryonic heart: an approach to development of the atrioventricular valves. Anat Rec 1992;234: 129–35.
[29] Wenink AC. Gittenberger-de Groot AC. Left and right ventricular trabecular patterns. Consequence of ventricular septation and valve development. Br Heart J 1982;48:462–8.
[30] Restivo A, Smith A, Wilkinson JL, et al. The medial papillary muscle complex and its related septomarginal trabeculation. A normal anatomical study on human hearts. J Anat 1989;163:231–42.
[31] Anderson RH, Ho SY. The architecture of the sinus node, the atrioventricular conduction axis, and the internodal atrial myocardium. J Cardiovasc Electrophysiol 1998;9:1233–48.
[32] Ho SY, Anderson RH, Sanchez-Quintana D. Atrial structure and fibres: morphologic bases of atrial conduction. Cardiovasc Res 2002;54:325–36.
[33] Sedmera D, Wessels A, Trusk TC, et al. Changes in activation sequence of embryonic chick atria correlate with developing myocardial architecture. Am J Physiol Heart Circ Physiol 2006;291:H1646–52.
[34] Lunkenheimer PP, Redmann K, Kling N, et al. Three-dimensional architecture of the left ventricular myocardium. Anat Rec A Discov Mol Cell Evol Biol 2006;288:565–78.
[35] Blausen BE, Johannes RS, Hutchins GM. Computer-based reconstructions of the cardiac ventricles of human embryos. Am J Cardiovasc Pathol 1990; 3:37–43.
[36] Sedmera D, Reckova M, DeAlmeida A, et al. Functional and morphological evidence for a ventricular conduction system in the zebrafish and Xenopus heart. Am J Physiol Heart Circ Physiol 2003;284: H1152–60.
[37] Jeter JR Jr, Cameron IL. Cell proliferation patterns during cytodifferentiation in embryonic chick tissues: liver, heart and erythrocytes. J Embryol Exp Morphol 1971;25:405–22.

[38] Rychterova V. Principle of growth in thickness of the heart ventricular wall in the chick embryo. Folia Morphol (Praha) 1971;19:262–72.

[39] Vrancken Peeters MP, Gittenberger-de Groot AC, Mentink MM, et al. The development of the coronary vessels and their differentiation into arteries and veins in the embryonic quail heart. Dev Dyn 1997;208:338–48.

[40] Hirokawa K. A quantitative study on pre- and postnatal growth of human heart. Acta Pathol Jpn 1972; 22:613–24.

[41] Waller BF, Smith ER, Blackbourne BD, et al. Congenital hypoplasia of portions of both right and left ventricular myocardial walls. Clinical and necropsy observations in two patients with parchment heart syndrome. Am J Cardiol 1980;46:885–91.

[42] Jenni R, Oechslin E, Schneider J, et al. Echocardiographic and pathoanatomical characteristics of isolated left ventricular non-compaction: a step towards classification as a distinct cardiomyopathy. Heart 2001;86:666–71.

[43] Finsterer J, Stollberger C. Do cypher gene mutations cause left ventricular noncompaction with subclinical myopathy? J Am Coll Cardiol 2004;44:1139 [author reply 1139–40].

[44] Ichida F, Tsubata S, Bowles KR, et al. Novel gene mutations in patients with left ventricular noncompaction or Barth syndrome. Circulation 2001;103: 1256–63.

[45] Pauli RM, Scheib-Wixted S, Cripe L, et al. Ventricular noncompaction and distal chromosome 5q deletion. Am J Med Genet 1999;85:419–23.

[46] Sasse-Klaassen S, Probst S, Gerull B, et al. Novel gene locus for autosomal dominant left ventricular noncompaction maps to chromosome 11p15. Circulation 2004;109:2720–3.

[47] Kwee L, Baldwin HS, Shen HM, et al. Defective development of the embryonic and extraembryonic circulatory systems in vascular cell adhesion molecule (VCAM-1) deficient mice. Development 1995; 121:489–503.

[48] Perez-Pomares JM, Phelps A, Sedmerova M, et al. Experimental studies on the spatiotemporal expression of WT1 and RALDH2 in the embryonic avian heart: a model for the regulation of myocardial and valvuloseptal development by epicardially derived cells (EPDCs). Dev Biol 2002; 247:307–26.

[49] Chen TH, Chang TC, Kang JO, et al. Epicardial induction of fetal cardiomyocyte proliferation via a retinoic acid-inducible trophic factor. Dev Biol 2002;250:198–207.

[50] Jouk PS, Usson Y, Michalowicz G, et al. Three-dimensional cartography of the pattern of the myofibres in the second trimester fetal human heart. Anat Embryol (Berl) 2000;202:103–18.

[51] Streeter DDJ. Gross morphology and fiber geometry of the heart. In: Berne RM, Sperelakis N, Geiger SR, editors. Handbook of physiology—section 2: the cardiovascular system. Bethesda (MD): Am Physiol Soc; 1979. p. 61–112.

[52] Tobita K, Garrison JB, Li JJ, et al. Three-dimensional myofiber architecture of the embryonic left ventricle during normal development and altered mechanical loads. Anat Rec A Discov Mol Cell Evol Biol 2005;283:193–201.

[53] Ostadal B, Schiebler TH. [The terminal blood bed in the heart of fish]. Z Anat Entwicklungsgesch 1971; 134:101–10 [in German].

[54] Tota B, Cimini V, Salvatore G, et al. Comparative study of the arterial and lacunary systems of the ventricular myocardium of elasmobranch and teleost fishes. Am J Anat 1983;167:15–32.

[55] Mikawa T, Borisov A, Brown AM, et al. Clonal analysis of cardiac morphogenesis in the chicken embryo using a replication-defective retrovirus: I. Formation of the ventricular myocardium. Dev Dyn 1992;193:11–23.

[56] Poelmann RE, Gittenberger-de Groot AC, Mentink MM, et al. Development of the cardiac coronary vascular endothelium, studied with antiendothelial antibodies, in chicken-quail chimeras. Circ Res 1993;73:559–68.

[57] Tomanek RJ. Formation of the coronary vasculature: a brief review. Cardiovasc Res 1996;31:E46-51.

[58] Nanka O, Valasek P, Dvorakova M, et al. Experimental hypoxia and embryonic angiogenesis. Dev Dyn 2006;235:723–33.

[59] Wikenheiser J, Doughman YQ, Fisher SA, et al. Differential levels of tissue hypoxia in the developing chicken heart. Dev Dyn 2006;235:115–23.

[60] Rongish BJ, Hinchman G, Doty MK, et al. Relationship of the extracellular matrix to coronary neovascularization during development. J Mol Cell Cardiol 1996;28:2203–15.

[61] Minot CS. On a hitherto unrecognised circulation without capillaries in the organs of Vertebrata. Proc Boston Soc Nat Hist 1901;29:185–215.

[62] Rychter Z, Ostadal B. Fate of "sinusoidal" intertrabecular spaces of the cardiac wall after development of the coronary vascular bed in chick embryo. Folia Morphol 1971;19:31–44.

[63] Gourdie RG, Harris BS, Bond J, et al. Development of the cardiac pacemaking and conduction system. Birth Defects Res C Embryo Today 2003; 69:46–57.

[64] Chuck ET, Freeman DM, Watanabe M, et al. Changing activation sequence in the embryonic chick heart. Implications for the development of the His-Purkinje system. Circ Res 1997;81:470–6.

[65] Reckova M, Rosengarten C, deAlmeida A, et al. Hemodynamics is a key epigenetic factor in development of the cardiac conduction system. Circ Res 2003;93: 77–85.

[66] Rentschler S, Vaidya DM, Tamaddon H, et al. Visualization and functional characterization of the developing murine cardiac conduction system. Development 2001;128:1785–92.

[67] Myers DC, Fishman GI. Toward an understanding of the genetics of murine cardiac pacemaking and conduction system development. Anat Rec 2004; 280A:1018–21.

[68] Sedmera D. Development of cardiac conduction system in mammals. Journal of Applied Biomedicine 2007;5:115–23.

[69] Hoogaars WM, Engel A, Brons JF, et al. Tbx3 controls the sinoatrial node gene program and imposes pacemaker function on the atria. Genes Dev 2007; 21:1098–112.

[70] Moskowitz IP, Pizard A, Patel VV, et al. The T-Box transcription factor Tbx5 is required for the patterning and maturation of the murine cardiac conduction system. Development 2004;131:4107–16.

[71] Kokubo H, Tomita-Miyagawa S, Hamada Y, et al. Hesr1 and Hesr2 regulate atrioventricular boundary formation in the developing heart through the repression of Tbx2. Development 2007;134:747–55.

[72] Lyons I, Parsons LM, Hartley L, et al. Myogenic and morphogenetic defects in the heart tubes of murine embryos lacking the homeo box gene Nkx2-5. Genes Dev 1995;9:1654–66.

[73] Harris BS, Spruill L, Edmonson AM, et al. Differentiation of cardiac Purkinje fibers requires precise spatiotemporal regulation of Nkx2-5 expression. Dev Dyn 2006;235:38–49.

[74] Jay PY, Harris BS, Maguire CT, et al. Nkx2-5 mutation causes anatomic hypoplasia of the cardiac conduction system. J Clin Invest 2004;113:1130–7.

[75] Gourdie RG, Wei Y, Kim D, et al. Endothelin-induced conversion of embryonic heart muscle cells into impulse-conducting Purkinje fibers. Proc Natl Acad Sci U S A 1998;95:6815–8.

[76] Takebayashi-Suzuki K, Yanagisawa M, Gourdie RG, et al. In vivo induction of cardiac Purkinje fiber differentiation by coexpression of preproendothelin-1 and endothelin converting enzyme-1. Development 2000;127:3523–32.

ELSEVIER
SAUNDERS

Heart Failure Clin 4 (2008) 247–259

HEART
FAILURE
CLINICS

Physiology in Phylogeny: Modeling of Mechanical Driving Forces in Cardiac Development

Anna Grosberg, PhD, Morteza Gharib, PhD*

California Institute of Technology (Caltech), Pasadena, CA, USA

In pursuing the evolutionary history, or phylogeny, of the heart one looks for common characteristics between the embryonic and adult hearts. One pronounced similarity is in the helical organization of the muscle fibers. The simple helical organization of the fibers has long been observed histologically [1]. Moreover, there is some evidence that the muscle fibers, unlike the collection of fibers that includes collagen, are in a double helical bundle. This has been observed in a controversial illustration where the collagen is removed off the heart by boiling [2,3]. Although the idea that such a band exists was formed on the basis of disputed histologic evidence, in recent diffusion tensor MR imaging studies done by Helm and colleagues [4] one can easily identify the band architecture (Fig. 1). This is significant, because this method images the actin, which is present in muscle fibers, but not in the collagen matrix or any other part of heart tissue.

By Ernst Haeckel's premise that ontogeny follows phylogeny, researchers use embryonic fish heart as a biologic model for the human embryonic heart [5,6]. By keeping track of the fluorescent myocardial cells, it is possible to create a picture of their movement during a heartbeat. The resulting looped movement is not symmetric, forming an oval for each cell. The long axis of these ovals has to be aligned with the direction of the fiber, because that is the major direction of the contraction. The directionality of the oval paths of the myocardial cells is not constant throughout the heart tube. The only way that a muscle fiber could have such a nonconstant direction as seen in the images is if it was helically arranged [7,8]. These fibers are not only helically shaped but they seem to be bundled into a band. Both the adult heart and the embryonic heart seem to be comprised of helical muscle bands. How are these two observations related?

Some hints from embryonic heart development

In the embryo, the heart muscle fibers start as a simple spiral, but as the embryo develops, the fibers transform into a more complex double helical structure. It is interesting to track how this development occurs, and how it is reflected in the fiber arrangement of the adult heart.

In general one can imagine a transformation, intriguing in its simplicity, which can be performed on the helix of the embryonic heart converting it to the double helix shape of the adult heart. This transformation is easy to perform on a ribbon (Fig. 2), but there is a world of difference between deforming ribbons and the actual heart muscle. How does nature achieve this transformation?

The development of the heart

The embryonic heart in the beginning stages of its development is a tube with two sulcus [9]. In humans, it starts beating on the 22 day after conception, and soon thereafter it starts to loop. The driving mechanism for this change of shape has not been fully established. The heart tube goes through a sequence of bending and twisting, first going into a "c" loop, then an "s" loop that is "matured," after which the main architecture of

* Corresponding author. California Institute of Technology, M/C 205-45, 1200 East California Boulevard, Pasadena, CA 91125.

E-mail address: mgharib@caltech.edu (M. Gharib).

1551-7136/08/$ - see front matter
doi:10.1016/j.hfc.2008.02.010

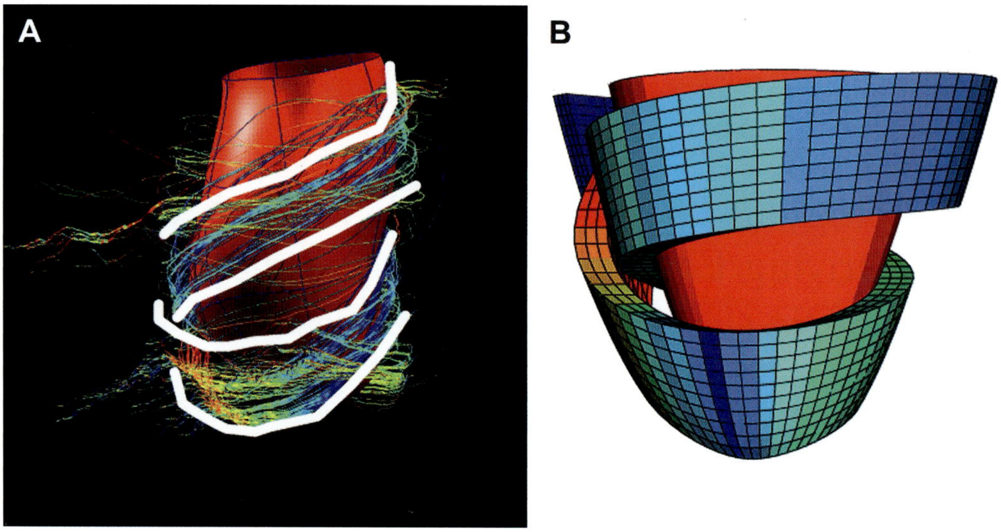

Fig. 1. Muscle fibers in the heart contrasted with the band model. (*A*) Dense MR image of the muscle fibers in the myocardium given by Dr. Helm. The muscle fibers are color-coded for the value of the pitch angle: blue, horizontal, to red, vertical. The red structure in the middle indicates the endocardial surface and represents the left ventricle volume. White lines are overlayed on the image to indicate where the band lies. The muscle fibers are more horizontal at the top band section, whereas at the left section of the bottom band they are more vertical and are accordingly colored yellow and red. (*B*) The double helix model, color coded in the same manner as the diffusion tensor MR images (blue for horizontal pitch angles, to red for vertical pitch angles). The model band repeats the same pattern as the muscle fibers in the diffusion tensor. MR images; the top portion of the band is dominantly horizontal, whereas the left section of the bottom portion of the band is going sharply up. The red structure inside the band is the modeled left ventricular volume.

the four-chamber heart is discernible [10,11]. By the eighth week some of the chamber walls are remodeled and the heart takes on the form of the four-chamber pump.

This looping has been experimentally modeled using an elastic tube [12]. It was observed that the tube on increasing twist deforms in the same way as the heart tube seen in direct images from chick embryos. Most importantly, the shape of the tube evolves in the same manner as the transformation of ribbon depicted in Fig. 2. The mechanical experiment of paper [12], however, starts at the "c" loop stage and explores the mode of rotation of the looping heart, not the driving forces necessary for such a deformation. Neither do these authors investigate the causes of the twist necessary to induce this transformation. Nevertheless, this experiment strongly suggests, that the shape change is governed by elastic mechanical properties of the material, rather than a specific genetically encoded biologic mechanism.

A basic observation

In support of the hypothesis of the dominant role of the mechanics in the heart's transformation, consider a simple tactile experiment. Take a rubber tube, such that the thumbs fit snugly at the ends, insert fingers into the tube and twist it; one can feel the stress on the fingers. Now, without untwisting, deform the tube to relieve the stress. It is remarkable how similar the resulting shape is to the "c" shape of the developing heart. This type of deformation is a well-known phenomenon in solid mechanics, where the structure bends to relieve stress caused by twist. Additionally, it is common in nature for stresses to play an important role in biologic growth and development (eg, in the growth of tree branches) [13]. From these arguments it is hypothesized that the stress from the twist causes the deformation in the embryonic heart. In the tactile experiment, however, one first needed to rotate the fingers to produce any change. What happens in the heart tube to induce the twist in the first place? In this light, it is curious that the heart begins to loop almost immediately after it starts beating. This is intriguing, because the contractions of the heart muscle are the only source of the force on the tube, not present before the looping was initiated. The next step is to look for the causes of the twist

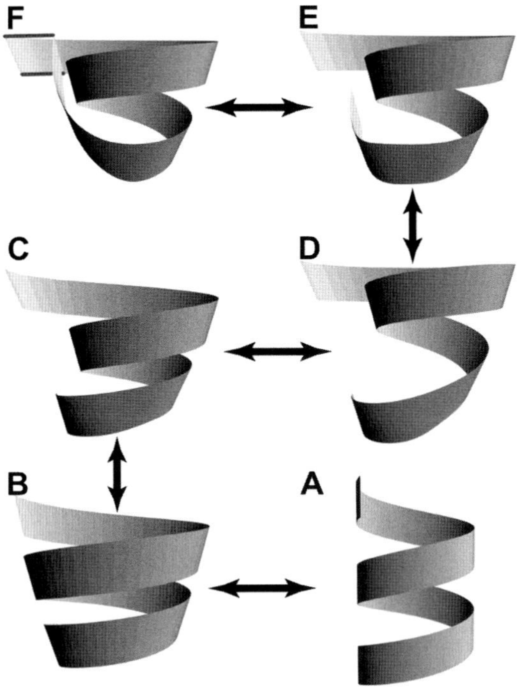

Fig. 2. A possible set of steps in the development from a spiral tube to a double helix band. (*A*) A spiral wound around a tube, like in an embryonic model. (*B*) A spiral wound around a tube that has a varying diameter. (*C*) The diameter of the tube changes such that the bottom and top loops of the spiral have a larger diameter than the middle loop. (*D*) The pitch angle of the bottom part of the band is changed to be more vertical. (*E*) The end of the spiral band is brought up toward the top end. (*F*) Both ends of the band are at the same level and can be connected to each other. This shape is the same as the double helix proposed by Torrent-Guasp as a heart model.

in the tube's response to the muscle fiber contractions.

Crane [14], writing on the general problems of biologic growth, pointed out that although the process in the whole can be too complex to produce an equation describing it, one can understand it if "the principles involved and something of the order of their importance" are known. In following his insight, it is postulated that for the property of heart function and development the leading order of importance belongs to the bundled helical arrangement of muscle fibers. This road-map is followed next and modeling tools are used to approach this question.

Modeling

Biologic pumping organs are complicated multiscale systems, and great efforts are directed at their computational modeling [15–19]. Despite the very significant resources applied and the impressive results achieved, it is currently an insurmountable challenge to computationally represent all the scales and aspects of these systems in their entirety. There exist neither a powerful enough computer, nor a sufficient understanding of the chemistry and control of muscle fibers to model complicated structures encompassing all the scales from the actin filaments up to the organ as a whole. At the same time, there is a great demand, especially from the medical community, for models that trade the microscopic details for predictive power [3,20]. In the authors' opinion, and according to the experience of the engineering field, models should be based on the insight into the biologically dominant features of the system. In such a situation it benefits one to be able to model the action of muscle without its intricate details. Although the popular cardiac models are based on the fact that the fibers inside the heart are helical [1], the notion that they bundle into a single band that is arranged into a double helix [2] has never been properly simulated. It is easy to fathom that such helical structures could be used to optimize the functional properties of the organ (eg, pumping). Here these macro-structures are modeled as applied to a problem of pumping. Meanwhile, knowing that a lot of times bandlike muscle fiber structures are results of self-assembly, watch for characteristics that are responsible for pushing the development of the tubular heart into the double helical arrangement. In that one can take advantage of how nature uses these larger-scale geometries and intricate dynamics to create wonderfully efficient mechanisms.

Two simple models of biologic pumps are presented: an embryonic fish and adult human hearts. Also considered are different possibilities of contracting the muscles that operate these pumps.

Methods

Geometry of the ribbon models

Embryonic tube heart

An embryonic heart is shaped like a tube, which is one of the simplest chambers one can enclose with a band of fibers. The fibers can be arranged circumferentially or longitudinally, or they can form a spiral wound about the tube. Mathematically, such bands can be easily described by a set of parametric equations, which are omitted here for the sake of brevity [21]. Using these equations one can vary the different parameters of the spiral and tube: pitch (fiber) angle, number of turns, tube radius, tube length, fiber length, cylinder volume, width, and thickness of the spiral band. The spirals with varying pitch angles are shown in Fig. 3; however, these parameters are not independent.

Adult heart

A more complicated structure that also involves helical muscle fibers is the human adult heart. There is histologic evidence that the fibers are arranged in a spiral band, as shown by Torrent-Guasp [2,3], who postulated that the heart muscle is a single band that starts from the pulmonary aorta, hugs the right ventricle, winds down to the apex as the descending segment, and then spirals up to the aortic valve as the ascending segment. It is more complicated in terms of mathematical presentation than a simple spiral, but the parametric equations can still be written down using the same mathematical tools [21]. The resulting structure can be seen in Fig. 4A, with the physiologic sections referenced in Fig. 4B. Fig. 4D shows how such a relatively simple band structure could be filled out to form a full two-ventricle heart.

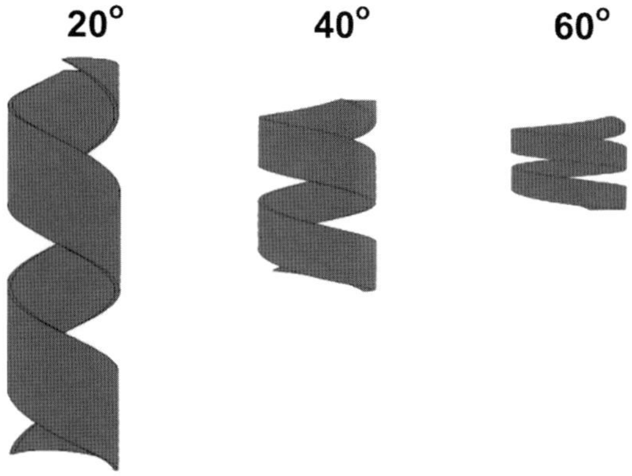

Fig. 3. Images of the spiral muscle band models for the embryonic heart. The numbers indicate the pitch (fiber) angle: 20 degrees, 40 degrees, and 60 degrees are shown. For all three spirals shown the radius of the tube is constant. The length of the band is also constant, and as a result the length of the tube varies with the pitch angle. The width of the band is taken to be half of the value that would have fully covered the surface of the tube, and as a result the width varies with the pitch angle.

Choosing the geometric parameters

In both geometric models of tubelike embryonic heart and a double helical adult heart, there is a range of parameters that can be varied. The choice of parameters here is based on physiologic observations, the goals of the simulations, and computational needs.

Embryonic tube heart

Number of turns. For the spiral wound about a tube to be deformable into a double helix it needs to make two complete rotations. The spiral makes two full turns. In the authors' model they specify it to go around another quarter of a turn, so that the boundaries do not impact the main body of the spiral.

Pitch angle. It is not possible to extract the pitch angle (fiber angle) from the images of the embryonic heart. The authors wanted the ability to vary the fiber angle. In the experiments the angle is varied between 5 and 80 degrees.

Radius of the tube. In the embryonic heart model the radius of the tube is known, but it is unclear how far up the tube the spiral fibers extend. The authors chose to keep the radius of the tube constant at 0.25 cm.

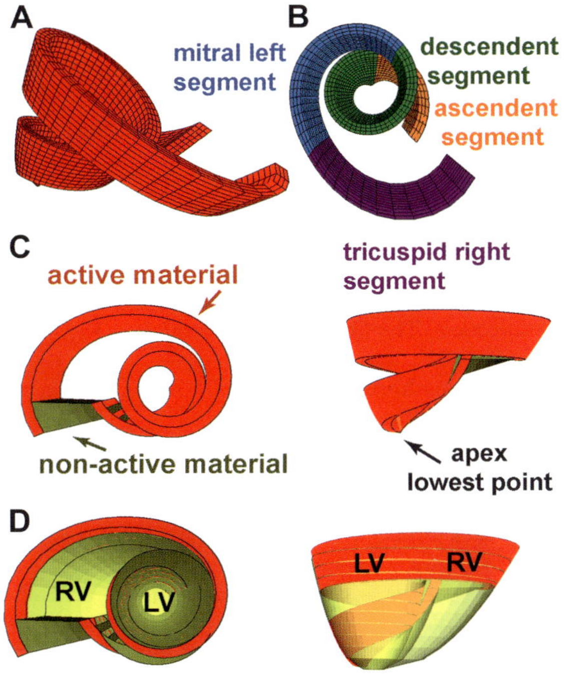

Fig. 4. Images of the double helical band model of the adult heart. The initial band shape and fitted volume shown from different points of view. (*A*) The double helical band. (*B*) The same band color-coded corresponding to physiologic segments. (*C*) The same band in different orientation, with labeled active and nonactive material, and the apex of the heart. (*D*) The fitted volumes for left ventricles (LV) and right ventricle (RV) are labeled on these pictures.

Length of the tube. Once both the number of turns of the spiral and the pitch angle are specified, the length of the tube is mathematically determined.

Fiber length. Once the previously mentioned parameters are chosen the fiber length is determined.

Band width. The choice of the parameters also defines the width of the band necessary to cover the whole surface of the tube. The authors chose for the width of the band to be limited to half of what covers the tube, to ensure that the material does not impinge on itself during twisting.

Band thickness. The thickness of the band is constant and small compared with the width (approximately one fifth of the width).

Adult heart

Number of turns. This parameter is dictated to be two turns by the model design.

Fiber angle. Unlike the pitch angle of the simple spiral, the fiber angle is not constant in the double helical arrangement. The authors took the information from the histologic studies done by Torrent-Guasp. As a result, the math description, although more cumbersome than in the case of the tube, is still known.

Long axis dimension. The long axis dimension is taken to be the same as in the normal adult heart, about 7 cm.

Basal radius. Again, the basal radius is taken to be the same as in the adult heart, about 3.5 cm.

Right heart size. The parameter controlling the size of the right heart was estimated so that the fitted right ventricle volume corresponds to the volume in a normal adult heart (about 130 mL).

Band width. To ease computation the band width is assumed to be a constant. The width is chosen such that the bottom of the mitral left segment does not impinge on the top of the descending segment (width approximately 2.5 cm).

Band thickness. The thickness of the band is constant and small compared with the width (thickness approximately 0.5 cm).

Material properties

The properties of the macrostructures of the organ's muscle are inevitably dictated by the muscle's building blocks. The muscle fibers contract along the length of the fiber; the muscle band that consists of a group of parallel muscle fibers contracts in the same direction. The fibers cannot contract much over 15% [22], and the band does not exceed this maximum shortening ratio at any point along its length. Although it is shortening in the fiber direction the band expands in the other two to conserve volume. The band can shorten as a whole, or parts of it can contract independently of each other. That means that the cells can act separately along the length of the band; the fibers in the width of the band can also contract at different times from each other. For simplicity, a linear elastic response is assumed while the material is not excited. The material is incompressible, so the maximal computationally possible Poisson ratio is chosen, $\nu = 0.48$ (an ideal incompressible material has $\nu = 0.5$). The choice of the Young's modulus is discussed later.

As regards the structure of the adult heart, it was necessary to hold it together with a nonactive material shown in Fig. 4C. The nonactive material was chosen to be four times softer than the active material (ie, the Young's modulus of the nonactive material is one fourth of the Young's modulus of the active material).

Boundary conditions

Unlike the heart inside a body, the models are not part of a whole organism. It is necessary to fix them in space. To do that one needs to constrain at least three degrees of freedom: the x – direction, y – direction, and z – direction.

Embryonic tube heart

It was found that the most meaningful results are obtained by fixing both ends of the tube. This allows one consistently to look at twisting and pumping in a range of different contraction schemes. If only one end of the tube is fixed, the other flaps about, which makes it hard to determine if there is any twist present.

Adult heart

To compare the dynamics of the double helical model with the heart's dynamics, the band is fixed to the model in space in the same manner as the heart. In the body, the heart's apex does not move up or down, whereas the top of the heart does not rotate. The band structure is fixed in the horizontal plane by the nonactive material, in the same manner as the heart is constrained by the vessels. The lowest point of the double helix is assumed to be the apex, and is constrained in the vertical direction (see Fig. 4C).

Excitation schemes

The simplest dynamic scheme is to excite all the cells at the same time and have the whole band contracting in sync. In this case the only periodicity is in time, so the authors call this a "uniform contraction."

The other choice is to excite a spatiotemporal wave contraction in the bands. In creating spatial waves, there are a lot of degrees of freedom. One can change the duration of the contraction, the length of the wave, the origin point of contraction, and so forth. Next are considered two examples of one-dimensional spatial-wave excitation.

To ease the explanation, label one end of the band α and the other β. A one-dimensional contraction wave is then described as originating from end α of the band and traveling to end β. This means that all the elements in width and thickness, the ones at the same centerline natural coordinate, contract and relax together.

For ease of comparison with the uniform contraction, where all the elements are contracted in sync, the authors create a wave that has the contraction front traveling from end α of the band to end β. Once the contraction front reaches the β end of the band, the relaxation front starts from the original α end. This means that there is one instance of time where the whole band is contracted. The authors call this the "long wave contraction."

Simulations are also run where the wave is shorter and the relaxation front starts before the contraction front reaches the β end. The authors call such a wave a "medium wave contraction."

For all the different types of contractions the maximal amplitude of enforced stress was adjusted such that at the given Young's modulus of the active material, the resulting strain does not exceed physiologic constraints discussed previously.

Computational methods

To enable spatiotemporal excitation it is necessary to allow different sections of the bands to contract independently. This creates a complex coupling between local small deformations and huge global shape responses, making it a challenging modeling problem. Another difficulty is that one is considering three-dimensional geometries. To combat these problems, the idea of finite elements is used. It is possible, with small quadrilateral elements, to build very complicated shapes. The finite element method also breaks down a complicated problem of the dynamics of a complicated system in response to deformation into a set of manageable equations. Because this set is very large, it behooves one to use the computing power available to solve it. The authors model these bands using a finite element package, ABAQUS, designed to handle such problems. In the finite element code ABAQUS built-in tools are used to "excite" each node independently, and when the nodes of an element are "excited," the element contracts in the direction of the longitudinal fiber direction.

Data analysis

Fortran and Matlab codes are used to extract and analyze the data from the simulations. For the purpose of this analysis the position of each node from the simulation is extracted. Using this information the volume is calculated. In case of the embryonic one-chamber tube model, the volume is approximated as a cylinder. During the deformation the diameter of the cylinder may vary as a function of the long axis. For the double helical, two-pumping chamber model of the adult heart, the left ventricle volume is approximated as nonaxisymmetric paraboloid. The shape of this paraboloid varies in the course of the beat.

These simulations do not model fluid. That means that it is unnecessary to model valves. Unless an actual pump has valves, it is very ineffectual. Indeed, in the absence of valves most of the blood pumped during a contraction flows back during relaxation. It is assumed that the valves are present. This assumption implies that if the volume of the chamber is increased, there is blood sucked into the pump from the inlet. When the volume of the chamber is decreased, the blood is forced out through the outlet. One can simply keep track of the volume that would fit inside the spiral to calculate the effectiveness of the pump.

To create a meter stick for the computational experiment the ejection fraction was calculated for each system as it deforms with time:

$$\mathrm{EF}(t) = \frac{V_{max} - V(t)}{V_{max}} \quad \textit{and} \quad \mathrm{EF}_{max} = \frac{V_{max} - V_{min}}{V_{max}} \tag{1}$$

where $V(t)$, V_{max}, and V_{min} are the volume at time t, maximum volume, and minimum volume of the chamber, respectively. This is the same formula that is used to find the ejection fraction in physiology for adult hearts, where $V_{max} = V_{end\ diasotolic}$ and $V_{min} = V_{end\ systolic}$.

To judge the dynamics of the simulations the visualization techniques available in a specialized software were used (ABAQUS CAE). For the tube model a wire-frame of the initial configuration is overlayed on the transformed configuration. This way it is possible to compare directly the original and deformed spiral shape. For the double helix adult heart model, a piece of very soft material that is fixed to the side of the simulated left ventricle was created. To make sure that this indicator does not impact the dynamics, it is made from a material that is two orders of magnitude softer than the material of the band (ie, the Young's modulus of the elastic indicator is one hundredth of the Young's modulus of the active material). Because the elastic indicator is attached along the length of the left ventricle, it indicates the amount of twist. If the elastic indicator deforms symmetrically there is no twist. If it deforms sideways, there has to be a twist present.

Results

The authors originally hypothesized that the cause of twisting in the embryonic tube heart is the response of the helical structure of the muscle fibers to muscle contractions. To test the hypothesis they created a spiral band wound about a tube. As the first simulation they induced a uniform periodic contraction. This means that at each heartbeat the spiral was uniformly contracted and then released.

No twist in a uniformly contracted spiral band

The fiber angle did not have appreciable impact on the dynamics throughout the range of meaningful values of 5 to 80 degrees. Fig. 5A shows a series of snapshots of the simulation for a representative fiber angle of 50 degrees. Initially, the muscle bands are relaxed (red); then they are

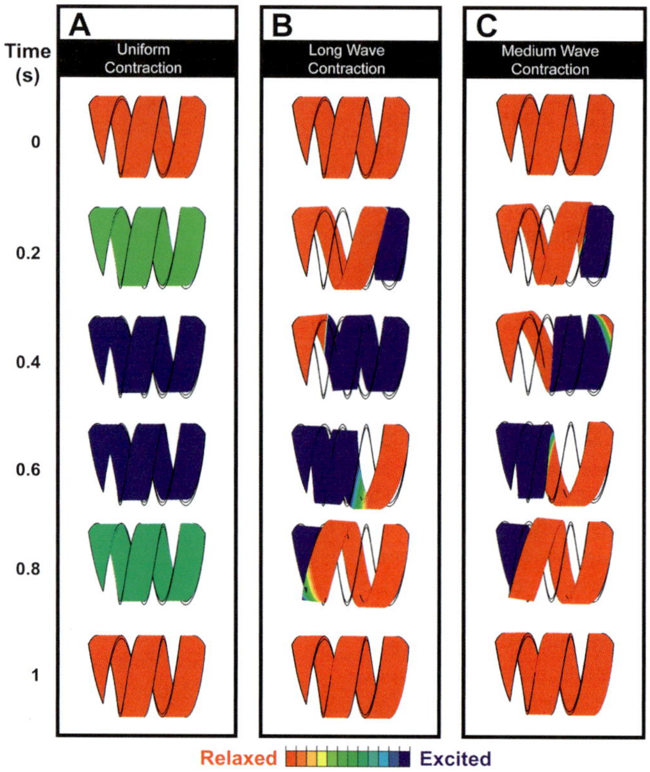

Fig. 5. Snapshots of the ABAQUS simulations at different time steps for the embryonic heart spiral model with a 50 degree pitch (fiber) angle. The left column indicates the time in seconds. Each snapshot shows the current configuration of the spiral. The colors indicate the level of excitation as shown in the panel at the bottom: blue, fully excited; red, relaxed. Each simulation starts at the relaxed state ($t = 0s$); goes through the contraction scheme and relaxation scheme; and ends back in the fully relaxed state ($t = 1s$). For comparison purposes, an outline of the initial shape of the spiral is overlayed on each picture as a thick black line. (*A*) Uniform contraction. Here the spiral smoothly contracts during $t = 0s - 0.4s$, and smoothly relaxes during $t = 0.6s - 1s$. The radius is smallest when the band is fully contracted $t = 0.4s - 0.6s$. There is no change in pitch angle as seen by comparing the current configuration with the outline of the initial shape. There is no twist in this simulation. (*B*) Long wave contraction. The contraction wave front starts at the right end ($t = 0.2s, 0.4s$) and travels through the band to the left end. The band is fully contracted at approximately $t = 0.5s$. The relaxation front starts at the left end of the band ($t = 0.6s, 0.8s$) and travels to the other end. The radius is reduced unsymmetrically along the length of the tube ($t = 0.4s - 0.6s$). The pitch angle is changed drastically as seen from comparing the current band to the outline of the initial configuration ($t = 0.2s - 0.8s$). This indicates that there is a twist in the tube. (*C*) Medium wave contraction. The contraction wave front starts at the right end ($t = 0.2s, 0.4s$) and travels through the band to the left end. The band is never fully contracted. The relaxation front starts at the left end of the band ($t = 0.6s, 0.8s$) and travels to the other end. The radius is reduced unsymmetrically along the length of the tube ($t = 0.4s - 0.6s$). The pitch angle is changed drastically as seen from comparing the current band with the outline of the initial configuration ($t = 0.2s - 0.8s$). This indicates that there is a twist in the tube.

gradually contracted until the elements reach the maximum allowable strain (blue); and then they are relaxed again. The outline of the original configuration is overlayed on each spiral band. The radius of the band at the maximum contraction ($t = 0.4s - 0.6s$) is smaller than the original radius. The snapshots of the simulation show how the spiral smoothly contracts about the central axis and then gradually releases. No perceptible twist is apparent in these images. The forces present are incapable of inducing a twist in the structure. The authors could have been disappointed by this result if they did not have an insight from modeling the adult heart.

Back to the future: adult heart model

To answer this quandary turn forward, in ontogeny time, to the adult heart. In the adult heart the contraction of the muscle fibers yields an intricate dynamics, the heart twists at each beat [23–25]. If one understands the origin of this twist, one can hope to understand the twist in the embryonic heart. One can draw conclusions about the dynamics of the embryonic heart from findings on the adult heart, because in both cases any movements are caused by the contraction of the muscle fibers.

In the adult heart the contraction is induced by the Purkinje network. This nerve network does not excite the whole myocardium at once. It is unlikely that the myocardium contracts all at once. As a result, the adult heart is subject to spatial-wave contractions instead of a uniform contraction.

Simulations of the adult heart

The idea of spatial-wave contractions is rarely considered in cardiac modeling. This is mostly because most cardiac models are so complex that it is a challenge to test such cases. For the authors' simplified model they were able to test such spatial-contraction patterns. Fig. 6 shows time snapshots of simulations with different excitation schemes. In each of the series of pictures the level of excitation is color coded, with red as relaxed and blue as fully excited. The excitation wave front starts at one end of the band and travels to the other. It is followed by a relaxation front moving in the same direction. One can vary the time between the contraction and relaxation fronts as one of the variables of the system. One of the possible wavelike contractions has the whole band fully contracted at some point in time (see Fig. 4B). It is also possible, however, that the spatial-contraction wave never contracts the band fully (see Fig. 4C). One may worry that the wave contraction negatively impacts the pumping ability.

How uniform versus spatial-wave contractions affect pumping ability: adult heart model

To ensure that pumping efficiency is not negatively affected the authors tested the double helix model of the adult heart under both a uniform contraction and a spatial-wave contraction. The results of these tests were judged by calculating the left ventricular ejection fraction. The use of this particular criteria is justified by the fact that a large amount of physiologic data is available for the left ventricular ejection fraction. To calculate the ejection fraction, the authors approximated the left ventricle as a paraboloid and calculated the volume at each time step. The ejection fraction is then simply given by equation (1).

The results for the simplified model easily match the physiologic data of maximal ejection fraction. The values in Table 1 show no drawback to having a spatial-wave contraction, as compared with a uniform contraction.

Different dynamics caused by spatial-waves

What is more fascinating is that the different contraction schemes produce different dynamics of the structure. Fig. 5 shows the snapshots of the three simulations side by side. The twist is easily visualized by keeping track of the elastic parabolic indicator fixed at the side of the structure's left ventricle. The piece of elastic material deforms in the same radial plane for the uniform excitation scheme ([see Fig. 5A]; $t = 0.2s - 0.8s$). For both the long and medium wave contraction, at some time step the indicator deforms out of the radial plane ([see Fig. 5B and C]; $t = 0.4s - 0.6s$). This means that the double helical structure twists in cases where the excitation is wavelike and does not in the case of a uniform excitation. This gives a hint that maybe a wave-type excitation in a tubular model could also be related to the twist.

Forward to the past: embryonic heart model

The authors tested a spatial-wave contraction scheme in the spiral wound about a tube. Fig. 5B and C show the time snapshots in which the contraction, represented in blue, starts at one end of the spiral and travels to the other end. The relaxation front, in red, follows the same pattern. As in the adult heart, the time between the excitation and relaxation front can be varied. In the uniform contraction scheme the whole spiral is contracted at once, which is not necessarily true for a spatial-wave contraction. The whole structure is contracted only if the two fronts are separated from each other by at least the length of the spiral.

How uniform versus spatial-wave contractions affect pumping ability: embryonic heart model

To ensure that the wave-form contraction does not affect pumping, the authors tracked the volume of the tube during the course of the beat. Looking at the snapshots of the uniformly contracting tube simulation, one would suspect that the volume should change just as smoothly as

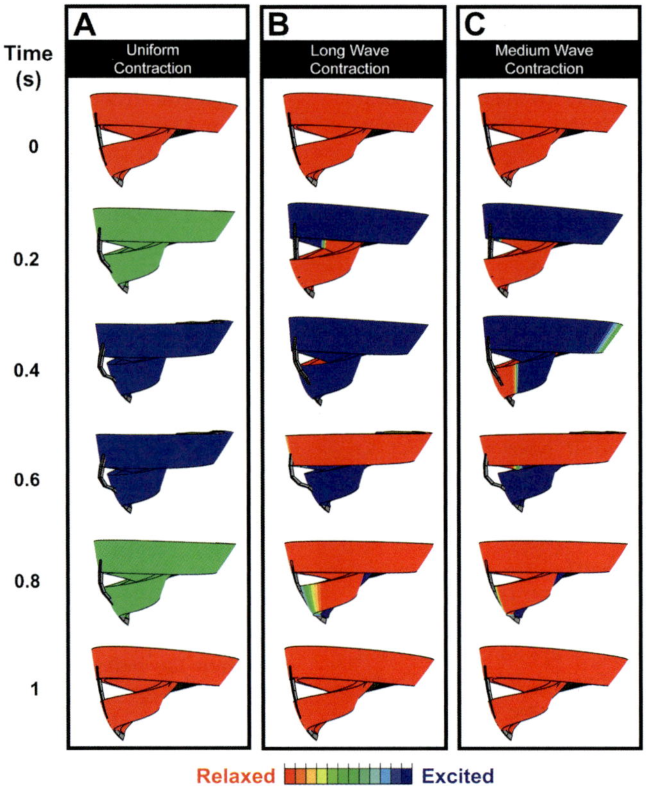

Fig. 6. Snapshots of the ABAQUS simulations at different time steps for the adult heart double helix model. The left column indicates the time in seconds. Each snapshot shows the current configuration of the double helix. The colors indicate the level of excitation as shown in the panel at the bottom: blue, fully excited; red, relaxed. Each simulation starts at the relaxed state ($t = 0s$); goes through the contraction scheme and relaxation scheme; and ends back in the fully relaxed state ($t = 1s$). From this point of view, the volume reduction can be seen in how the top and bottom parts of the band come together during the contraction. A soft elastic material piece, indicated in dark gray, is fixed to the side of the left ventricle. (*A*) Uniform contraction. Here the double helix smoothly contracts during $t = 0s - 0.4s$, and smoothly relaxes during $t = 0.6s - 1s$. There is no twist of the left ventricle as indicated by ends of the gray material piece having a symmetric vertical position on the helical band. (*B*) Long wave contraction. The contraction wave front starts at right heart end ($t = 0.2s, 0.4s$) and travels through the band. The band is fully contracted at approximately $t = 0.5s$. The relaxation front starts at the right ventricle end of the band ($t = 0.6s, 0.8s$) and travels to the other end. The gray elastic material does not deform symmetrically ($t = 0.4s - 0.6s$). This indicates that there is a twist of the left ventricle. (*C*) Medium wave contraction. The contraction wave front starts at right heart end ($t = 0.2s, 0.4s$) and travels through the band. The band is never fully contracted. The relaxation front starts at the right ventricle end of the band ($t = 0.6s, 0.8s$) and travels to the other end. The gray elastic material does not deform symmetrically ($t = 0.4s - 0.6s$). This indicates that there is a twist of the left ventricle.

Table 1
The ejection fraction values for double helical pumps under different excitation patterns

		Contraction type (%)		
	Physiologic (%)	Uniform	Medium wave	Long wave
Maximal ejection fraction	50–60	54	54	53

the contraction (see Fig. 5A). That is the case as seen in Fig. 7.

As a matter of principle, it is possible for the spatial-wave contraction to affect pumping beneficially. Indeed, the spatial-wave contraction can induce not only simple shrinking, but also suction. In the plot of a representative fiber angle spiral undergoing a wave contraction the volume increases, then sharply decreases (see Fig. 7A). This means that initially more fluid is sucked in and then a larger amount is ejected, larger than is

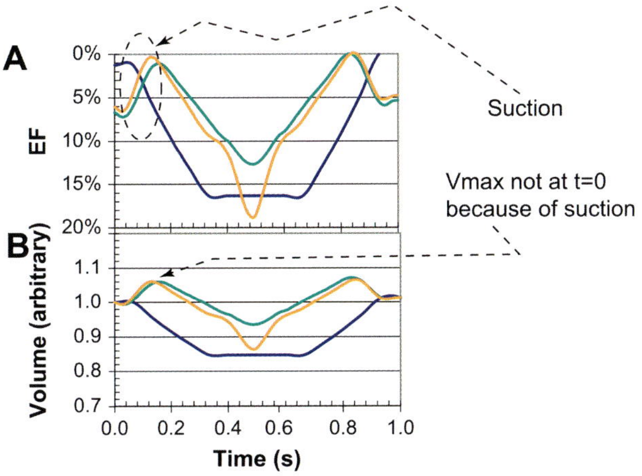

Fig. 7. (*A*) Plot of normalized volume of the tube chamber versus time. In case of wave-type contractions, the volume initially increases ($t = 0.04s - 0.15s$), because of suction. The volume is normalized over the initial value, and as a result the maximum volume in the case of wave contractions is at approximately $t = 0.15s$, as indicated by the arrow. (*B*) Plot of ejection fraction versus time. The ejection fraction of the long wave contraction is greater than that of the uniform contraction, because of suction. The period of suction is circled with a dotted line. Blue, uniform contraction; green, medium wave contraction; orange, long wave contraction.

otherwise possible. The subsequent increase in volume does not produce back flow because of the valves. In the snapshots in Fig. 5B and C it is possible to see qualitatively the cause of this suction. In the spatial-wave contraction, the part of the spiral that is contracting pulls on the piece that is still relaxed. In coming to mechanical equilibrium, part of the helix opens up, to reduce the stress on the band. Is this suction effect sufficiently beneficial to offset the fact that the whole band is not contracted at the same time?

For each contraction scheme the maximal ejection fraction at different fiber angles was compared. Equation (1) was used to calculate the ejection fraction of these pumping tubes. Table 2 shows the ejection fraction for spirals with different fiber angles undergoing different contraction schemes.

Even a spatial-wave contraction that does not contract the whole spiral is not a significant detriment to the pumping efficiency of the tube. Indeed, at some fiber angles a spatial-contraction scheme is beneficial to the effective pumping. This shows that the spatial-wave does not negatively impact the pumping efficiency. So, did it produce twist?

Evidence of twisting in a spiral undergoing a spatial-wave contraction

The snapshots in Fig. 5B and C qualitatively show that there is an asymmetry in how the spiral deforms. Unlike the deformations in response to a uniform excitation, for both wave excitation patterns the deformed shape is significantly offset from the original outline. The same mechanism that causes suction produces this radical deformation. In a tube, this deformation corresponds to a twist, to accommodate the change in pitch angle of parts of the spiral.

This begs the question: maybe the characteristic of leading importance is the wavelike contraction, and not the helical shape as originally claimed? If one had induced the propagating wave contraction in a simple tube with either longitudinal fibers or circumferential fibers the

Table 2
The ejection fraction values for tubular pumps with different pitch (fiber) angles under different excitation patterns

	Contraction type (%)		
Pitch angle	Uniform	Medium wave	Long wave
5	24	18	18
10	23	19	24
20	9	7	10
30	11	7	9
40	13	7	11
50	17	13	19
60	21	21	29
70	23	30	36
80	20	34	38

forces would have been in the axial or circumferential directions, respectively. As a result, the pumping efficiency would be reduced, because there would be no suction effect. In the longitudinal fiber case the length of the tube decreases, without opening up any part of the tube. In the radial fiber case, the radius of the tube simply decreases unsymmetrically, but no twist occurs. This model shows that only the combination of the helical structure and the spatial-wave type contraction scheme produces the twist necessary for further development. That is the main result of this study.

In summary, as Kemp [26] observed in his treatise on "spirals of life," helical designs in living creatures are generally appreciated for their static structure, rather than the active functional benefits they bring. There are many examples in nature where there is a helical muscle structure, ranging from worms to embryonic fish hearts [5,27,28]. It is shown here that the helical structure cannot be the sole cause of the mechanical twist necessary for development. If the contraction of the spiral is smooth and symmetric, it cannot lead to twist.

In the adult heart the twisting dynamics are well documented. It is also well known that the adult heart is excited in a complicated pattern. By modeling spatiotemporal excitation waves and simple temporal excitation in the adult heart model it is shown that the twist is only possible if the excitation is in the form of spatial-waves. Additionally, it is shown that no negative effects on pumping efficiency are brought about by wavelike contractions.

By applying this knowledge to the embryonic heart the authors demonstrate twisting of the spiral structure. The spiral tube's pumping ability is also not impacted by switching from a uniform excitation to a spatiotemporal excitation.

In light of these results one can form a better understanding of the development history of the heart. In the embryonic tube heart the fibers are organized helically. As it starts to beat the excitation pattern is not uniform, but is instead wavelike. The stress produced by the twisting of the tube under these conditions forces the tube to bend. Thus begins the road of phylogeny, changing the simply spiraled muscle fibers into a double helix structure of the adult heart.

References

[1] Streeter DD Jr, Spotnitz HM, Patel DP, et al. Fiber orientation in the canine left ventricle during diastole and systole. Circ Res 1969;24:339–47.

[2] Torrent-Guasp F, Kocica MJ, Corno AF, et al. Towards new understanding of the heart structure and function. Eur J Cardiothorac Surg 2005;27(2): 191–201.

[3] Buckberg GD, Weisfeldt ML, Ballester M, et al. Left ventricular form and function: scientific priorities and strategic planning for development of new views of disease. Circulation 2004;110(14):e333–6.

[4] Helm P, Beg MF, Miller MI, et al. Measuring and mapping cardiac fiber and laminar architecture using diffusion tensor MR imaging. Ann N Y Acad Sci 2005;1047(1):296–307.

[5] Forouhar AS, Liebling M, Hickerson A, et al. The embryonic vertebrate heart tube is a dynamic suction pump. Science 2006;312(5774):751–3.

[6] Liebling M, Forouhar AS, Wolleschensky R, et al. Rapid three-dimensional imaging and analysis of the beating embryonic heart reveals functional changes during development. Dev Dyn 2006; 235(11):2940–8.

[7] Moghaddam AN. Measurement and analysis of structure and function of myocardium in embryonic and adult heart, in option of bioengineering. Pasadena (CA): California Institute of Technology; 2006.

[8] Nasiraei-Moghaddam A, Liebling M, Forouhar AS, et al. A lagrangian approach reveals the active and passive regions in the embryonic zebrafish heart. Annals of Biomedical Engineering, submitted for publication.

[9] Larsen WJ. Development of the heart, in human embryology. Philadelphia: WB Saunders Company; 1997 p. 131–55.

[10] Bartman T, Hove J. Mechanics and function in heart morphogenesis. Dev Dyn 2005;233:373–81.

[11] Harvey RP, Rosenthal N. Heart development. San Diego (CA): Academic Press; 1999.

[12] Männer J. On rotation, torsion, lateralization, and handedness of the embryonic heart loop: new insights from a simulation model for the heart loop of chick embryos. Anat Rec A Discov Mol Cell Evol Biol 2004;278A(1):481–92.

[13] Mattheck C. Design in nature: learning from trees. New York: Springer; 1998.

[14] Crane HR. Principles and problems of biological growth. The Scientific Monthly 1950;70(6):376–89.

[15] Sallin EA. Fiber orientation and ejection fraction in the human left ventricle. Biophys J 1969;9(7): 954–64.

[16] Peskin CS, McQueen DM. A general method for the computer simulation of biological systems interacting with fluids. Symp Soc Exp Biol 1995;49: 265–76.

[17] Kovács SJ, McQueen DM, Peskin CS. Modelling cardiac fluid dynamics and diastolic function. Philosophical Transactions of the Royal Society A: Mathematical, Physical and Engineering Sciences 2001;359(1783):1299–314.

[18] Vendelin M, Bovendeerd P, Engelbrecht J, et al. Optimizing ventricular fibers: uniform strain or

stress, but not ATP consumption, leads to high efficiency. Am J Physiol Heart Circ Physiol 2002;283: 1072–81.

[19] Costa KD, Hunter PJ, Rogers JM, et al. A three-dimensional finite element method for large ventricular myocardium. Transactions of the ASME 1996; 118:452–72.

[20] Sengupta PP, Korinek J, Belohlavek M, et al. Left ventricular structure and function, basic science for cardiac imaging. J Am Coll Cardiol 2006;48(10): 1988–2001.

[21] Dubrovin BA, Fomenko AT, Novikov SP. Modern geometry: methods and applications. In: Axler S, Gehring FW, Ribet KA, editors. Springer series in Soviet mathematics, graduate texts in mathematics. 2nd edition. New York: Springer-Verlag; 1992. p. 61–8.

[22] Humphrey JD. Cardiovascular solid mechanics. New York: Springer; 2002.

[23] Moon MR, Ingels NB Jr, Daughters GT II, et al. Alterations in left ventricular twist mechanics with inotropic stimulation and volume loading in human subjects. Circulation 1994;89(1):142–50.

[24] Beyar R, Yin FCP, Hausknecht M, et al. Dependence of left ventricular twist-radial shortening relations on cardiac cycle phase. Am J Physiol 1989;257: H1119.

[25] Yun KL, Niczyporuk MA, Daughters GT II, et al. Alterations in left ventricular diastolic twist mechanics during acute human cardiac allograft rejection. Circulation 1991;83(3):962–73.

[26] Kemp M. Spirals of life: D'Arcy Thompson and Theodore Cook, with Leonardo and Durer in retrospect. Physis: Rivista Internazionale di Storia della Scienza 1995;32(1):37–54.

[27] Clark RB, Cowey JB. Factors controlling the change of shape of certain Nemertean and Turbellarian worms. Journal of Experimental Biology 1958;35: 731–48.

[28] O'Reilly JC, Ritter DA, Carrier DR. Hydrostatic locomotion in a limbless tetrapod. Nature 1997; 386(6622):269–72.

ELSEVIER
SAUNDERS

Heart Failure Clin 4 (2008) 261–272

HEART
FAILURE
CLINICS

The Myocardial Band

Manel Ballester, MD[a,*], Ana Ferreira, MD[b], Francesc Carreras, MD[c]

[a] *University of Lleida, Barcelona, Spain*
[b] *Hospital Royo Villanova, Zaragoza, Spain*
[c] *Hospital de la Santa Creu i Sant Pau, Barcelona, Spain*

The complexity of ventricular myocardial fiber distribution has appealed investigators for a long time. Since Lower's initial description of the helical transmural overlapping pattern of ventricular myocardial fibers, several investigators in the last four centuries have tried to decipher a unique ruled-based assignment that, in the words of Franklin Pain Mall (1862–1917), "..may be applied equally well to all the ventricular myocardial fibers, showing them together in a coherent, common architectural plan" [1]. In fact, the ultimate reason for ventricular myofiber orientation has eluded a rationale explanation for its existence and its relevance to cardiac function.

Francisco (Paco) Torrent-Guasp (1931–2005), a Spanish cardiologist working in Dènia, Alicante, through careful myocardial dissection studies spanning half a century [2–11] eventually discovered that the complex structure of the ventricular myocardium is due to a double-loop helical orientation of a single muscular band that extends from the pulmonary artery to the aorta, with a 180-degree twist in its middle part (Fig. 1) [12–14]. The band is deemed to be a consequence of changes in the circulatory system through evolution (Fig. 2A), evolving to an extravasation of blood into a self-contained pumping structure that constitutes the ventricles (Fig. 2B). Once the myocardial band is unveiled, the enigma of fiber orientation appears obvious and the inevitable result of its helical structure.

* Corresponding author. Lluis Jover 40, 08340 Vilassar de Mar, Barcelona, Spain.

E-mail address: mballesterr@comll.cat (M. Ballester).

Form determines function, and once the band anatomy was clear to Torrent-Guasp [12], he predicted myocardial mechanics before the first magnetic resonance descriptions appeared in the literature [15–17] and suggested that the ventricular myocardium works as an agonist-antagonist unit [18].

This article focuses on unfolding the band following the guidelines previously established by Torrent-Guasp [18], describes the segments of such bands and their intricate relationship to form an anatomically and functionally nonhomogeneous myocardium, and outlines the function that derives from such anatomy, with an emphasis on agonist-antagonist interaction and systolic ventricular filling [19].

Naked-eye myocardial fiber visualization and local orientation

When the myocardium is macroscopically inspected, small bundles of tissue identified as "myocardial fibers" are observed. These fibers are, in fact, the result of several myocytes wrapped in a spongelike scaffold formed by connective tissue, blood vessels, and nerves which have a precise local orientation. The main (predominant) course of the myocardial fibers can easily be followed without any tool after boiling a heart to soften the collagen structure; however, when no points of reference are used, myofiber dissection inevitably leads one to follow some fibers for a short course until dissection is made impossible. Torrent-Guasp discovered certain areas where the courses of bundles of fibers crossed each other in different planes (cleavage planes). Knowledge of these planes provides landmarks for manual dissection and is the clue to

1551-7136/08/$ - see front matter
doi:10.1016/j.hfc.2008.02.011

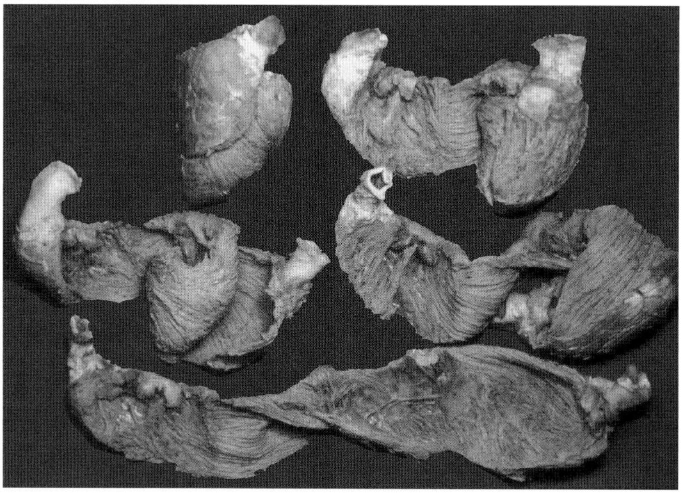

Fig. 1. Stages of the manual unfolding of the ventricular myocardium into a single myocardial band that suffers a 180-degree twist in its middle portion. In the extended myocardial band, the myocardial fibers can be followed from the pulmonary artery to the aorta. (*From* Torrent-Guasp F. Estructura y función del corazón. Rev Esp Cardiol 1998;51:92; with permission.)

a systematic unfolding of the ventricular band. When the band is unfolded, myocardial fibers are easily identified and followed from the pulmonary artery to the aorta.

Before a description is made of the unfolding procedure, it must be pointed out that the term *band* is used not to describe a discrete, well-defined, bundle of muscle in the way that skeletal muscle is arranged.

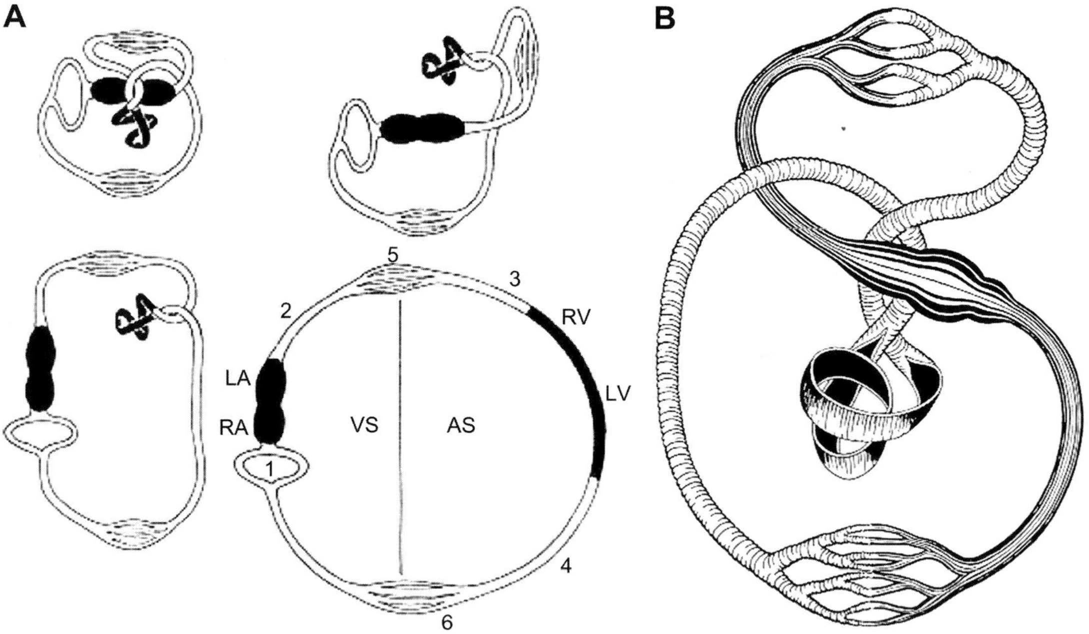

Fig. 2. (*A*) Proposed phylogenetical explanation of the evolution of the circulatory system from the fish to humans, according to Francisco Torrent-Guasp. AS, arterial segment; LA, left atrium; LV, left ventricle; RA, right atrium; RV, right ventricle; VS, venous segment. (*B*) In this drawing by Torrent-Guasp, the extravasation of the blood contents into a self-contained complex helical modification of a part of the vessel to form the right and left ventricles is shown. The triangle-shaped opening and closing of the modified part at the level of the pulmonary artery and aorta (both ends of the myocardial band) can be observed at dissection.

Indeed, clear-cut boundaries or anatomic planes are not observed, but a functional (vectorial) arrangement of fibers lying on an optimal direction to exert their function as a continuous medium is found.

Unfolding the ventricles

After boiling the heart, atria can easily be separated from the ventricles (Fig. 3). Fig. 4 depicts the successive stages of unfolding the ventricles. Once fat is removed from the epicardial surface, the pulmonary artery and aorta are separated. The first step is to remove the superficial fibers bridging the anterior interventricular sulcus (aberrant fibers). In this way, the right ventricular free wall can be dissected and moved aside (see Fig. 4A, B). The right ventricular free wall is now exposed, and its fibers inevitably lead to the posterior border of the wall in close contact with the left ventricular mass (see Fig. 4C). Gently pushing the right ventricular fibers following their predominant direction opens the path for these fibers to encircle the left ventricle up to the root of the aorta (see Fig. 4D–I). At this moment, the strong attachment of band by the left aortic fibrous trigon must be cut (see Fig. 4J). In this way, the basal loop is unfolded. Once the basal loop is freed from its attachment to the aortic root, fibers suddenly change their orientation and dive from the epicardium to the endocardium in a helical fashion (descendant segment). This basal twist and change in orientation at the base of the left ventricle is responsible for the 180-degree twist visible in its middle portion when the band is extended (see Fig. 1). The dissection then proceeds at another part of the heart, at the level of the cleavage plane formed by the horizontal fibers of the descendant segment and the vertical ones that follow to reach the aorta (see the arrows in Fig. 4K). Careful dissection of this plane (see Fig. 4L–P), after cutting the right aortic trigone, allows entering the left ventricular cavity (see Fig. 4Q) and untwisting the helical ascendant part of the band (see Fig. 4R, S) to its full length (see Fig. 4T).

Segmental band distribution

The distribution of the myocardial segments constituting the myocardium in 29 calf hearts is shown in Fig. 5. This distribution was systematically accomplished by the unfolding technique described previously and by painting the entire surface of each segment with different colors: the right segment (blue) from the origin of the pulmonary artery to the posterior limit of the right ventricle, the left segment (red) to the point where the twist of the band starts, the descendant segment (yellow) from the middle twist of the band to where the ascending trajectory starts, and the ascendant segment (green) from this point up to the aortic root.

After the painted myocardial preparations were left to dry, the band was folded and glued

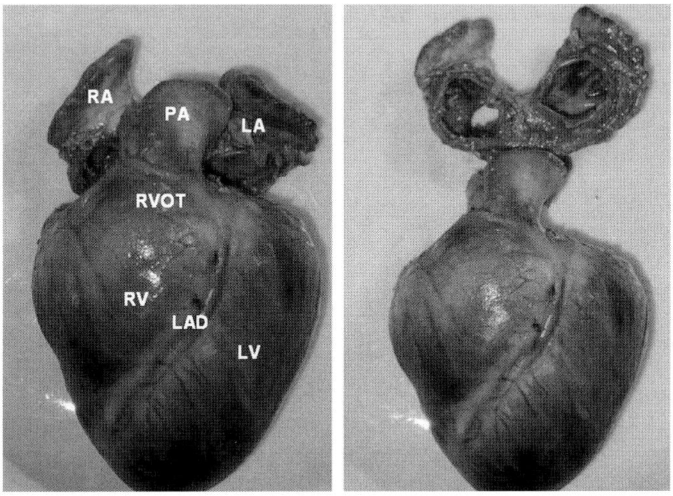

Fig. 3. Before dissection of the ventricles and after boiling the entire heart, the atria are easily separated from the ventricles. Note that both atria are in continuity (impossible to dissect one from the other), and that the two perforations correspond with the tricuspid and mitral valve ventricular orifices. LA, left atrium; LAD, left anterior descending coronary artery; LV, left ventricle; PA, pulmonary artery; RA, right atrium; RV, right ventricle; RVOT, right ventricular outflow tract.

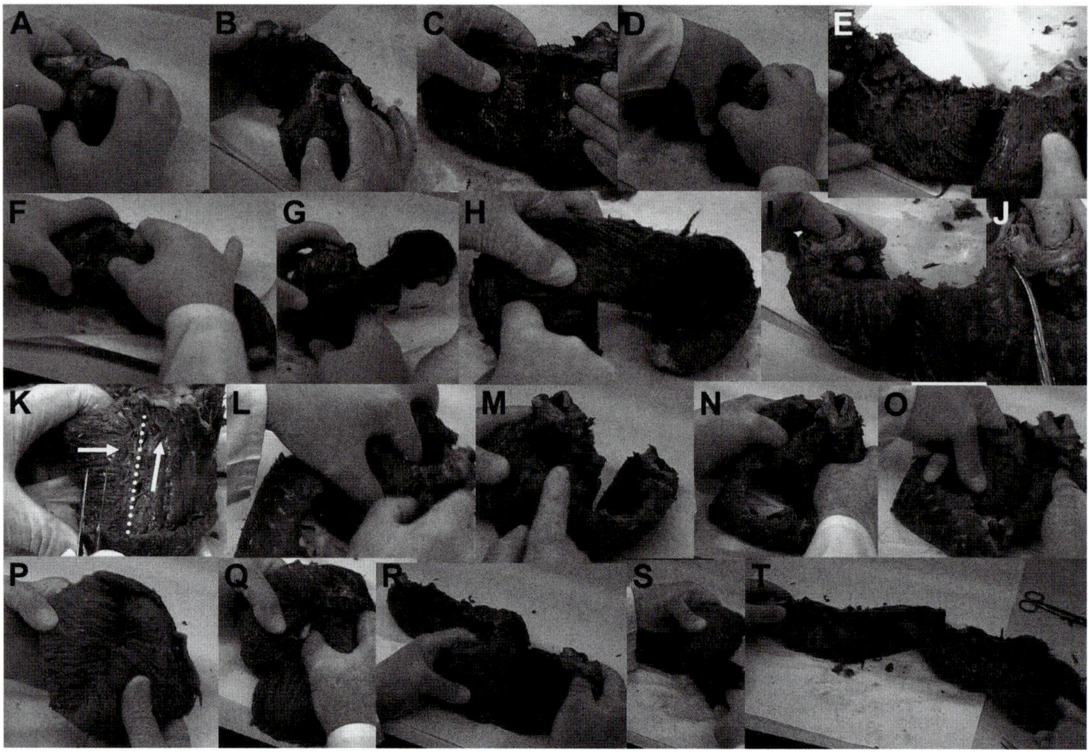

Fig. 4. (*A–T*) Successive stages of unfolding the ventricles to unveil the myocardial band (see text for description).

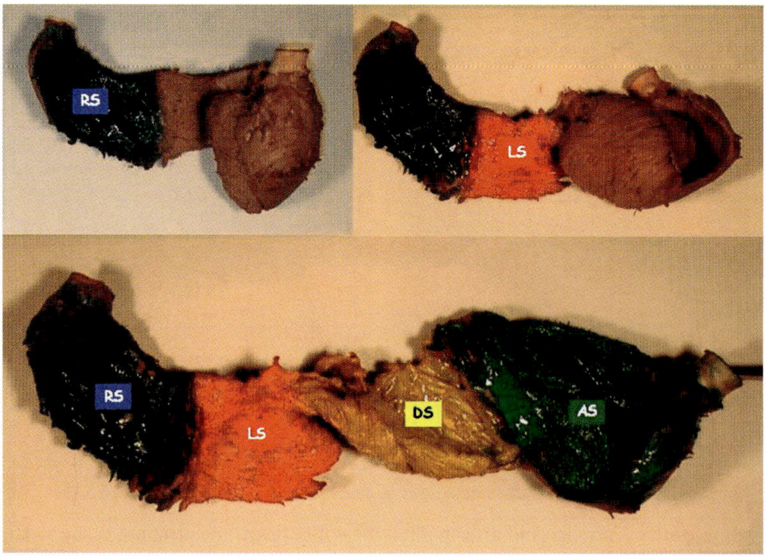

Fig. 5. Scheme of the colored band segments. The right ventricle (blue) and upper portion of the left ventricle (red) form the basal loop. The descendant (yellow) and ascendant (green) segments form the apical loop. AS, ascendant segment; DS, descendant segment; LS, left segment; RS, right segment.

to its original position and the hearts sliced in planes similar to those obtained in standard imaging: long-axis slices (7 hearts), four-chamber sections (7 hearts), and short-axis slices (basal, midventricular, and apical) (6 hearts). After slicing the hearts, the exposed myocardium of the different segments of the band was manually painted taking as reference the color of its surface. The percentage contribution of each segment to the myocardial thickness in each plane was measured.

After exclusion of five hearts because the unfolding could not be performed successfully, the distribution of each of the segments of the myocardial band in the ventricular walls in the remaining 21 was determined (Figs. 6–9). In the long-axis section (see Fig. 6), the right segment (blue) was well delineated and constituted 100% of the thickness of the free wall of the right ventricle. The left segment (red) occupied a small area in the most posterobasal portion of the free wall of the left ventricle and overlaid the ascendant segment (green). At the level of the midseptum, the ascendant and descendant segments contributed to septal thickness. The posterior wall of the left ventricle was occupied in its basal regions by the left segment and by the ascendant segment in the midventricular and apical regions.

In the four-chamber section (see Fig. 7), the descendant segment occupied the inner surface of the left ventricle and was surrounded by the ascendant segment. In the lateral wall, the proportion occupied by the ascendant segment contrasted with the small contribution of the basal segment.

In the short-axis section (see Fig. 8), a complex distribution of the band segments was observed. At the base of the heart (see Fig. 8, top), the right and left segments were in continuity and enclosed both descendant and ascendant segments. In the middle portion of the ventricles (see Fig. 8, middle), the ascendant segment wrapped around the descendant almost 360 degrees; at this section, the basal loop was barely seen. At the level of the apex, the segmental distribution was similar to the middle portion of the ventricles (see Fig. 8, bottom).

Table 1 discloses the contribution of each segment to the left ventricular thickness. Therefore, the left ventricular myocardium is not a homogenous structure but is formed by different overlapping ventricular segments that constitute the myocardial walls.

Segmental function: twist-untwist

The unique anatomy of the reciprocal helical configuration of the ventricular myocardial band determines the way the ventricles exert their double function—ejection and suction of the blood (see Fig. 9A). Torrent-Guasp suggested that ventricular electromechanical activation is anistropically propagated following the myocardial band and takes place in the following sequence: right ventricular segment and left ventricular segment (basal loop) → descendant segment → ascendant segment

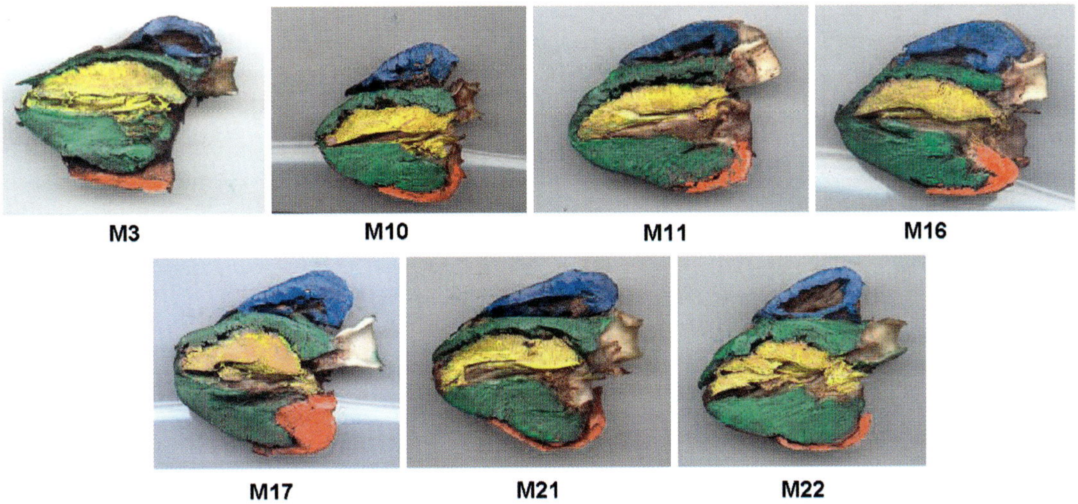

Fig. 6. Long-axis sections of seven colored porcine hearts. Colors indicate right segment (blue), left segment (red), descendant segment (yellow), and ascendant segment (green).

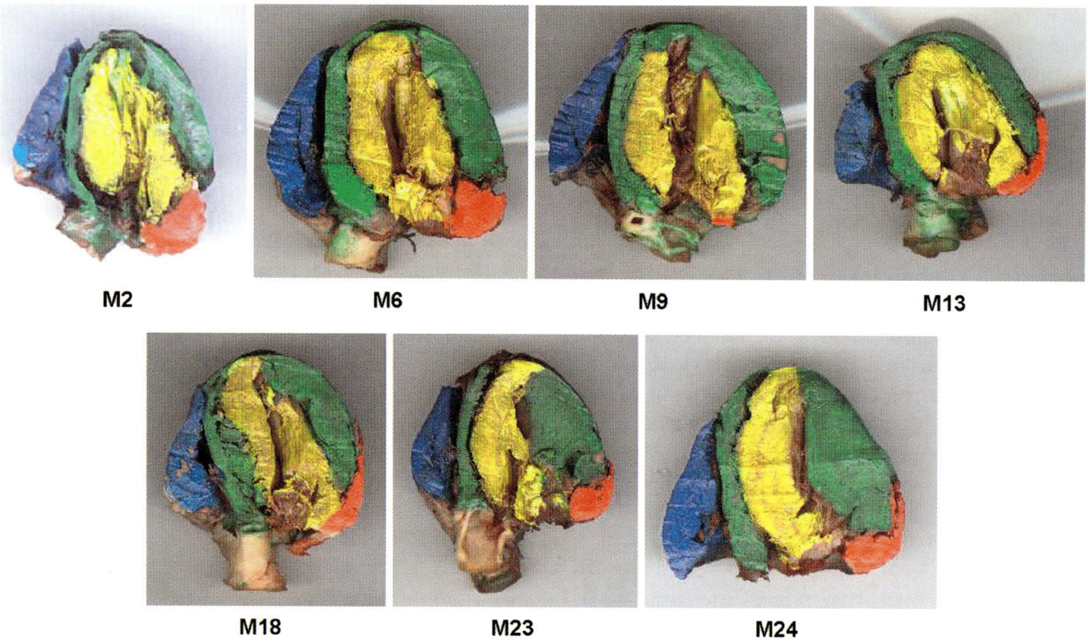

Fig. 7. Four-chamber sections of the colored hearts.

(apical loop) [12–14]. Recent Fourier analysis of the sequence of ventricular mechanical activation has confirmed a base (right and left) to apex sequence of activation [20,21].

After contraction of the basal loop has taken place, subsequent contraction of the descendant segment pulls the basal loop downward and toward the apex, thereby shortening the longitudinal axis of the ventricular cavities, reducing its volume, and twisting the base clockwise and the apex anticlockwise to give way to ventricular ejection (see Fig. 9A, right). Contraction of the ascendant segment follows, which generates a rapid upward displacement of the base of the heart that

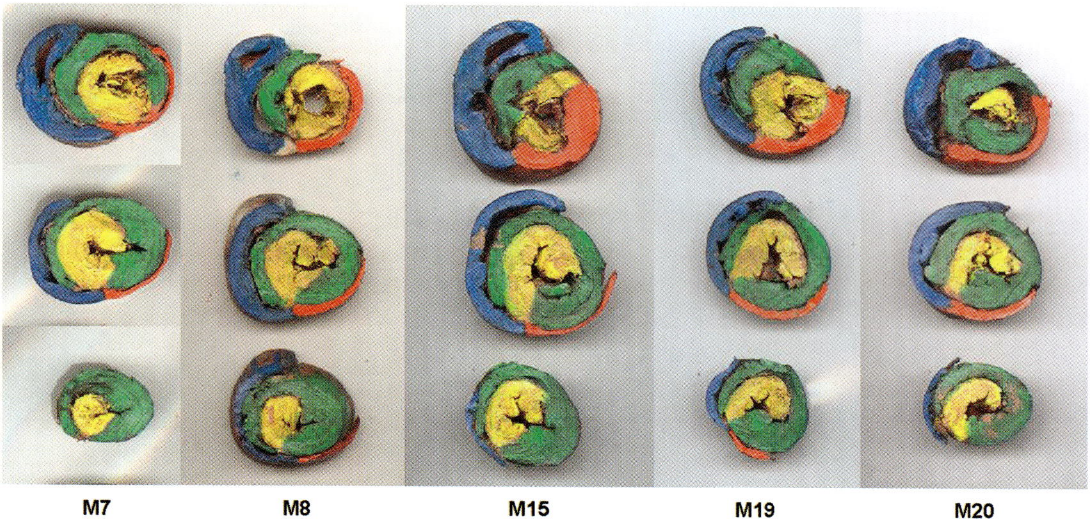

Fig. 8. Short-axis sections of the colored porcine hearts. Top, basal section; middle, midventricular section; bottom, apical sections.

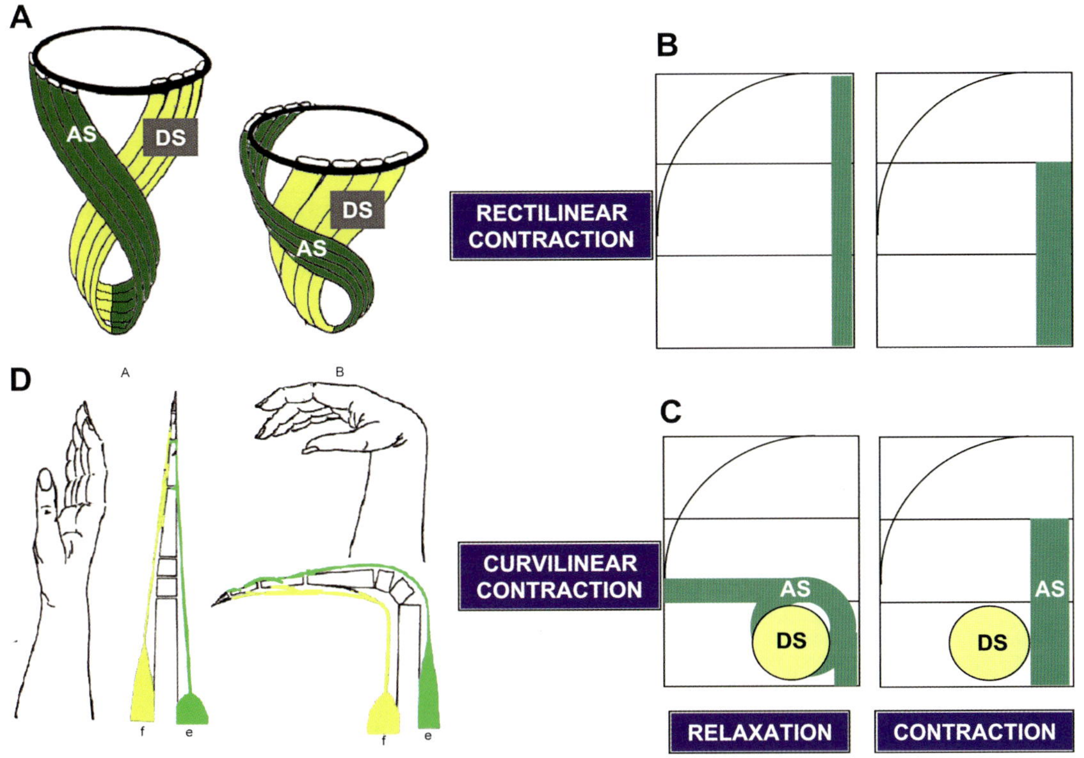

Fig. 9. (*A*) Torrent-Guasp's proposed twist and untwist ventricular function [18,19]. Left drawing, diastole; right drawing, systole. AS, ascendant segment (green); DS, descendant segment (yellow). (*B*) Scheme of a muscular rectilinear contraction (ie, biceps). When the muscle contracts, it thickens and shortens. (*C*) In a curvilinear contraction, the muscle behaves in the same way, but when leaning on a neighboring structure, the motion causes elevation of the muscle. (*D*) Contraction of the forearm in which an agonist-antagonist unit operates to contract and extend the hand. Torrent-Guasp proposed that this mechanism underlies the upward movement of the ascendant segment that causes the ventricular cavity to increase its longitudinal axis and ultimately suck the blood and fill the ventricle. AS, ascendant segment; DS, descendant segment; e, extensor muscle; f, flexor muscle.

increases the ventricular longitudinal axis and volume (see Fig. 9A, left) and untwists the ventricles. This sequence has been tested in experimental studies using microcrystals placed at the endocardium, along the descendant myofibers, and the epicardium, following the ascendant myofibers, where simultaneous initial activation of both segments but a late prolongation of the activity of the ascendant segment was observed [22].

Several imaging modalities and experiments support the twist-untwist ventricular mechanics initially proposed by Torrent-Guasp [23–26]. The first evidence was provided by tagging MR studies [27,28] where torsion and untorsion dynamics were described [15–17], but no interpretation as to the nature of this motion was provided. A recent report using Doppler tissue imaging allowed noninvasive quantification of ventricular torsion, which closely correlated with MRI studies [29]. A recent modality of ultrasound studies, speckled tracking echocardiography [30–32], has provided a unique means to tag speckles from the B-mode, which are natural acoustic markers that can be selectively identified and followed in consecutive frames during the heart cycles. This technique has shown that, at an apical level, the left ventricle rotates counterclockwise as viewed from apex, whereas the base rotates clockwise. This gradient of left ventricle rotation between the two levels creates a "wringing" motion.

The myocardium as an agonist-antagonist unit and systolic ventricular filling

It was suggested by Torrent-Guasp [18] that descendant and ascendant segments of the apical

Table 1
Percentage occupation of each of the segments of the ventricular myocardial band in conforming the ventricular walls in each of the sections

A. Long-axis section

	Basal septum		Midseptum		Apical septum		Posterobasal		Posterobasal		Posteromedial		Posteroapical
Parameter	Des	Asc	Asc	Des	Asc	Des	Left	Asc	Left	Asc	Asc	Left	Asc
Mean	39.30	60.69	34.03	65.96	40.84	59.15	80.82	19.17	16.62	83.37	89.81	10.18	100.00
Min	21.05	34.88	20.00	45.00	22.22	40.54	32.43	.00	8.70	70.00	81.25	.00	100.00
Max	65.12	78.95	55.00	80.00	59.46	77.78	100.00	67.57	30.00	91.30	100.00	18.75	100.00

B. Four-chamber section

	Basal septum		Basal septum		Midseptum		Apical septum		Basal lateral		Lateral basal		Midlateral		Lateral apical	
Parameter	Asc	Des	Asc	Des	Asc	Des	Asc	Des	Left	Des	Left	Des	Des	Asc	Des	Asc
Mean	86.34	13.65	36.66	63.33	34.49	65.50	34.88	65.11	53.24	46.75	55.90	44.07	9.63	90.36	.00	100.00
Min	55.56	.00	23.08	36.36	23.53	40.74	23.81	50.00	.00	.00	.00	.00	.00	69.23	.00	100.00
Max	100.00	44.44	63.64	76.92	59.26	76.47	50.00	76.19	100.00	100.00	100.00	100.00	30.77	100.00	.00	100.00

C. Short-axis section

Basal

	Septum		Lateral			Anterior		Posterior	
Parameter	Asc	Des	Left	Asc	Des	Asc	Des	Left	Des
Mean	60.08	39.91	52.06	21.90	26.03	32.28	67.71	45.74	54.26
Min	41.67	25.00	20.00	.00	.00	16.67	53.33	28.57	.00
Max	75.00	58.33	100.00	71.43	66.67	46.67	83.33	100.00	71.43

Midventricular

	Septum		Lateral			Anterior		Posterior		
Parameter	Asc	Des	Left	Asc	Des	Asc	Des	Left	Asc	Des
Mean	31.34	68.65	14.29	75.13	10.56	37.01	62.98	28.71	47.54	23.73
Min	23.53	53.33	10.53	38.10	.00	24.00	50.00	23.81	19.05	.00
Max	46.67	76.47	16.67	86.67	47.62	50.00	76.00	33.33	71.43	57.14

Apical

	Septum		Anterior		Posterior			Lateral
Parameter	Asc	Des	Asc	Des	Asc	Des	Left	Asc
Mean	31.97	68.02	39.09	100.00	48.02	40.92	11.05	100.00
Min	21.05	57.14	20.00	100.00	.00	.00	.00	100.00
Max	42.86	78.95	63.16	100.00	84.62	83.33	20.00	100.00

Abbreviations: Asc, ascendant segment; Des, descendant segment; Left, left segment; Min, minimum; Max, maximum.

loop act as an agonist-antagonist muscle contraction unit, the first being responsible for systole and the latter for diastole. The way in which contraction of the ascendant segment of the band can lead to long-axis lengthening of the heart, ventricular volume expansion, and, ultimately, suction of blood is intriguing. The key question is how a contraction of a segment may give rise to elongation of the ventricles. Normally, contraction of a rectilinear muscle, such as the biceps, leads to shortening (see Fig. 9B). When a muscle adopts a curvilinear spatial configuration (ie, that of the forearm that leans against the bones of the wrist), contraction also leads to shortening, but the distal part of the muscle becomes elevated (see Fig. 9C, D). An elegant model proposed by Torrent-Guasp to show how a curvilinear contraction works in the heart is shown in Fig. 10. Contraction of

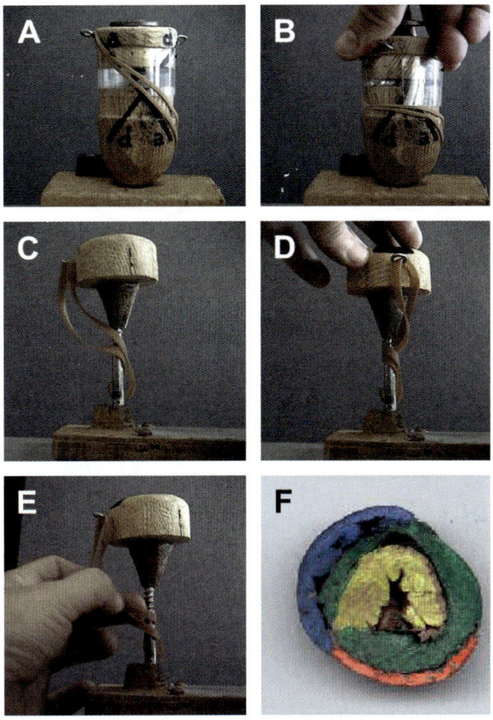

Fig. 10. (*A*) A simple model devised by Torrent-Guasp to explain how contraction of the ascendant segment (represented by a rubber band) can elevate the basal loop. The descendant segment is drawn as a black line. (*B*) Manual simulation of contraction of the descendant segment twists the base and elongates the ascendant segment, which now adopts a more horizontal position. When released, the base untwists and both segments recover their original position as in (*A*). (*C*) When the apex is removed, (*D*) contraction of the descendant segment brings the basal loop down but no untwisting action follows. (*E*) Only if the ascendant segment leans against a structure (ie, a finger, as shown in the frame) is the untwisting action recovered. (*F*) The structure that allows untwisting is the contracted mass of the descendant (yellow) segment, which is surrounded 360 degrees by the ascendant segment.

the descendant segment (systole) forces the ascendant segment to elongate and spatially adopt a more horizontal configuration that changes its orientation to a more vertical one when contraction of the ascendant segment (diastole) takes place.

Contraction of the ascendant segment requires this segment to lean against another structure; otherwise, this untwist motion is not possible (see Fig. 10C–E). Such structure is provided by the contracted descendant segment, around which the ascendant segment wraps around almost 360 degrees (see Fig. 10F).

The descendant and ascendant myocardial segments, responsible for both systole and diastole, are in anatomic continuity and sequentially activated. The reciprocal helical distribution and 360-degree wrapping around one to another allow the entire agonist-antagonist contraction unit to work in an extraordinary fashion to elicit both functions. The similarities between the myocardial antagonist unit and the forearm are shown in Fig. 11.

Implications

Once the helical anatomy is observed and its subsequent function comprehended, it becomes difficult to interpret the existing literature that has provided the basis of contemporary cardiology. There are several fields in which the impact is presumed to be of importance.

In the assessment of systolic ventricular function, the angle between the descendant fibers and the ascendant ones seems to be crucial for efficient systolic function [33,34]. In a similar way to the helical angle of a screw, the wider the angle, the more efficient the torsion dynamics and ejection. In dilated cardiomyopathy, the more horizontal angle of the fibers due to ventricular remodeling favors subsequent impairment of cardiac function; therefore, in the surgical treatment of heart failure, not only the size of the ventricle but also the fiber angle should be taken into account. The near future possibility of imaging online the myocardial fiber dynamics through resonance tensor diffusion imaging [35] opens the way to research and the development of adequate surgical strategies.

Over the past 20 years, noninvasive evaluation of diastolic function has relied on echo-Doppler analysis of how blood volume enters the ventricle, which largely depends on its loading conditions. One approach is to evaluate the degree of ventricular untwist that occurs during diastole [36], either by speckle tracking echocardiography [30] or velocity vector imaging, a new ultrasound technique that is angle independent and thus provides an avenue to evaluate short-axis mechanics of the left ventricle [37]. Sampling of the descendant myocardial band segment responsible for systole and of the ascendant band responsible for diastole has recently been performed by Vannan and colleagues [38]. The results revealed that normal and hypertensive patients disclose a similar peak twist velocity (1.9 ± 0.2 versus 2.3 ± 0.2 cm/s), whereas untwist is significantly less in hypertensive patients (1.7 ± 0.1 versus 1.1 ± 0.1 cm/s), suggesting that early diastolic dysfunction can be

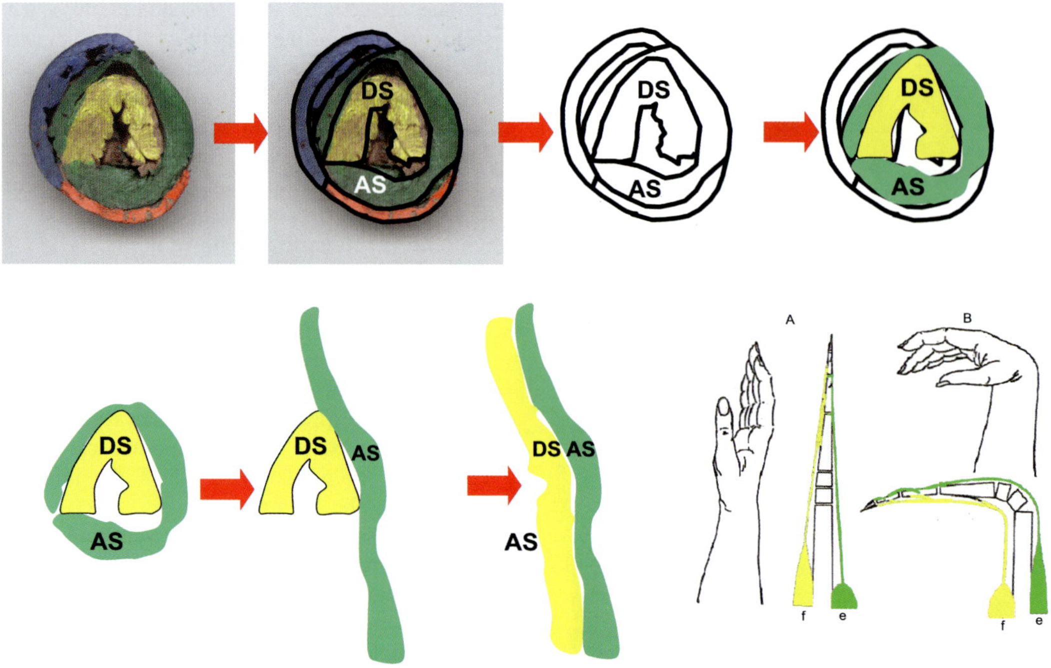

Fig. 11. Similarities between the agonist-antagonist mechanics of the ventricle and that of the forearm. Flexion and extension of the hand are due to the interaction of both sets of forearm muscles. The reciprocal helical structure of the descendant and ascendant segments of the ventricle makes systole similar to flexor contraction of the forearm and diastole similar to its extension.

ascribed to the generation of less force of the ascendant segment. This finding might have important implications in terms of the early diagnosis of diastolic dysfunction and therapy.

In this respect, the anatomy of the band might explain why diastolic dysfunction occurs before systolic alteration of function. Table 1 shows the thickness of the descendant segment, much greater than that of the ascendant segment. Early diastolic dysfunction before systolic dysfunction seen in diseases such as hypertension and other entities could be explained by damage-associated hypertrophy [39] first involving the thinner ascendant segment and later the more robust descendant segment.

In surgery for heart failure, it seems appropriate once the helical conformation of the ventricle is known, to plan surgery in such a way as to spare the helical ventricular anatomy. In an initial study by Torrent-Guasp and colleagues [40,41], four theoretic possibilities of surgically reducing left ventricular volume without impairing the helical structure of the ventricles were considered. The most logical approach seems to spare the apical loop (small volume and the true motor of the ventricle) and reduce the basal loop; however, new initiatives are needed to convert these theoretic possibilities into practical surgical approaches.

In resynchronization therapy, an explanation of why some patients respond to the device implantation whereas others fail to improve is not forthcoming. The issue is not that the left ventricle should contract simultaneously (most of the indexes developed are aimed at the detection of this phenomenon); rather, what is crucial is the sequence of contraction of the descendant and ascendant segments. In fact, knowledge of the natural sequence of electromechanical ventricular activation [21,42] should open the way to study the effects of selective stimulation of the segments of the band on ventricular function, and should provide a rationale for ventricular pacing protocols. In this respect, two recent articles using microcrystals selectively placed in the descendant and ascendant segments of the band have shown the hemodynamic disruption caused by right or left ventricular pacing [43]. This disruption is not solved by atrio-biventricular pacing, which compares less favorably (QRS complex, systolic and diastolic function, and cardiac index) with a more physiologic high septal pacing. With the latter mode of stimulation, the dynamics between descendant and ascendant segments are close to normal [44].

Other implications that follow the new anatomy and ventricular function relate to the interpretation of ECG. Electrical propagation of the impulse starts at the endocardial level and proceeds to the epicardium via the Purkinje system in a radial way; however, the Purkinje system in humans only exists at the subendocardium and is not found intramyocardially [45]. In addition, the nonhomogeneous nature of the ventricular anatomy (see Fig. 8) is unlikely to convey the electrical impulse in a nonanistropic fashion from the endocardium, perpendicularly crossing different ventricular segments to reach the epicardial surface. It seems likely that the explanation for the early subendocardial and late subepicardial electrical activation is due to its orderly propagation via first the descendant (subendocardial) segment and later the ascendant (subepicardial) segment. These considerations prompt reinterpretation of the ECG patterns, certainly an immense field for research.

In the same way, the cardiac cycle should be explained in the light of the new anatomy and function and should include the twist and untwist motion and its relationship with the mechanical and acoustic events. Specially important is a description of muscular movements during isovolumic contraction and relaxation [30,36].

The paradigmatic change in ventricular anatomy and function prompts research in every field of cardiology [46]. In the words of Dr. James L. Cox, "It is such a dramatic change from the understanding of the heart's physiology that we can almost go back and start repeating the experiments of the last 50 years with this new knowledge and see how we interpret these experiments now" (for more information, see www.helicalheart.com).

References

[1] Kocica ML, Corno AF, Carreras-Costa F, et al. The helical myocardial band: global, three-dimensional, functional architecture of the ventricular myocardium. Eur J Cardiothorac Surg 2006;9(Suppl 1): S21–40.

[2] Torrent-Guasp F. El ciclo cardiaco: considerationes criticas sobre la interpretación clásica y nuevas ideas sobre el mismo. Madrid (Spain): Diana Artes Graficas; 1954. p. 13–45.

[3] Torrent-Guasp F. [Sobre morfología y funcionalismo cardiacos. I Comunicación]. Rev Esp Cardiol 1966; 19:48 [in Spanish].

[4] Torrent-Guasp F. [Sobre morfología y funcionalismo cardiacos. II Comunicación]. Rev Esp Cardiol 1966; 19:56 [in Spanish].

[5] Torrent-Guasp F. [Sobre morfología y funcionalismo cardiacos. III Comunicación]. Rev Esp Cardiol 1966; 19:72 [in Spanish].

[6] Torrent-Guasp F. [Sobre morfología y funcionalismo cardiacos. IV Comunicación]. Rev Esp Cardiol 1967; 20:1 [in Spanish].

[7] Torrent-Guasp F. [Sobre morfología y funcionalismo cardiacos. V Comunicación]. Rev Esp Cardiol 1967; 20:14 [in Spanish].

[8] Torrent-Guasp F. Estructuración macroscópica del ventrículo izquierdo. (I) Mitad apexiana. Rev Esp Cardiol 1972;1:68–81.

[9] Torrent-Guasp F. Estructuracion macroscopica del ventriculo izquierdo. (II) Mitad basal. Rev Esp Cardiol 1972;2:109–18.

[10] Torrent-Guasp F. El músculo cardiaco. Madrid (Spain): Fundación Juan March; 1972.

[11] Streeter DD, Powers WE, Ross MA, et al. Three-dimensional fiber orientation in the mammalian left ventricular wall. In: Baan H, Noordergraaf A, Raines J, editors. Cardiovascular system dynamics. Cambridge (MA): MIT Press; 1978. p. 73–7.

[12] Torrent-Guasp F. La estructuración macroscópica del miocardio ventricular. Rev Esp Cardiol 1980; 133:265–87.

[13] Torrent-Guasp F. Estructura y función del corazón. Rev Esp Cardiol 1998;51:91–102.

[14] Torrent-Guasp F, Ballester M, Buckberg GD, et al. Spatial orientation of the ventricular muscle band: physiologic contribution and surgical implications. J Thorac Cardiovasc Surg 2001;122:389–92.

[15] Torrent-Guasp F, Buckberg GD, Clemente C, et al. The structure and function of the helical heart and its buttress wrapping. I. The normal macroscopic structure of the heart. Semin Thorac Cardiovasc Surg 2001;13(4):301–19.

[16] Lorenz CH, Pastorek JS, Bundy JM. Delineation of normal left ventricular twist throughout systole by tagged cine magnetic resonance imaging. J Cardiovasc Magn Reson 2000;2:97–108.

[17] Moore CC, Lugo-Olivieri CH, McVeigh ER, et al. Three-dimensional systolic strain patterns in the normal human left ventricle: characterization with tagged MR imaging. Radiology 2000;214:453–66.

[18] Henson RE, Song SK, Pastorek JS, et al. Left ventricular torsion is equal in mice and humans. Am J Pathol 2000;278:H1117–23.

[19] Torrent-Guasp F. La mecánica agonista–antagonista de los segmentos descendente y ascendente de la banda miocárdica ventricular. Rev Esp Cardiol 2001;54(9):1091–102.

[20] Torrent-Guasp F, Kocica MJ, Corno A, et al. Systolic ventricular filling. Eur J Cardiothorac Surg 2004;25(3):376–86.
[21] Ballester-Rodés M, Flotats A, Torrent-Guasp F, et al. Base-to-apex ventricular activation: Fourier studies in 29 normal individuals. Eur J Nucl Med Mol Imaging 2005;32:1481–3.
[22] Ballester-Rodés M, Flotats A, Torrent-Guasp F, et al. The sequence of regional ventricular motion. Eur J Cardiothorac Surg 2006;29(Suppl 1):S139–44.
[23] Castella M, Buckberg GD, Saleha S, et al. Structure function interface with sequential shortening of basal and apical components of the myocardial band. Eur J Cardiothorac Surg 2005;27:980–7.
[24] Carreras F, Ballester M, Pujadas S, et al. Morphological and functional evidences of the helical heart from non-invasive cardiac imaging. Eur J Cardiothorac Surg 2006;29(Suppl 1):S50–5.
[25] Buckberg GD, Mahajan A, Jung B, et al. MRI myocardial motion and fiber tracking: a confirmation of knowledge from different imaging modalities. Eur J Cardiothorac Surg 2006;29(Suppl 1):S165–77.
[26] Sengupta PP, Korinek J, Belohlavek M, et al. Left ventricular structure and function: basic science for cardiac imaging. J Am Coll Cardiol 2006;48: 1988–2001.
[27] Sengupta PP, Krishnamoorthy VK, Korinek J, et al. Left ventricular form and function revisited: applied translational science to cardiovascular ultrasound imaging. J Am Soc Echocardiogr 2007;20(5):539–51.
[28] Rademakers FE, Buchalter MB, Rogers WJ, et al. Rotational deformation of the canine left ventricle measured by magnetic resonance tagging: effects of catecholamines, ischaemia and pacing. Cardiovasc Res 1994;28:629–35.
[29] Rademakers FE, Bogaert J. Left ventricular myocardial tagging. Int J Card Imaging 1997;13:233–45.
[30] Notomi Y, Setser RM, Shiota T, et al. Assessment of left ventricular torsional deformation by Doppler tissue imaging: validation study with tagged magnetic resonance imaging. Circulation 2005;111(9): 1141–7.
[31] Notomi Y, Lysyansky P, Setser RM, et al. Measurement of ventricular torsion by two-dimensional ultrasound speckle tracking imaging. J Am Coll Cardiol 2005;45(12):2034–41.
[32] Helle-Valle T, Crosby J, Edvardsen T, et al. New noninvasive method for assessment of left ventricular rotation: speckle tracking echocardiography. J Am Coll Cardiol 2005;45:2034–41.
[33] Amundsen BH, Helle-Valle T, Edvardsen T, et al. Noninvasive myocardial strain measurement by speckle tracking echocardiography: validation against sonomicrometry and tagged magnetic resonance imaging. J Am Coll Cardiol 2006;47:789–93.
[34] Sallin EA. Fiber orientation and ejection fraction in the human ventricle. Biophys J 1969;9:954–64.
[35] Ingels NB Jr. Myocardial fiber architecture and left ventricular function. Technol Health Care 1997;5: 45–52.
[36] Schmid P, Jaermann T, Boesiger P, et al. Ventricular myocardial architecture as visualised in postmortem swine hearts using magnetic resonance diffusion tensor imaging. Eur J Cardiothorac Surg 2005;27: 468–74.
[37] Foster E, Lease KE. New untwist on diastole: what goes around comes back. Circulation 2006;113: 2477–9 [editorial].
[38] Vannan MA, Pedrizzetti G, Li P, et al. Effect of cardiac resynchronization therapy on longitudinal and circumferential left ventricular mechanics by velocity vector imaging: description and initial clinical application of a novel method using high-frame rate B-mode echocardiographic images. Echocardiography 2005;22:826–30.
[39] Vannan MA, Li P, Wang J, et al. Isolated diastolic dysfunction is a velocity vector imaging. J Am Coll Cardiol, in press.
[40] Pons-Lladó G, Ballester M, Borrás X, et al. Myocardial cell damage in human hypertension. J Am Coll Cardiol 2000;36(7):2198–203.
[41] Torrent-Guasp F, Caralps-Riera JM, Ballester M. Cuatro propuestas para la remodelación ventricular en el tratamiento quirúrgico de la miocardiopatía dilatada. Rev Esp Cardiol 1997;50:682–8.
[42] Torrent-Guasp F, Ballester M, Caralps-Riera JM, et al. Spatial orientation of the ventricular muscle band and approach to partial ventriculotomy in heart failure. In: Narula J, Virmani R, Ballester M, et al, editors. Heart failure: pathogenesis and treatment. London: Martin Dunitz; 2002. p. 685–93.
[43] Wyman BT, Hunter WC, Prinzen WP, et al. Mapping propagation of mechanical activation in the paced heart with MRI tagging. Am J Physiol 1999; 276:H881–91.
[44] Liakopoulos OJ, Tomioka H, Buckberg GD, et al. Sequential deformation and physiological considerations in unipolar right or left ventricular pacing. Eur J Cardiothorac Surg 2006;29S:S188–97.
[45] Tomioka H, Liakopoulos OJ, Buckberg GD, et al. The effect of ventricular sequential contraction on helical heart during pacing: high septal pacing versus biventricular pacing. Eur J Cardiothorac Surg 2006; 29(Suppl 1):S198–206.
[46] Coghlan HC, Coghlan AR, Buckberg GD, et al. The structure and function of the helical heart and its buttress wrapping. III. The electrical spiral of the heart: the hypothesis of the anisotropic conducting matrix. Semin Thorac Cardiovasc Surg 2001;13: 333–41.
[47] Buckberg GD, Weisfeldt ML, Ballester M, et al. Left ventricular form and function: scientific priorities and strategic planning for development of new views of disease. Circulation 2004;110:e333–6.

ELSEVIER
SAUNDERS

Heart Failure Clin 4 (2008) 273–288

HEART
FAILURE
CLINICS

Models Versus Established Knowledge in Describing the Functional Morphology of the Ventricular Myocardium

Paul P. Lunkenheimer, MD[a,*], Klaus Redmann, MD[a], Peter Niederer, MD[b], Peter Schmid, MD[b], Morten Smerup, MD, PhD[c], Jörg Stypmann, MD[a], Sabine Däbritz, MD[d], Kai Rothaus, MD[a], Robert H. Anderson, MD[e]

[a]*University of Münster, Münster, Germany*
[b]*ETH and University of Zürich, Zürich, Switzerland*
[c]*University Hospital, Århus, Denmark*
[d]*University Hospital Münster, Münster, Germany*
[e]*Imperial College, London, UK*

The progress made in the practice and knowledge of cardiology during the twentieth century has been impressive. At the same time, the approaches of those persons exploring the morphologic and physiologic aspects have proven to be incoordinate. Morphologists, being relatively unfamiliar with complex cardiac function, have not always described their observations in a fashion that is useful to persons exploring cardiodynamics [1–4]. Physiologists have provided detailed accounts of the bioelectrical activity of the myocardium [5,6], its pattern of motion [7–13], its capacity to develop tension [14–20], and, more recently, its molecular biologic activity [21–24]; however, they have been less concerned about the correlation between function and morphology. Mathematical models for the dynamics and energetics of the ventricular walls have been developed on the basis of simplistic structural assumptions [25–27].

Perhaps because of the intricate pattern of ventricular motion, many researchers exploring the anatomic arrangement of the ventricular myocytes have sought discrete anatomic units within an overall three-dimensional meshwork, ignoring the fact that the heart, in essence, is a modified blood vessel. It is unrealistic to expect its architecture to replicate the arrangement seen in skeletal muscles, where there is discrete packing, for example, of the muscles within the forearms providing the precision for the fine movements of the hand and fingers. Those persons seeking discrete subunits argue that the notion of a continuum does not readily explain the twisting movements of the ventricles seen during their emptying and filling. Many investigators have suggested that the ventricular walls are compartmented in the form of bands [28–30], nested shells [4,31], sheets [26,32], spirals [4,11,28–30], toroidal pretzels [33], tracts [3], and discrete layers [2,3]. Despite their protestations of the existence of subunits, none of these investigators has provided evidence of any fibrous structures enclosing their alleged compartments. This is hardly surprising, because no such compartments exist.

This work was supported by Deutsche Forschungsgemeinschaft, Ernst und Berta Grimmke Stiftung, Karl und Lore Klein Stiftung, BMBF, and the British Heart Foundation.

* Corresponding author. Experimental Thoraco-vascular Surgery, University of Münster, Domagkstr. 11, 48129 Münster, Germany.

E-mail address: lunkenhe@uni-muenster.de (P.P. Lunkenheimer)

1551-7136/08/$ - see front matter
doi:10.1016/j.hfc.2008.02.012

Although ventricular architecture remains a controversial topic, understanding the morphologic, physiologic, and clinical aspects of diseases of the heart and determining the optimal therapeutic approaches can be greatly facilitated by the provision of appropriate models. Unfortunately, existing models for ventricular mural stress remain founded on the original hypotheses of Frank [8]. He claimed that all forces generated by the ventricular walls acted exclusively as constrictors, denying the ability of the myocardium to generate dilating forces. In this review, the authors show that the heterogeneous distribution of tension throughout the ventricular walls is able to produce antagonistic functions within the myocardium [34,35]. At different times during the cardiac cycle, the meshwork is able to generate initially forces that are mostly constricting and yet subsequently produce predominant dilating actions [34]. The balance between these forces sustains, first, emptying during ventricular systole and only at the end of systole favors dilatory effects.

Controversies relating to subunits within the ventricular walls

The essence of ventricular contraction is to provide global constriction. Such conformational change also involves a biphasic countertwisting of the base relative to the apex [36–38], a degree of systolic straightening of the apex toward the sternum, with the base of the ventricular mass used as a fulcrum, and a systolic descent of the apical trabecular component of the ventricles, concomitant with a comparable systolic descent of the plane of the atrioventricular valves [7]. The latter motion is seen particularly in emergency situations, such as when venous return is critically impaired. Thickening of the individual myocytes during their contraction is insufficient to account for the increase in thickness of the ventricular walls [39]. Furthermore, the existence of discrete movements during ventricular constriction may seem to require the presence of anatomic units sequestrated within the overall ventricular mass. Nonetheless, the architecture of the ventricular walls as revealed by histologic examination rules out the possibility for the existence of such sequestrated anatomic subunits. Histologic studies show that the functional unit of the myocardium is the myocyte. Each myocyte is attached up to 15 times to its neighbors, with the resulting meshwork supported in a matrix of fibrous tissue. Because the individual myocytes have greater length than width, there is an obvious orientation to their packing (Fig. 1).

This arrangement permits the packed myocytes to be removed by gross dissection, with the long axis of the units removed paralleling the orientation of the contained myocytes (Fig. 2) [2,3,40–42]. No obviously hierarchically ordered fibrous structures are found that bind together the parts that are removed. In particular, there is no ordered arrangement of the supporting fibrous matrix that permits the distinction of "fibers," "fascicles," or "sheets" (Fig. 3). In reality, the markedly asymmetrical structure of the ventricular cone (see Fig. 2) is able, by itself, to sustain the disparate movements of the ventricular mass seen during contraction and relaxation [43].

Does diffusion tensor MRI provide evidence of the alleged subunits within the ventricular walls?

The problem with any form of anatomic dissection is that, of necessity, it is destructive. Only by removal of the epicardial elements is the dissector able to demonstrate the orientation of the long axis of the aggregated myocytes making up the deeper parts of the ventricular mass. To reveal these deeper layers, it is also necessary for the dissector to destroy the linkages between the myocytes, of necessity, producing artifacts. Such artifacts can now be avoided by the use of diffusion tensor MRI [44], or by new histologic techniques making use of polarized light [33].

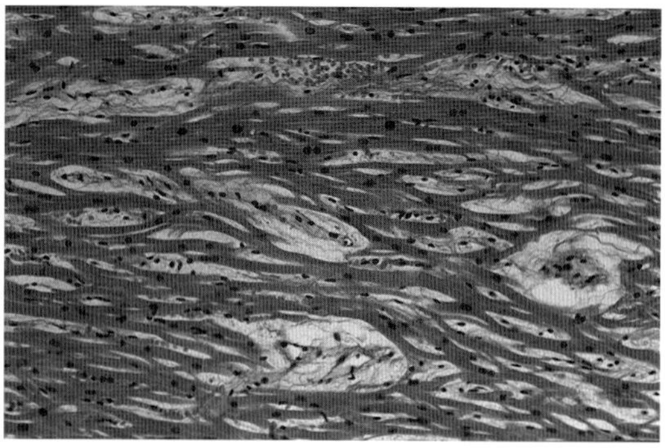

Fig. 1. This histologic section of porcine ventricular myocardium, spread by experimentally induced edema, reveals the prevailing longitudinal alignment of the myocytes. Each myocyte is joined to its neighbors in end-to-end fashion, with additional side branches to adjacent cells. The overall effect is to produce a three-dimensional meshwork.

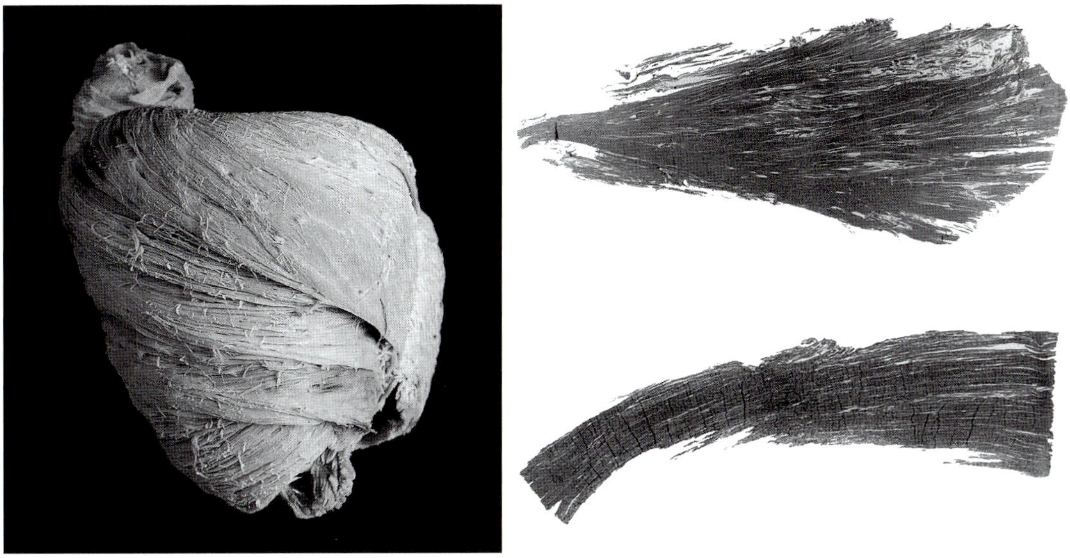

Fig. 2. The arrangement of the myocytes aggregated together within the three-dimensional mesh has been revealed by destructive peeling of successive layers, starting at the epicardial surface at the left ventricle's base and extending toward the endocardium near the apex (left). There is a gradual shift in the overall "grain" of the aggregated myocytes. Sections of the blocks of tissue removed during the process of peeling show that the grain matches the long axis of the aggregated myocytes (right). Note that the angulation of the epicardial myocytes (near the base) is opposite that of those closest to the endocardium (near the apex), with the myocytes in the midportion of the walls orientated in circular fashion (left).

Diffusion tensor MRI makes it possible to track the infinite continuum of the myocytic chains (Fig. 4).

The interregional connections exposed by tracking the aggregated myocytic chains confirm the continuity of a myocardial mesh throughout the ventricular walls. This arrangement guarantees that the contractile forces are transmitted in a spatially coordinated fashion. Whether the pathways are surrogates of a far-reaching interregional interaction remains to be determined. Brutsaert [17] has long since suggested an interregional transfer of forces to be an essential tool in controlling global ventricular contractility.

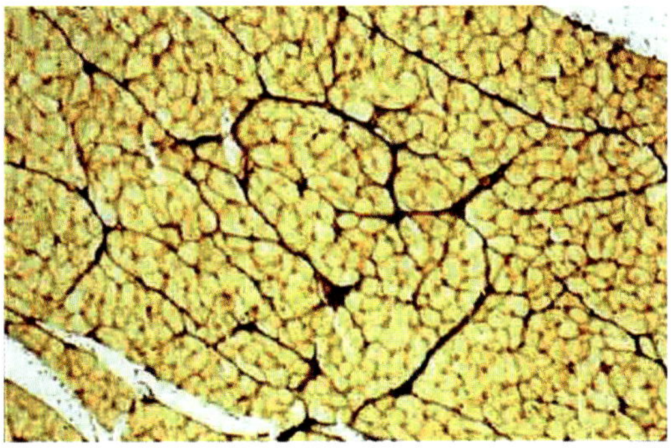

Fig. 3. The supporting fibrous matrix in this section has been revealed by staining with silver. Note that each myocyte is enclosed by an endomysial layer. Thickened areas, known as perimysial strands, bind together multiple myocytes but without any regular arrangement. The perimysial parts of the fibrous matrix, when evaluated in serial sections, do not form radial sheets as has been claimed by some investigators [32] on the base of electron microscopic studies, nor do they permit the demonstration of a "unique myocardial band" as claimed by others [28,29,30].

What of sheets, lamellas, and harmonica-like gaps?

Researchers investigating the second and third eigenvectors revealed by diffusion tensor MRI have interpreted the findings to suggest that the myocytes are aggregated together in more or less radial fashion, with their axes arranged in variable directions [45]. This phenomenon, if validated, is of great significance to those who assume systolic mural thickening to be the consequence of radial erection in a fanlike fashion of preformed lamellar sheets [26,32,46]. Nevertheless, histologic studies have failed to confirm any organized arrangements of the fibrous matrix extending in radial fashion from epicardium to endocardium (see Fig. 3). The components of the matrix are aggregated in

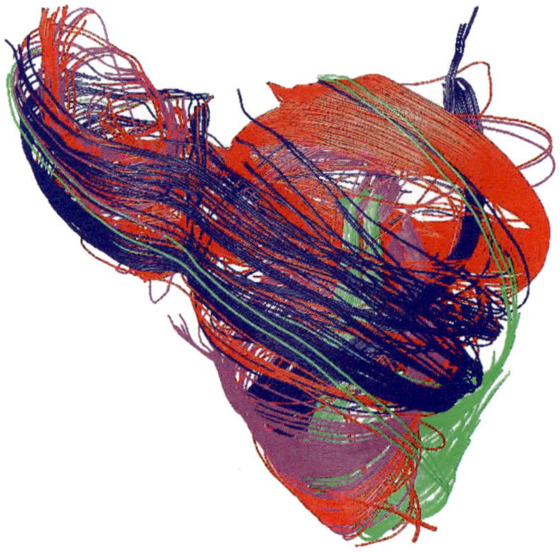

Fig. 4. The diverse nature of the changes of aggregated myocytes within the ventricular walls revealed by diffusion tensor MRI. Note the resemblance to the dissection shown in Fig. 2. Note also the tracking of myocytes from the left to the right ventricle.

heterogeneous fashion and variably aligned, producing gaps between the myocytes [47]. This arrangement suggests some kind of compartmentation of the myocytes, but the gaps observed do not continue in structured fashion through the full thickness of the ventricular walls (Fig. 5) [48,49].

The ventricular myocardial mass modeled as a continuous rope

By dint of its three-dimensional weave, it is possible to unravel the ventricular mass once its supporting matrix of fibrous has been destroyed, such as by heat denaturation. The form of the bandlike item thus produced is determined exclusively by the intention of the prosector. Torrent-Guasp [28,29] chose to unravel the ventricular mass to show that the myocytes take their origin from the pulmonary trunk and insert at the aorta (Fig. 6). It is equally possible to unravel the myocardial mass starting from the inferior interventricular groove [2,3]. The question is not whether the ventricular mass can be unraveled but, rather, whether the band thus produced has any functional significance. According to Torrent-Guasp, both the conduction of the excitatory wave and the transmission of force exclusively follow the long axis of the purported band. Only in restricted parts of the dissected band are the myocytes aligned strictly parallel to its long axis (Fig. 7).

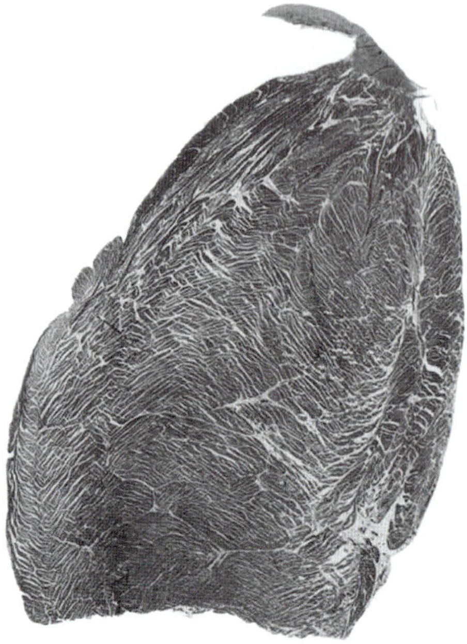

Fig. 5. This longitudinal section through the base of a porcine left ventricle exposes a multitude of gaps between the aggregated myocytes, albeit, with the gaps aligned in random directions. It is not possible to recognize organized sheets extending in radial fashion from epicardium to endocardium.

The simplistic concept fails to take into account the extensive circular layer of myocytes occupying not only the parietal wall of the left ventricle but also the septum. These myocytes make up the "triebwerkzeug" described by Krehl [13] and have been demonstrated by several others examining the ventricular mass using either dissection or histology [2,4,12,31,33,40–42,48–60]. Neither Torrent-Guasp [28,29] nor any of his current followers [30] have taken note of the obvious fact that the triebwerkzeug forms a compact and closed ring. Instead, they divide the ring into two continuous and serial loops, hence, double its length. In their search for mechanisms underscoring active late systolic ventricular dilation, Torrent-Guasp and colleagues [29] also proposed several illusive biomechanical activities, such as the cobra-like erection of his purported ascending limb of an apical loop, the interaction of the alleged basal and apical loops in buttress fashion, and, ultimately, the dilating effect of his so-called "aberrant fibers." All three proposed mechanisms neglect the simple physical axiom that any

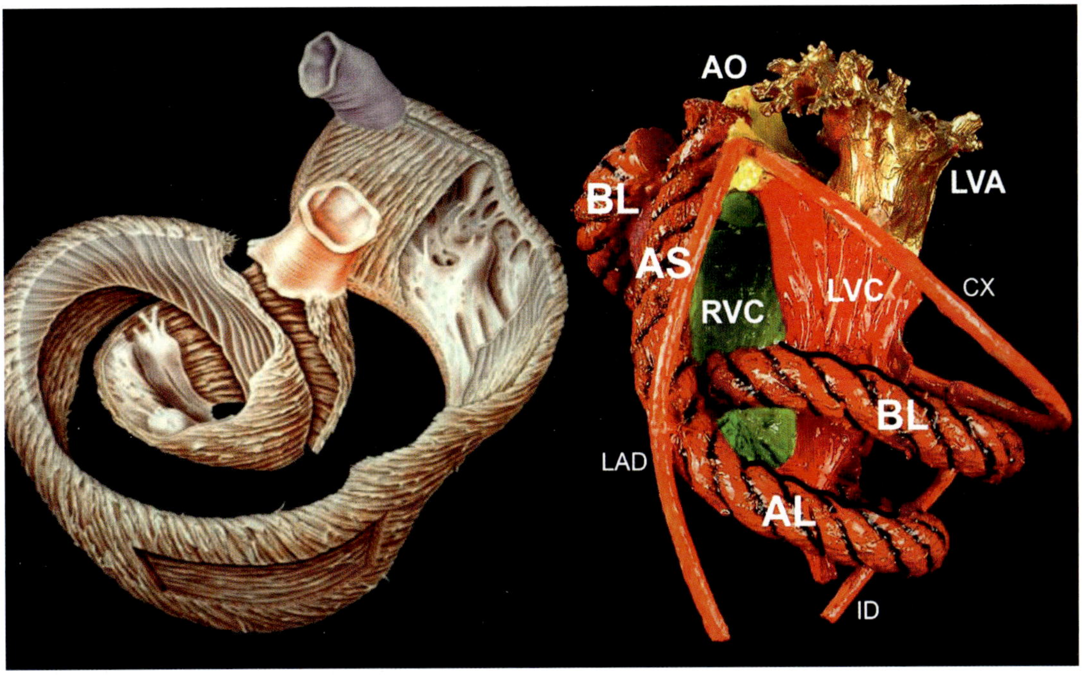

Fig. 6. The cartoon shows the "unique myocardial band" (left) commencing at the aorta (red) and extending to the pulmonary trunk (blue) that Torrent-Guasp was able to dissect from the ventricular mass. In an initial version of this concept, Torrent-Guasp proposed the band to be a rope (right), suggesting a continuous epi-to-endocardial and endo-to-epicardial pathway of alignment of the myocytes. AL, apical loop; AS, ascending segment of the apical loop; BL, basal loop; CX, circumflex coronary artery; ID, inferior descending coronary artery; LAD, left superior descending coronary artery; LVC, left ventricular cavity; RVC, right ventricular cavity. The presumed ropelike biventricular continuum in this image is wrapped about casts of the bovine right (green) and left (red) ventricles, seen from the obtuse margin. Note the regular repetition of an endo-epicardial alignment of the myocytic grain resulting from the purported ropelike basic structure.

structure having a hollow center, with the myocytes aligned tangential to the epicardial surface as assumed by Torrent-Guasp, can do no more while contracting than sustain its move toward its concavity.

Clinical applications of the band model

The authors have shown in experiments on normal pigs that during sequential sequestration of different mural segments using a sucker device, in contrast to the apical compartment, the basal circumference is particularly sensitive to the induced deformation. Surgeons have argued in favor of resecting the ventricular base to provide a reduction in ventricular radius, presumably prompted by the unproven hypothesis put forward by Torrent-Guasp and colleagues [29], namely, the need to preserve the purported left ventricular apical loop. Suma and his colleagues [61,62] in Japan compromised between directing their surgical resections at the purported basal and apical loops, choosing to resect a particularly small segment from the ventricular equatorial zone, and extended it only minimally toward the base and apex. These procedures resulted in a minimal reduction of left ventricular diameter with a small increase in ejection fraction. Irrespective of the reasons for adopting this approach, the results obtained do not match those published by European surgeons [62–65] who apply more standard procedures [66,67] for achieving reduction of ventricular radius. In similar fashion, the approach to reduction of ventricular radius proposed by the group working at the Cleveland Clinic [67,68] produced results inferior to those using the initial approach suggested by Batista, and set back the more widespread adoption of this useful tool in the surgical armamentarium for treatment of the failing heart.

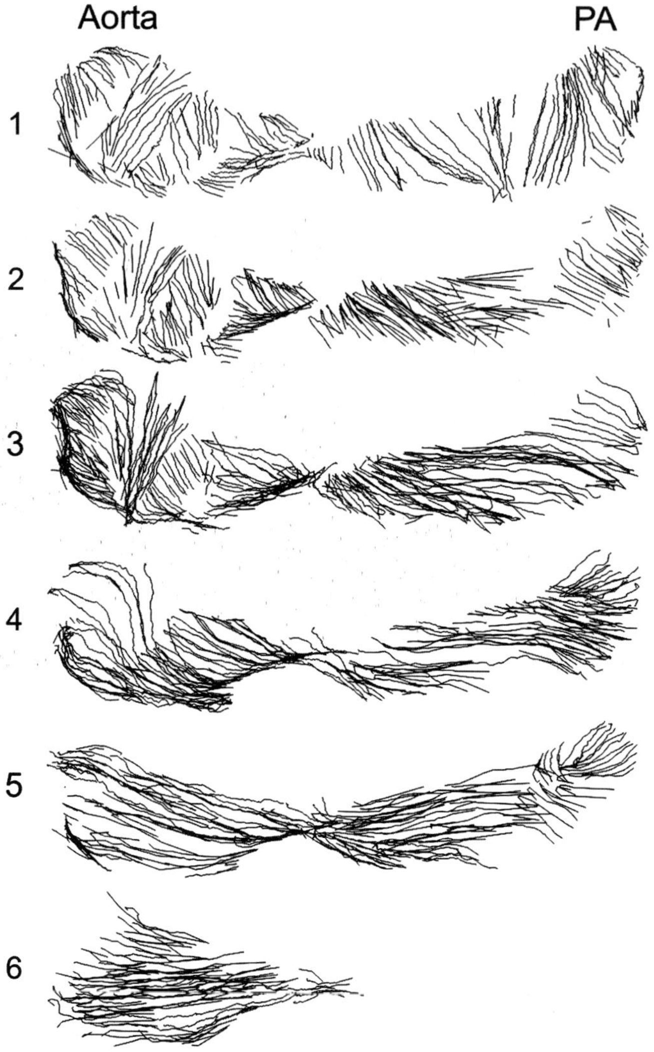

Fig. 7. The ventricles have been dissected to produce the "unique band" postulated by Torrent-Guasp, and the band has then been peeled to show the orientation of the aggregated myocytes passing from the subepicardial (left) to the subendocardial (right) surfaces. As can be seen, there is no uniformity in packing of the myocytes unless one assumes that the band consists of a rope contorted on itself.

Persons seeking to modify surgical procedures on the basis of ventricular architecture should appreciate that the spiraling motion of the myocardial mass is not produced because of the presence of individual anatomic subunits existing within the walls. Instead, it is a consequence of the overall action of the myocardial mass, which is inseparably composed of interweaving and ubiquitous tangential and intruding components. Wherever the surgeon places an incision or resects part of the wall, the process destroys helical, tangential, and intruding components of the myocardial spatial net. Partial left ventriculectomy, in its original version [66,69,70], has been tolerated in satisfactory fashion by a great number of patients whenever it has proved possible to reduce the diameter of the left ventricle while at the same time preserving coronary arterial perfusion of the remaining myocardium and ensuring mitral valvar competence [63–65]. A paramount factor constraining the uniform excellence of this approach has been the impairment of ventricular mural motion by preexisting fibrotic tethering [71]. Nonetheless, the concept of partial left ventriculectomy as introduced by Batista [66,69,70] serves to show that the continuum of the myocardial mass can readily be interrupted and reunited by interposition of an extended scar, a process which destroys or resects extended myocardial components previously assumed to be inseparable.

This clinical experience is not in line with established knowledge about the vulnerability of the myocardium as defined by experiments in electrophysiology [5,6]. The area of myocardium damaged by the extended resection amounts to 20 to 65 cm^2 depending on the length of the incision and the thickness of the wall from which the sequestered area has been taken. Although this extended wound should be prone to act as an arrhythmogenic substrate, the patients rarely sustain life-threatening arrhythmias [63]. Another surprising finding is the persistence of adequate ventricular constriction, resulting in a consistent improvement in global ventricular function, even though the original technique published by Batista [66,69,70] resected essential parts of the specific conducting system localized within the ventricular apex. The reason for this unexpected tolerance remains unexplained.

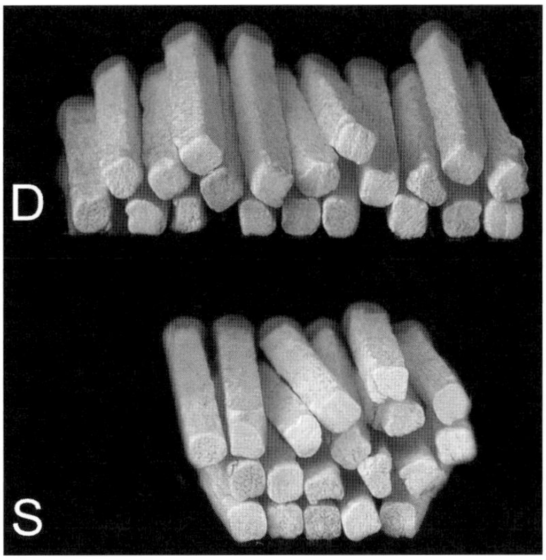

Fig. 8. Matchsticks can be used to illustrate the postulated repacking of the myocytes within the ventricular walls during systolic contraction. Matches aligned in two or three layers during diastole (upper panel) are compressed during systole from both sides so that they are superimposed to form three to four layers (lower panel).

How do we account for systolic mural thickening?

As each myocyte shortens by about one sixth during ventricular contraction, it thickens in the mean by no more than around one twentieth. The ventricular walls, in contrast, increase in thickness by three fifths during systole [39]. To explain the thickening of the ventricular walls, it is necessary to postulate rearrangements of the individual myocytes relative to each other within the thickness of the walls. As has been shown by Hort [47] and Spotnitz and colleagues [39], the myocytes during systolic contraction realign themselves within the thickness of the wall, increasing essentially the number of cross-sections of myocytes superimposed during systole (Fig. 8).

The true architecture of the ventricular walls

The mammalian ventricular myocardium is organized in the form of a three-dimensional mesh. The pattern is dictated by the coupling and branching of the myocytes with their neighbors, not only in end-to-end but also in lateral fashion [31,39,55,72–74]. The myocytes are aggregated together within a mesh, with the aggregated cells having no obviously defined beginning and end. Numerous small gaps of arbitrary size and orientation are interspersed throughout the mesh, and branchings and linkages between individual myocytes are rare or absent at these sites. In macroscopic terms, the ventricular muscle mass has a well-organized spatial architecture, and several investigators have emphasized the marked local heterogeneities [48,54–56]. Thus far, it has been difficult to provide a comprehensive three-dimensional picture of the entirety of the ventricular mass because of the inability to section in orthogonal planes all of the myocytes in their long axis [31,39,48,54].

Throughout this discussion thus far, the authors have intentionally avoided describing the components making up the ventricular walls as "fibers," because there are no discrete anatomic units within the walls other than the aggregated myocytes and no entities deserving of the title "fiber." It is true that, when applying the peeling procedure [2,3,50,52,54], the ventricular wall can be dismantled to reveal the overall long axis of the aggregated myocytes; however, the removed myocytes are not naturally bound together in length or in thickness (see Fig. 2).

When assessed relative to the equatorial plane of the ventricular mass, it is well established that the orientation in long axis of the aggregated myocytes turns in a characteristic fashion with increasing depth within the ventricular wall, with the variation of these myocytes measured relative to the equator being known as the helical angle [31,54,55,74,75]. Less attention has been paid to changes in angulation of the myocytes relative to the epicardial and endocardial surfaces, the so-called angle of "intrusion" [56] or imbrication [31]. As initially stated by Frank [8], it is presumed that virtually all of the myocytes are orientated with their long axes tangential to the epicardial surfaces. To assess the precise angle of any myocyte intruding within the ventricular walls, it is necessary to examine representative numbers parallel to their long axis throughout the mural thickness. To achieve this, the authors developed a novel technique for sectioning the ventricular wall using circular knives [56]. We have now measured the angles of intrusion using histology [56] and subsequently diffusion tensor MRI [58,59], seeking to relate the structure of the three-dimensional mesh with its function. We harvested semicircular sections from the ventricular wall, with the changing angulation of the circular knife compensating for the depth-related turn of the predominant long axis of the myocytes upon the radial axis. Wherever the myocytes are sectioned longitudinally, their deviation from a strictly tangential alignment, in other words, their angle of intrusion, is clearly exposed. Our measurements revealed a coherent orthotropic three-dimensional arrangement (Fig. 9).

We also demonstrated local heterogeneities within the global ventricular organization. For example, in all slices harvested from the basal level, positive angles prevailed in three fifth of the segments measured, with values varying between 0 and 45 degrees, whereas negative angles of intrusion in the same range of subtended angles were found in one third. In the slices removed from the apex, in contrast, more than half of segments intruded in a positive direction and only two fifths in a negative one. In more than nine tenths of all linear segments measured, we found evidence of myocytes intruding into the left ventricular wall at angles ranging from zero to ± 45 degrees, with three tenths subtending angles between zero and ± 7.5 degrees, thus being aligned quasi-tangentially, and one quarter subtending angles between ± 7.5 and 15 degrees. A concentration of myocytes intruding at high negative angles was found in the equatorial slices [59].

The prevalence of negative angles of intrusion in the greater portion of the left ventricular cone complies with the time-honored model of a spiraling structure. Nonetheless, the spiraling myocytes are intricately interwoven with other myocytes that show less intrusion, being aligned more in longitudinal or circumferential fashion. The overall spiraling myocardial architecture is inseparably incorporated into the entirety of the myocardial body. This feature invalidates any attempt to divide the ventricular wall in functional subunits. The myocytes act together so as to generate ventricular constriction and twisting while also eventually restoring ventricular width [34,56]. Any attempt to average the extent of the heterogeneities in angulation simply disguises their structural significance.

Because the ventricular mesh is composed of myocytes supported by a fibrous matrix, the two having different mechanical properties, each

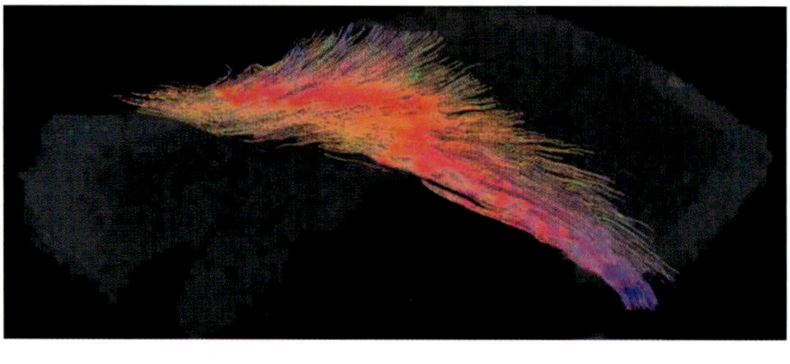

Fig. 9. Diffusion vector imaging of the myocytic orientation in a semicircular slice harvested from the subbasal left ventricular superior wall of a porcine heart which exposes only those structures that run parallel to the section plane. The epicardial surface is the upper border of the slice and the endocardial the lower border of the slice. The septal end of the slice is on the left, and the right end of the slice is near the obtuse margin; therefore, the transmural slice is seen from the apex.

myocyte faces a double site of interaction. The overall structure of the myocardial mesh revealed by histology suggests an unimpeded axial and spatial transmission of contractile forces between contiguous myocytes. Their loading is generally understood to be determined by hemodynamic resistance to ventricular emptying. If we are to properly explain cardiodynamics, we must also account for the impact of the supporting fibrous matrix; therefore, we invoke a twofold anchorage of each myocyte (Fig. 10).

Like the myocytes, the connective tissue is also arranged as a continuum, which is densely interlaced like felt [48,76–81]. The overall arrangement is that of frequently branching tunnels which house the continuous chains of myocytes (see Fig. 10). The fibrous matrix thus formed is scarcely distensible. Its restricted freedom of motion is determined by the direction of alignment of collagenous fibers and by their degree of curling in systole or diastole. Because the fibrous matrix is spatially interlaced, its potential for reshaping in one direction necessarily depends on concomitant passive deformation in the other directions. The systolic increase in mural thickness must be accompanied by a corresponding decrease in ventricular length or diameter, with the increase in mural thickness being matched in volume with the decrease in the other dimensions of the ventricular walls.

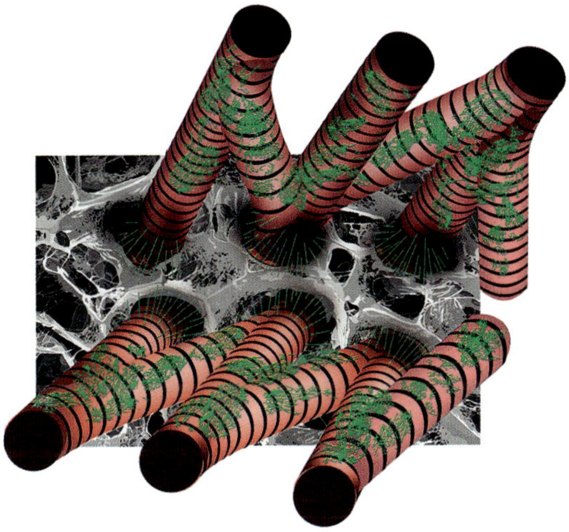

Fig. 10. Topography of the entanglement of the myocytic continuum (red) with its sustaining and rigid fibrous matrix (gray). The branching myocytes (red) are housed in a spatially arranged system of frequently branching tunnels in the densely netted, hence, feltlike fibrous matrix (gray). The myocytes are densely suspended by radiating struts (green). Those struts confine the freedom of the myocytes to glide within their supporting tunnels. Their axial gliding is ultimately confined by the frequent occurrence of spandrels, each of which separates two branches of the tunnel where it divides. The impediment to displacement is key to the spatial deviation of contractile forces across the ventricular walls. Where gliding is impeded by the fibrous matrix, contractile forces are transferred from the myocardial to the fibrous compartment. From then on, the deviation of forces is determined by the direction of freedom of motion of the fibrous matrix rather than by that of the spatial netting of the myocytes themselves.

The collagenous scaffold is not a system of branching channels in which endless chains of myocytes slide freely. Instead, the many sarcomeres making up the individual myocytes are each linked to their tunnel-like fibrous conducts by a rim of struts that radiate from the circumference of each sarcomere. Caulfield and Borg [77] have long suggested that the struts are taut during diastole and slack during systole, implying that the fibrous matrix limits the diastolic expansion of the myocytes rather than their systolic shortening. This assumption is in contrast to the experimental finding of Lamberts and colleagues [83], who showed that acute enzymatic degradation of the struts enhanced systolic contractile forces without affecting primarily diastolic compliance. The authors opine that the struts are involved both in intercepting and ultimately deviating the direction of contractile forces of the myocytes and in controlling their diastolic extension. We also suggest that, in the myocardium, the scarcely distensible collagenous fibrous matrix is the primary point of incidence for load engendered by the contraction of the aggregated myocytes.

Myocardial fibrosis is an insidious disease

When the myocardium becomes fibrotic as a consequence of disease, the mechanics of the connective tissue are altered in significant fashion. Circumscribed accumulations of scar tissue and irregularly thickened strands of collagen intrude and eventually septate the ventricular walls to a much greater extent than normal [77–82]. In the setting of disease, the fibrous matrix no longer behaves as one interdependent unit. Multifocal scars of variable size and shape act as pathologic fixed points dispersed in irregular fashion between epicardium and endocardium and between base and apex, because these points are firmly anchored within the fibrous scaffold via starlike strands of collagen (Fig. 11).

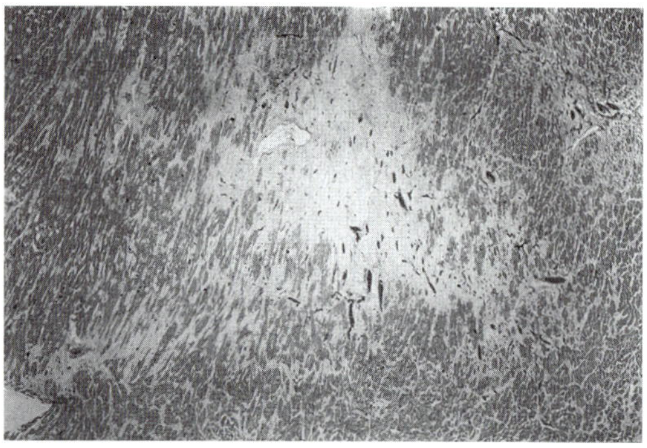

Fig. 11. Starlike microfocal scars seen in a histologic section of human myocardium from a patient who died of septic shock having undergone catecholamine treatment during intensive care.

Because their suspension is not distensible, they remain motionless during the cardiac cycle. The myocardium itself responds with hypertrophy, with the myocytes being thicker in the environs of the scar. This perifocal hypertrophy reflects the hopeless fight of the myocardial component of the mesh against its petrified suspension. The share of expenditure of contractile energy is wasted and, hence, does not contribute to hemodynamic performance. Ultimately, the contractile forces generated by the aggregated myocytes fall victim to their embedment and tethering in the mesh of indistensible connective tissue.

Cardiodynamics confirming the prevalence of an intrinsic antagonism

When considered in its entirety, the ventricular mass is activated almost synchronously with only minor delays in circumscribed areas. The duration of this activation, in contrast, largely varies with the mode of contraction of each individual myocyte [14–19]. Myocytes aligned tangentially contract and shorten during the short period of ejection at a decreasing maximal force. These myocytes, acting exclusively to produce ventricular constriction, are unloaded, with the ventricular radius decreasing concomitant with mural thickening [34]. In other words, they obey the law of Laplace. In contrast to these myocytes, it is now known that up to two fifths of the overall population is inclined within the ventricular wall toward the endocardium or epicardium. Furthermore, the angle of the transmural force vector they produce is augmented by their engagement within the supporting matrix of fibrous tissue. One force vector in the vector parallelogram thus produced acts against systolic mural thickening and against systolic ventricular constriction (Fig. 12).

The authors have shown using needle probes (Fig. 13) [34] that, as afterload increases during systolic contraction, the developed force increases measurably (Fig. 14). We consider this mode of contraction to be auxotonic. Such auxotonic contraction is typically delayed within the cardiac cycle, with the active state of the myocyte being prolonged while its distance of shortening is particularly short (see Fig. 14) [14–19]. The population of myocytes producing auxotonic contraction does not follow the law of Laplace. There is nothing special about these myocytes in terms of their structure. Indeed, all myocytes have the potential to contract in auxotonic fashion depending on the afterload to which they are submitted. The peak of auxotonic force is a function of the angle of intrusion. Auxotonic end-systolic force declines

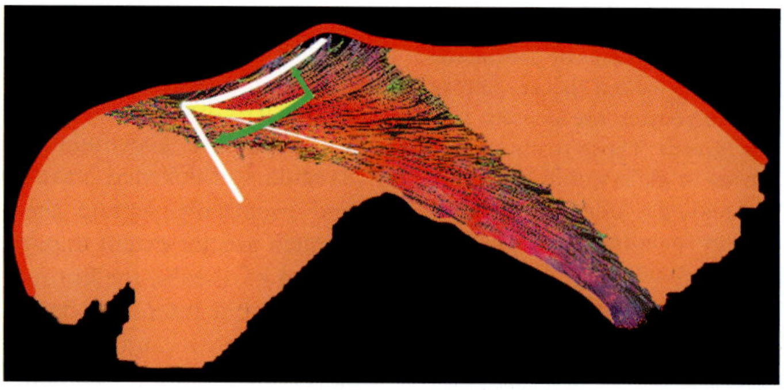

Fig. 12. The cartoon takes the situation shown in Fig. 9 but with the vector parallelogram of forces superimposed. The force vector shown in yellow results from two opposing forces shown in green, a small one acting in a radial direction and a dominant one acting in a tangential direction. The small resulting vector does not reach the level of inclination of 45 degrees, shown by the fine white beam, this being the value to be exceeded so as to produce a prevailing dilatory force.

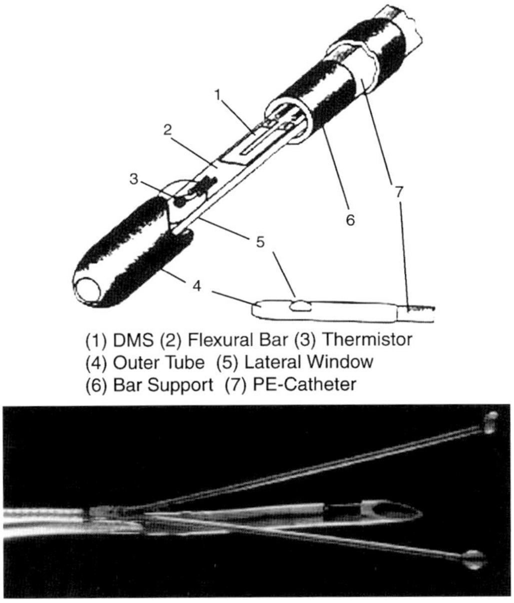

Fig. 13. Needle force probe shown in the upper panel exposing its components, where DMS is the strain gauge. The lower panel shows the probe at the tip of a catheter with two lateral wires which support the probe and keep it in place. The needle itself is inserted into the ventricular wall with the lateral (black) window aligned at a right angle to the long axis of the focal striation of myocytes.

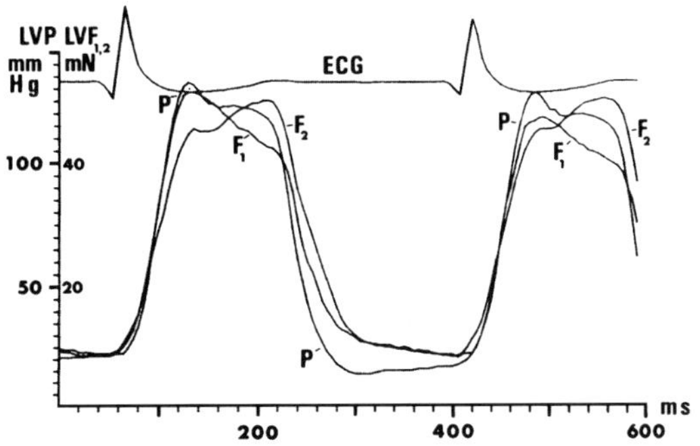

Fig. 14. Superimposed signals of the left ventricular pressure (P), electrocardiogram (ECG), left ventricular unloaded type of force (F_1), and auxotonic force (F_2).

in the dilated, properly filled, and thin-walled ventricle, but increases in the constricted, poorly filled, and thick-walled ventricle [34]. In technical terms, the heart functions as a synchronous bidirectional generator of force. In an exactly timed periodicity, the direction of generation of force is reversed just like an alternating thrust actuator. The mechanism that switches the direction of effective force is inherent in systolic mural thickening itself. Forces generated by the tangentially oriented population of myocytes rapidly vanish as these myocytes are free to shorten. Contractile forces generated in obliquely intruding structures, in contrast, continue to increment as they are hindered in their shortening. Their active state outlasts that of the tangentially aligned myocytes. This disparate mode of contraction ultimately reverses the prevailing direction of effective forces from a tangential to a radial orientation, with this late systolic reversal generating the initial thrust of early diastolic ventricular dilation along with elastic rebound [55]. The authors' studies using histologic [57] and diffusion tensor imaging [59,60] of sections of myocardium cut with circular knives have revealed a widely variable ratio of tangential to obliquely intruding populations of myocytes throughout the ventricular walls. Each region generates its typical pattern of antagonism (Fig. 15) [34].

The authors interpret the resulting disparate segmental mural motion to provide control of a time-dependent inward motion. Such bidirectional and, hence, mutually tempered contraction ensures an unimpeded intracavitary flow of blood from the mitral to the aortic valve. The ratio of tangential to obliquely intruding myocytes determines the proportions of unloading as opposed to auxotonically contracting myocytes, with the latter ratio determining the onset, amount, duration, and termination of the inward motion and thickening of each mural segment. Intracavitary flow, which is twisted on itself [84] simply because of the overall arrangement of the myocardial mesh, is molded by an exactly timed pattern of sequential and quantitatively controlled inward motion of the squeezing walls.

The rigid support provided for the myocytes by the supporting fibrous matrix ultimately explains why unloading and auxotonic forces do not equalize, although both signals exist close to each other within the myocardial continuum [34]. Even during major conformational changes of the ventricle, resulting alterations in auxotonic forces have hardly any appreciable impact on the unloading signals measured in neighboring populations of myocytes. Likewise, experimentally distorted forces mediated by the local application of suction on circumscribed sites of the left ventricular epicardial surface, when measured by needle force probes, are rarely found to be transmitted further than 2 cm from the site of disturbance.

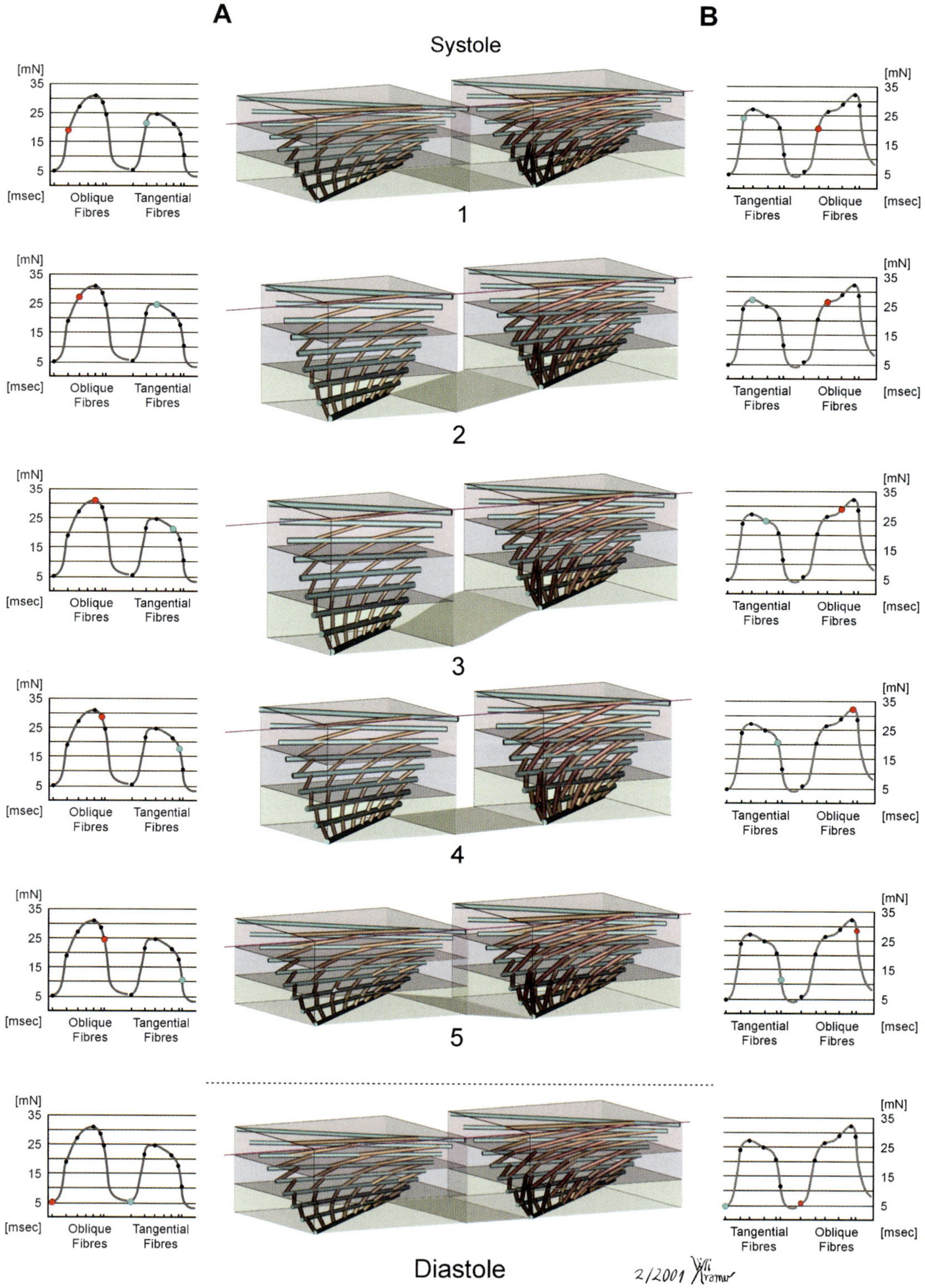

Fig. 15. The segmental contraction at (*A*) is fast, short, and at a high level of mural thickening, being almost unimpeded by a small number of obliquely intruding connections of myocytes. In contrast, at (*B*) the transmural netting is more pronounced. Mural thickening is delayed, confined, and lasts longer, being tempered by intrinsic antagonism. The forces recorded in the two segments are displayed on both sides.

The authors infer that the global changes in ventricular conformation are essentially shaped by the freedom of motion of the supporting fibrous matrix. The pattern of alignment of the aggregated myocytes interferes only within the limitations of the constraints of the fibrous matrix in which the myocytes are suspended.

To summarize our proposed correlation of structure with function, ventricular mural segments do not exist as anatomically defined entities because, in the normal heart, there is no evidence of anatomic segmentation of the ventricular walls. Nonetheless, regional mural motion is known to show marked individuality, which can deteriorate focally in the setting of disease and which can benefit from focal surgical therapy. Surgery designed to reduce the ventricular radius has proven that, in particular regions of the ventricular walls, segments can be resected without critically disadvantaging global ventricular function [63–67,69,70]. This rule holds true as long as resection is adequately sized, coronary arterial perfusion of the remaining myocardium is preserved, and any concomitant valvar disease is corrected; the ventricle has a preoperative diameter of more than 7 cm; and preexisting fibrosis has not critically confined systolic mural thickening of the remaining myocardium [72].

The presence of intrinsic antagonism invalidates current diagnostics in cardiology

Any antagonistic or bidirectional generation of force must call into question current concepts for routine diagnosis. According to the concepts outlined previously, intracavitary pressure, ejection fraction, cardiac output, and derived measures such as maximal velocity of rise in left ventricular pressure and outflow velocity are no more than resultants of two opposing forces working throughout the cardiac cycle. The instantaneous ratio of constrictive to dilatory forces depends on the ventricular size because mural thickness varies depending on the mean filling of the cardiac cavities. More importantly, this ratio undergoes inestimable alterations in the diseased and structurally remodeled ventricle.

Pharmacologic control of the intrinsic antagonism

It is an established quality of myocytes contracting auxotonically that their active state

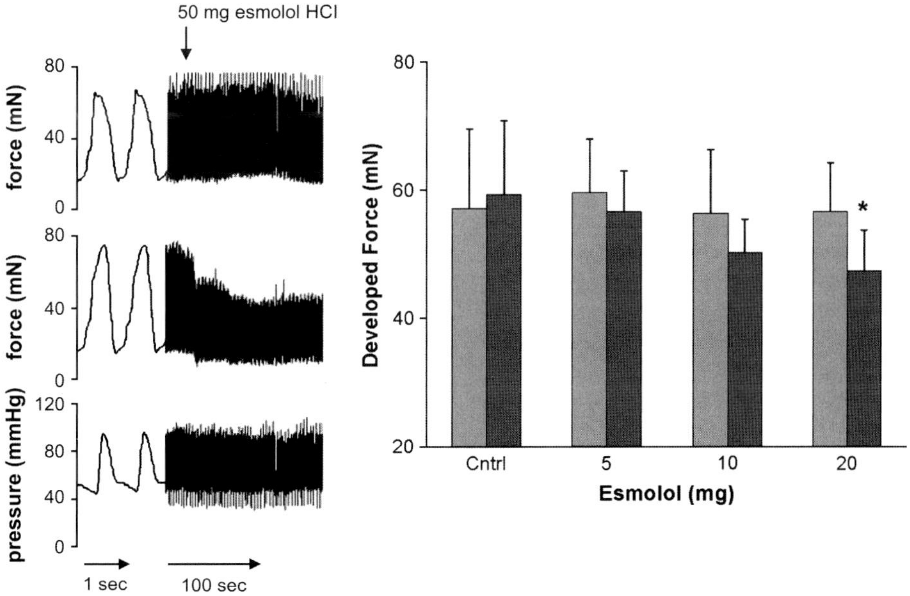

Fig. 16. A single dose of 50 mg of esmolol injected intravenously during cardiac surgery while local forces are measured in two sites of the left ventricular myocardium (left) shows that the first site engenders an unloaded type of force which remains unaltered, while the second site engenders an auxotonic force which drops by about two fifths on medication. The pressure measured in the radial artery remains unaffected. The right panel shows the mean change of developed unloading (light gray) and auxotonic (dark gray) forces with increasing doses (5, 10, 20 mg) of esmolol given intravenously in 10 patients during cardiac surgery (significance, $P = .05$).

persists longer than that of myocytes contracting in the unloaded fashion [14–19]. Another feature of auxotonic contraction is its striking sensitivity to inotropic stimulation in positive and negative directions [34]. This pharmacologic selectivity means that any imbalance in the internal antagonism can be treated by modulating the ratio of constrictive to dilatory forces. This modulation can be brought about by beta-blockade at low dosage [35] or by barbiturates [34]. In these settings, auxotonic forces decrease up to two fifths, whereas the unloading type of contraction remains unimpaired (Fig. 16).

At higher dosages, both types of forces are negatively damped. At low dosage, when auxotonic forces decline, there are no measurable hemodynamic alterations (see Fig. 16). On the other hand, positive inotropy selectively augments auxotonic forces more than the unloading type of contraction. Taking into consideration the prevalence of such intrinsic antagonism, the pathognomonic potential of myocardial hypertrophy is systematically misunderstood [85]. Such a hypertrophic disorder, together with fibrosis, underscores a critical imbalance in myocardial antagonism which ultimately leads to dilation of the cavities of the failing ventricles. The authors question whether any solely positive or compensatory effect of myocardial hypertrophy could act independently of the augmenting intrinsic antagonism. Instead, the pharmacologic damping of the dilatory auxotonic component of the antagonistic dualism by the use of negative inotropic drugs, such as beta-blockade, could be considered the treatment of choice [35].

References

[1] Lower R. Tractatus de corde. London: J Allestry; 1669.
[2] Pettigrew JB. On the arrangement of the muscular fibres in the ventricular portion of the heart of the mammal (Croonian lecture). Proceedings of the Royal Society of London 1860;10:433–40.
[3] Mall FP. On the muscular architecture of the ventricles of the human heart. Am J Anat 1911;11:211–78.
[4] Robb JS, Robb RC. The normal heart, anatomy and physiology of the structural units. Am Heart J 1942; 23:455–67.
[5] Lab JM. Mechanoelectric feedback (transduction) in heart: concepts and implications. Cardiovasc Res 1996;32:3–14.
[6] Marban E, Robinson SW, Wier WG. Mechanism of arrhythmogenic delayed and early after depolarizations in ferret ventricular muscle. J Clin Invest 1986;78:1185–92.
[7] Böhme W. Über den aktiven Anteil des Herzens an der Förderung des Venenblutes. Ergeb Physiol 1936;38:252–338.
[8] Frank O. Isometrie und Isotonie des Herzmuskels. Z Biol 1901;41:14–34.
[9] Gibson DG, Prewitt TA, Brown DJ. Analysis of left ventricular wall movement during isovolumic relaxation and its relation to coronary artery disease. Br Heart J 1976;38:1010–9.
[10] Hammermeister KE, Gibson DG, Hughes D. Regional variation in the timing and extend of left ventricular wall motion in normal subjects. Br Heart J 1986;56:226–35.
[11] Ingles NB Jr. Myocardial fiber architecture and left ventricular function. Technol Health Care 1997;5: 45–52.
[12] Keith A. The functional anatomy of the heart. Br Med J 1918;1:316–63.
[13] Krehl L. Beiträge zur Kenntnis der Füllung und Entleerung des Herzens. Abhandlungen d. math.-physischen Classe d. Königl. Sächs. Ges. d. Wiss. Hierzel Leipzig 1891;17:341–83 [in German].
[14] Brady AJ. Onset of contractility in cardiac muscle. J Physiol 1966;184:560–80.
[15] Brady AJ. Active state in cardiac muscle. Physiol Res 1968;48:570–600.
[16] Brutsaert DL, Sonnenblick EH. Force-velocity-length-time relation of the contractile elements in heart muscle of the cat. Circ Res 1969;24:137–49.
[17] Brutsaert DL. Nonuniformity: a physiologic modulator of contraction and relaxation of the normal heart. J Am Coll Cardiol 1987;9:341–8.
[18] Jewell BR, Wilkie DR. An analysis of the mechanical components in frogs striated muscle. J Physiol 1958;143:515–40.
[19] Jewell BR, Wilkie DR. The mechanical properties of relaxing muscle. J Physiol 1960;152:30–47.
[20] Noble MIM, Hefner LL, Browen RE. Force-velocity relation of cat cardiac muscle studied by isotonic and quick-release techniques. Circ Res 1969;24:821–33.
[21] Scoote M, Williams AJ. The cardiac ryanodine receptor (calcium release channel): emerging role in heart failure and arrhythmia pathogenesis. Cardiovasc Res 2002;56:359–72.
[22] Hasenfuss G, Pieske B. Calcium cycling in congestive heart failure. J Mol Cell Cardiol 2002;34: 951–69.
[23] Molkentin JD, Dorn IG II. Cytoplasmic signaling pathways that regulate cardiac hypertrophy. Annu Rev Physiol 2001;63:391–426.
[24] Strehler EE, Treiman M. Calcium pumps of plasma membrane and cell interior. Curr Mol Med 2004;4: 323–35.
[25] Bovendeerd PHM, Huyghe JMRJ, Arts T, et al. Influence of endocardial-epicardial crossover of muscle fibers on left ventricular wall mechanics. J Biochem 1994;27:942–51.
[26] Costa KD, Takayama Y, McCulloch AD, et al. Laminar fibre architecture and three-dimensional

systolic mechanics in canine ventricular myocardium. Am J Physiol 1999;276:H595–607.

[27] Hunter PJ, McCulloch AD, Nielsen PMF, et al. A finite element model of passive ventricular mechanics. Computational Methods in Bioengineering 1988;9:387–97.

[28] Torrent-Guasp F. La estructuración macroscópica del miocardio ventricular. Rev Esp Cardiol 1980; 33:265–98 (Juan March Foundation, Madrid, 1973).

[29] Torrent-Guasp F, Kocica MJ, Corno F, et al. Towards new understanding of the heart structure and function. Eur J Cardiothorac Surg 2005;27(2): 191–201.

[30] Buckberg GD, Clemente C, Cox JL, et al. The structure and function of the helical heart and its buttress wrapping. IV. Concepts of dynamic function from the normal macroscopic helical structure. Semin Thorac Cardiovasc Surg 2001;13:342–57.

[31] Streeter DD Jr. Gross morphology and fiber geometry of the heart. In: Berne RM, Sperelakis N, editors. Handbook of physiology: the cardiovascular system. Washington DC: American Physiologic Society; 1979. p. 61–112.

[32] LeGrice IJ, Smaill BH, Cahi LZ, et al. Laminar structure of the heart: ventricular myocyte arrangement and connective tissue architecture in the dog. Am J Physiol 1995;269:H571–82.

[33] Jouk PS, Usson Y, Michalowicz G, et al. Three-dimensional cartography of the pattern of myofibres in the second trimester fetal human heart. Anat Embryol (Berl) 2000;202:103–18.

[34] Lunkenheimer PP, Redmann K, Florek J, et al. The forces generated within the musculature of the left ventricular wall. Heart 2004;90:200–7.

[35] Lunkenheimer PP, Redmann K, Cryer CW, et al. Beta-blocker at low doses restoring the physiological balance in myocytic antagonism. Eur J Cardiothorac Surg 2007;32(2):225–30.

[36] Buchhalter MB, Weiss JL, Rogers WJ, et al. Non-invasive quantification of left ventricular rotational deformation in normal humans using magnetic resonance imaging myocardial tagging. Circulation 1990;81:1236–44.

[37] Rademakers FE, Buchalter MB, Rogers WJ, et al. Dissociation between left ventricular untwisting and filling. Circulation 1992;85:1572–81.

[38] Shapiro EP, Rademakers EF. Importance of oblique fiber orientation for left ventricular wall deformation. Technol Health Care 1997;5:21–8.

[39] Spotnitz HM, Spotnitz WD, Cottrell RS, et al. Cellular basis for volume related wall thickness changes in the rat left ventricle. J Mol Cell Cardiol 1974;6: 317–31.

[40] Lev M, Simkins CS. Architecture of the human ventricular myocardium. Lab Invest 1956;5:396–409.

[41] Lunkenheimer PP, Redmann K, Dietl KH, et al. The heart's fibre alignment assessed by comparing two digitizing systems: methodological investigation into the inclination angle towards wall thickness. Technol Health Care 1997;5:65–77.

[42] Sanchez-Quintana D, Garcia-Martinez V, Hurle JM. Myocardial fiber architecture in the human heart. Acta Anat (Basel) 1990;138:352–8.

[43] Dorri F, Niederer P, Lunkenheimer PP. A finite element model of the left ventricular systole. Comput Methods Biomech Biomed Engin 2006;9:319–41.

[44] Basser PJ, Matiello J, LeBihan D. MR diffusion tensor spectroscopy and imaging. Biophys J 1994;66: 259–67.

[45] Helm P, Beg MF, Miller MI, et al. Measuring and mapping cardiac fiber and laminar architecture using diffusion tensor MR imaging. Ann N Y Acad Sci 2005;1047:296–307.

[46] Harrington KB, Rodriguez F, Chang A, et al. Direct measurement of transmural laminar architecture in the anterolateral wall of the ovine left ventricle: new implications for wall thickening mechanics. Am J Physiol Heart Circ Physiol 2005;288:H1324–30.

[47] Hort W. Strukturdynamik des Myokard. Bd 22/I: Pathologische Anatomie des Herzens und seiner Hüllen. In: Doerr W, Seifert G, Uehlinger E, editors. Spezielle pathologische Anatomie. Berlin: Springer; 1993. p. 201–36.

[48] Feneis H. Das Gefüge des Herzmuskels bei Systole und Diastole. Gegenbauers Morphologisches Jahrbuch 1944/45;89:371–406.

[49] Anderson RH, Ho SY, Redmann K, et al. The anatomical arrangement of the myocardial cells making up the ventricular mass. Eur J Cardiothorac Surg 2005;28:517–25.

[50] Dorri F, Niederer P, Redmann K, et al. An analysis of the spatial arrangement of the myocardial aggregates making up the wall of the left ventricle. Eur J Cardiothorac Surg 2007;31:430–7.

[51] Anderson RH, Becker AF. The orientation of fibres within the ventricular mass. In: Anderson RH, Becker AF, editors. Cardiac anatomy. London: Churchill Livingstone; 1980. p. 5.14–26.

[52] Fernandez-Teran MA, Jurle JM. Myocardial fibre architecture of the human heart ventricles. Anat Rec 1982;204:137–47.

[53] Grant RP. Notes on the muscular architecture of the left ventricle. Circulation 1965;32:301–8.

[54] Greenbaum RA, Ho SY, Gibson DG, et al. Left ventricular fibre architecture in man. Br Heart J 1981; 45:248–63.

[55] Bettendorf-Bakman DE, Schmid P, Lunkenheimer PP, et al. A finite element study relating to the rapid filling phase of the human ventricles. J Theor Biol 2006;238(2):303–16.

[56] Hort W. Quantitative histologische Untersuchungen am wachsenden Herzen. Virchows Arch 1953;323: 223–42.

[57] Lunkenheimer PP, Redmann K, Kling N, et al. Three-dimensional architecture of the left ventricular myocardium. Anat Rec 2006;288(Part A):565–78.

[58] McLean M, Protheroe J. Determination of relative fiber orientation in heart muscle: methodological problems. Anat Rec 1992;232:459–65.

[59] Schmid P, Jaermann T, Boesiger PP, et al. Ventricular myocardial architecture as visualised in postmortem swine hearts using magnetic resonance diffusion tensor imaging. Eur J Cardiothorac Surg 2005;27:468–71.
[60] Schmid P, Lunkenheimer PP, Redmann K, et al. Statistical analysis of the angle of intrusion of porcine ventricular myocytes from epicardium to endocardium using diffusion tensor magnetic resonance imaging. Anat Rec 2007;290:1413–23.
[61] Suma H, Tanabe H, Uejima T, et al. Selected ventriculoplasty for idiopathic dilated cardiomyopathy with advanced congestive heart failure: midterm results and risk analysis. Eur J Cardiothorac Surg 2007;32:912–6.
[62] Isomura T, Horii T, Suma H, et al. Septal anterior ventricular exclusion operation (pacopexy) for ischemic dilated cardiomyopathy: treat form not disease. Eur J Cardiothorac Surg 2006;29:S245–50.
[63] Angelini GD, Tryn S, Mehta D, et al. Left ventricular-volume reduction for end-stage heart failure [letter]. Lancet 1997;(9076):350.
[64] Konertz W, Khoynezhad A, Sidiropoulos A, et al. Early and intermediate results of left ventricular reduction. Eur J Cardiothorac Surg 1999;15(Suppl 1): S26–30.
[65] Lunkenheimer PP, Redmann K, Cryer CW, et al. Late ventricular structure following partial left ventriculectomy: a case report. Ann Thorac Surg 2000; 69(4):1257–9.
[66] Batista R. Partial left ventriculectomy—the Batista procedure. Eur J Cardiothorac Surg 1999;15 (Suppl 1):S12–9 [discussion: S39–43].
[67] Batista RJV, Verde J, Nery P, et al. Partial left ventriculectomy to treat end-stage heart disease. Ann Thorac Surg 1997;64:634–8.
[68] Fukamachi K, McCarthy PM, Starling RC, et al. Effects of partial left ventriculectomy on cardiac performance [letter]. Circulation 1998;98(19):2101–2.
[69] Redmann K, Lunkenheimer PP, Dietl KH, et al. Immediate effects of partial left ventriculectomy on left ventricular function. J Cardiothorac Surg 1999;13: 453–62.
[70] Batista RJV, Santos JLV, Takeshita N, et al. Partial left ventriculectomy to improve left ventricular function in end-stage heart disease. J Card Surg 1996;11: 96–7.
[71] McCarthy PM, Starling RC, Wongj J, et al. Early results with partial left ventriculectomy. J Thorac Cardiovasc Surg 1997;114:755–63.
[72] Frazier OH, Gradinac S, Segura AM, et al. Partial left ventriculectomy: which patients can be expected to benefit? Ann Thorac Surg 2000;69:1836–41.
[73] Karlon WJ, Covell JW, McCulloch AD, et al. Automated measurement of myofiber disarray in transgenic mice with ventricular expression of ras. Anat Rec 1998;252:612–25.
[74] Humphrey JD, McCulloch AD. The cardiovascular system: anatomy, physiology and cell biology. In: Holzapfel GA, Ogden RW, editors. Biomechanics of soft tissue in cardiovascular systems. New York: Springer; 2003. p. 1–4.
[75] Anderson RH, Ho SY, Sanchez-Quintana D. Heuristic problems in defining the three-dimensional arrangement of the ventricular myocytes. Anat Rec 2006;288(Part A):579–86.
[76] Anderson RH, Sanchez-Quintana D, Redmann K, et al. Structural and functional correlates of the three-dimensional arrangement of the myocytes making up the ventricular walls. J Cardiothorac Surg, in press.
[77] Caulfield JB, Borg TK. The collagen network of the heart. Lab Invest 1979;40:364–71.
[78] Pearlman ES, Weber KT, Janicki JS, et al. Muscle fiber orientation and connective tissue content in the hypertrophied human heart. Lab Invest 1982; 46:158–64.
[79] Weber KT, Brilla CG, Janicki JS. Structural remodeling of myocardial collagen in systemic hypertension: functional consequences and potential therapy. Heart Fail 1990;29:129–37.
[80] Weber KT. Cardiac interstitium in health and disease: the fibrillar collagen network. J Am Coll Cardiol 1989;13:1637–52.
[81] Hort W. Untersuchungen zur funktionellen Morphologie des Bindegewebsgerüstes und der Blutgefäße der linken Herzkammerwand. Virchows Archiv fur Pathologische Anatomie 1960;33:565–81.
[82] Linzbach AJ. Heart failure from the point of view of quantitative anatomy. Am J Cardiol 1960;5: 370–81.
[83] Lamberts RR, Maurice JJ, Willemsen MF, et al. Acute and specific collagen type I degradation increases diastolic and developed tension in perfused rat papillary muscle. Am J Physiol Heart Circ Physiol 2004;286:H889–94.
[84] Mächler H, Reiter G, Perthel M, et al. Influence of a tilting prosthetic mitral valve orientation on the left ventricular flow—an experimental in vivo magnetic resonance imaging study. Eur J Cardiothorac Surg 2007;32:102–7.
[85] Strauer BE. Kraft-Geschwindigkeits-Beziehungen der isotonischen Relaxation bei myokardialer Hypertrophie und Insuffizienz. Z Kardiol 1973;62: 220–7.

ELSEVIER
SAUNDERS

Heart Failure Clin 4 (2008) 289–301

HEART
FAILURE
CLINICS

Toward Patient-Specific Myocardial Models of the Heart

Maxime Sermesant, PhD[a,b,*], Jean-Marc Peyrat, MSc[a], Phani Chinchapatnam, PhD[c], Florence Billet, MSc[a], Tommaso Mansi, MSc[a], Kawal Rhode, PhD[b], Hervé Delingette, PhD[a], Reza Razavi, MD[b], Nicholas Ayache, PhD[a]

[a]*Institut National de Recherche en Informatique et en Automatique, Sophia Antipolis, France*
[b]*St Thomas' Hospital, London, UK*
[c]*University College London, London, UK*

Integrating computational models of the heart with clinical data can open up ways to improve diagnosis, treatment planning, and interventions for cardiovascular diseases. It provides a consistent, biophysically based framework for the integration of the fragmented and heterogeneous clinical data currently available. Obtaining patient-specific computational models of the cardiac physiology could help diagnosis by providing physically meaningful cardiac indices. Moreover, once validated, models can have a predictive use and guide in patient management and therapy planning. For example, these computational models provide an excellent basis to optimize the design of implantable devices for improved therapy. However, the application of this modeling research has yet to be translated into the clinical environment, mainly because of the difficulty of validating these models with in vivo data, and efficiently personalizing them.

There is a growing body of literature on the functional imaging of the heart, for example with the measurement of electrical activity, deformation, flows, fiber orientation [1–4], and on the modeling of the electrical and mechanical activity of the heart [5–9]. Many of these models are direct computational models, designed to reproduce in a realistic manner cardiac activity, often requiring high computational costs and the manual tuning of a very large set of parameters.

The proposed approach is to design models that are directly related to the phenomena observed in clinical data. Although the models used here are often simplified when compared with the very detailed models available in the literature, the authors try to select a level of modeling compatible with reasonable computing times and involving a limited number of parameters, thus allowing the identification of the model parameters from clinical measurements of a specific patient, through the resolution of the inverse problem (Fig. 1).

There are still many challenges in achieving a patient-specific electromechanical model of the heart, but some parts can already be personalized, as demonstrated here. The authors will present this work in three sections concerning the anatomy, the electrophysiology, and the biomechanics. But the first challenge in this area is to obtain patient data on these different parts, and integrate them in the same spatio-temporal coordinates.

Clinical data acquisition and fusion

The construction, testing, and personalization of biophysical models rely on the ability to fuse

* Corresponding author. INRIA, Asclepios project, 2004 route des Lucioles, 06 902 Sophia Antipolis, France.
E-mail address: maxime.sermesant@inria.fr (M. Sermesant).

1551-7136/08/$ - see front matter
doi:10.1016/j.hfc.2008.02.014

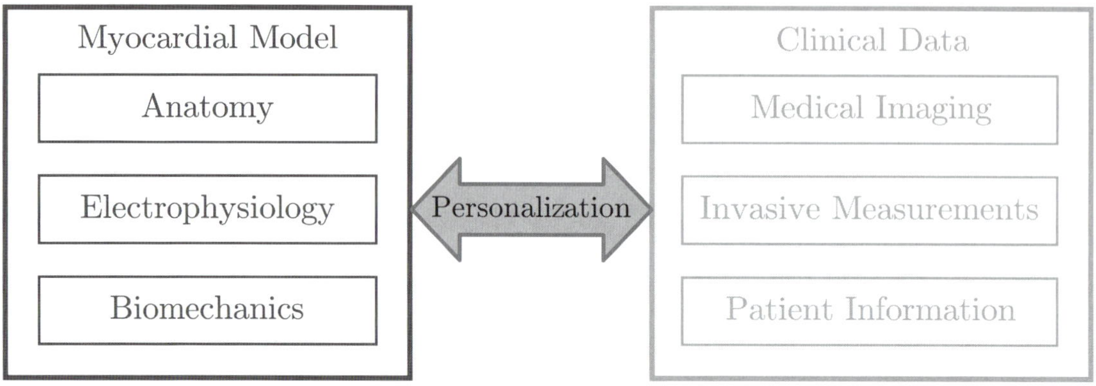

Fig. 1. Global scheme of the model building blocks and of the clinical data used to personalize it.

data from a variety of sources. For cardiac modeling, the fusion of anatomic, mechanical, and electrical data is of primary interest. This fusion must be both in the spatial and temporal domains. High quality cardiac anatomic data can be obtained from both computerized tomography (CT) and magnetic resonance imaging (MRI). MRI can also be used to obtain functional data, such as myocardial wall motion and blood flow. Electrical data can be obtained from catheter-based measurements that are guided using X-ray fluoroscopy.

Spatial fusion of these different data requires an effective image registration strategy. The authors' solution has focused on the use of the X-ray/MR (XMR) hybrid imaging system that allows the seamless collection of both MRI and X-ray-based data (Fig. 2). The authors have developed a real-time registration solution [10] that allows the spatial integration of MRI-based anatomic and functional data with X-ray-based catheter data, such as intracardial electrical and pressure signals. For the temporal integration, the electrocardiogram gives information on the heart rhythm that makes possible the synchronization of the different datasets.

Myocardial anatomy

In the authors' approach, only the compact biventricular myocardium is considered. As the valves are not modeled, the papillary muscles are not simulated, and only the atria and arteries as

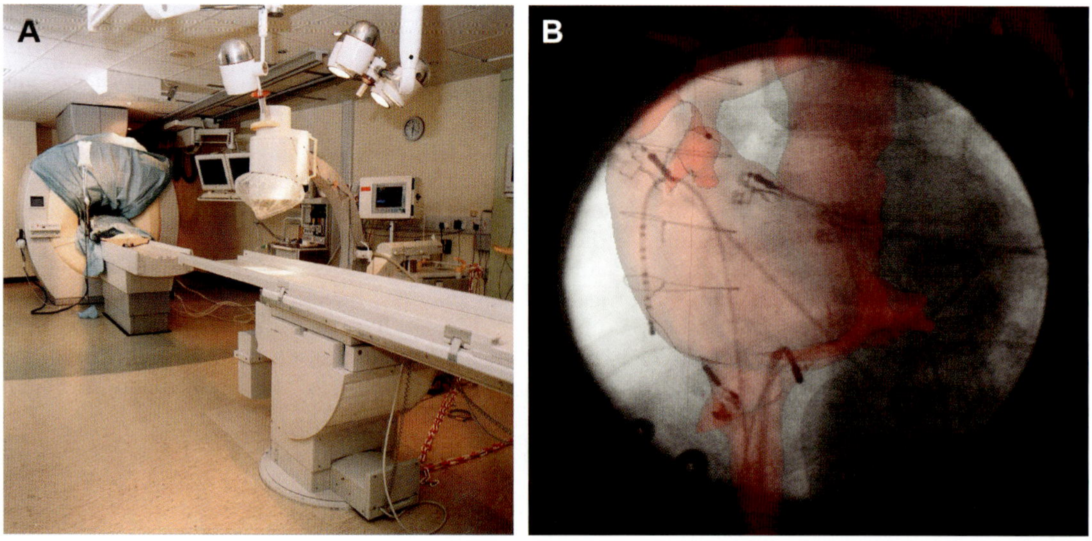

Fig. 2. (*A*) XMR suite with the MR scanner and the X-ray C-arm. (*B*) Catheters in place during an atrial flutter ablation and overlay of the MR-derived anatomy (*in red*) of the right side of the heart.

before-load and after-load boundary conditions are integrated.

Patient-specific myocardial shape

The authors have developed a method to create a biventricular mesh adapted to the three-dimensional (3D) image of the heart of a given patient. There is important literature on cardiac image analysis for the segmentation of the heart from medical images [11–21]. The idea is not to be exhaustive but to present a generic pipeline where most of the approaches can fit. The full pipeline relies both on intensity-based algorithms and deformable models [22]. The workflow is to extract from the images a preliminary segmentation of the blood pools and then to adjust the mesh geometry. Deformable models evolve under the influence of both external forces, computed from the preliminary segmentation, and internal forces, computed from the laws of mechanics.

More precisely, the pipeline consists of three main steps, detailed below: image filtering, to enhance image quality and correct possible artifacts; intensity-based labeling, to get a first segmentation of the ventricular cavities; and model-based segmentation, to get the final 3D myocardial shape (Fig. 3).

Image filtering

To increase the robustness of the algorithm on routine cardiac MRI, prone to acquisition artifacts (noise, slice misalignment, motion artifacts), the images must first be processed to facilitate automatic labeling. First, intensity inhomogeneities caused by magnetic field variations can be attenuated using, for instance, the N3 algorithm [23], which estimates image intensity variations using a nonparametric approach. Next, a histogram-based algorithm can be applied to enhance image contrast (remove extrema quantiles). Finally, image signal-to-noise ratio can be improved by using anisotropic filtering, where nonlinear partial differential equations (PDE) are used to smooth the noise while preserving the edges [24].

Intensity-based labeling of left and right blood pools

A first extraction of the ventricular blood pools is achieved by relying on a region-growing approach. For each ventricle, the user interactively places a few control points to define the valve annuli and initial seeds inside the cavities. The algorithm automatically expands the seeds, covering the voxels with similar intensities. In order to enforce the right topology, smooth the borders, and propagate along the time sequence, a deformable surface is then used. The Marching Cubes algorithm [25] provides a 3D surface representing the preliminary segmentation. Then the endocardial surfaces can be extracted from each image of the sequence: the mesh is immersed into the second frame and forces are applied to deform it toward the new endocardial boundaries [13]. An internal force ensures its smoothness while a region-based external force makes it evolve according to the image gray-level intensities. Afterward, the resulting surface is embedded into the following frame and deformed, and so forth until the end of the sequence. Thus, the labeling of both left and right blood pools in each cardiac phase is finally obtained.

Myocardium segmentation

The epicardium is hardly visible in most of the standard clinical MR sequences. Thus, it is first delineated with an interactive tool. The user places a few control points inside, on, and outside the epicardium. A 3D surface is generated in real-time, as the user adds, removes, or moves control points, using variational implicit surfaces and radial basis functions [26]. From the epicardial and endocardial surfaces, a binary image corresponding to the myocardium is created. A volumetric mesh is finally deformed under the influence of internal and external forces. The material properties of the muscle are used in the

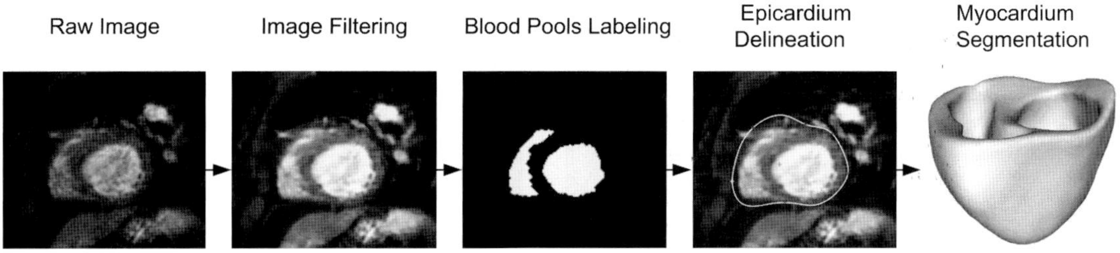

Fig. 3. Global scheme of the segmentation pipeline. Different algorithms can be used for each step of this process.

internal forces to ensure the smoothness and the incompressibility of the myocardial mesh [22]. Results of this pipeline are presented in Fig. 4.

Myofiber orientations

In the compact myocardium, the muscle fiber orientations play a crucial role in cardiac electrophysiology and electromechanics. Thus, their introduction in the model is important. However, there is currently no accurate in vivo measurement of these orientations at high resolution [27], so investigators have to mainly rely on prior knowledge.

The complete 3D reconstruction of fiber orientations from histologic sections [28], and more recently its direct 3D acquisition on ex vivo hearts with diffusion tensor MRI (DT-MRI) [29], have been used for a more realistic description of the myofiber architecture. However, they still come from a single subject and thus do not take into account any intersubject variability. In order to improve these models by building an average fiber architecture (Fig. 5) and by measuring its variability, the authors computed a statistical atlas of DT-MRIs from a small database of nine canine hearts [30], which is available on the World Wide Web (http://www-sop.inria.fr/asclepios/data/heart/). The authors performed a groupwise nonrigid registration of the cardiac geometries to an average geometry (see Fig. 5A). Then the DT-MRIs were properly transformed to fit the average geometry in which the average (see Fig. 5B) and covariance of diffusion tensors at each voxel was computed.

Because there is a direct link between the fiber orientations and the primary eigenvector of diffusion tensors, the authors derived the fiber orientation variability from the analysis of the covariance of the diffusion tensors. The results showed a strong coherence within the canine population. Thanks to the exceptional access to an ex vivo human cardiac DT-MRI data set, its comparison with the canine population showed good interspecies similarities [30]. The use of an average model from different species makes sense for a more realistic and generic prior knowledge on fiber orientations. Because it is known that some pathologies have an impact on the fiber architecture, there may be local adjustment to perform on these orientations when simulating these pathologies. This could be done, for example, with synthetic models built with analytic laws describing general trends of fiber orientations observed in different studies [31]. However, the influence of this variability in terms of the electrical and mechanical behavior of the heart is currently studied based on biomechanical simulations.

Myocardial electrophysiology

Electrophysiology model

Modeling the cell electrophysiology (EP) has been an active research area since the seminal work of Hodgkin and Huxley [32]. At the organ level, it involves a cell membrane model embedded into a set of PDEs representing a continuum. The approaches can be divided into three categories, in decreasing order of computational complexity:

- Biophysical: semilinear evolution PDE with ionic models (up to 50 equations for ions and channels) [33–37]
- Phenomenologic: semilinear evolution PDE with mathematical simplifications of biophysical models (bidomain, monodomain) [38–40]

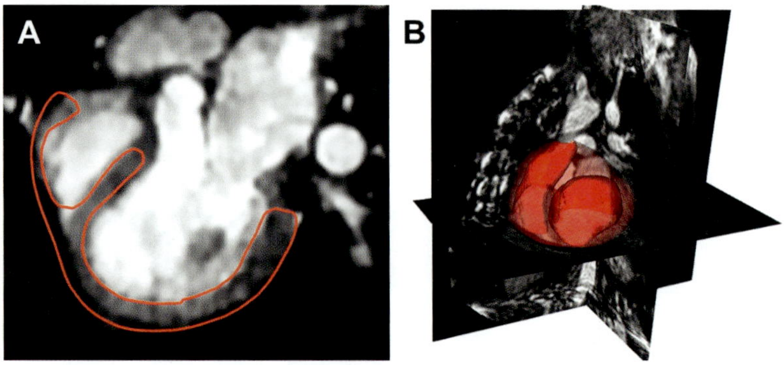

Fig. 4. Results of myocardium segmentation using the presented pipeline. (*A*) Intersection between the final segmentation (*in red*) and the MR image. (*B*) 3D visualization of the final mesh within the MR volume.

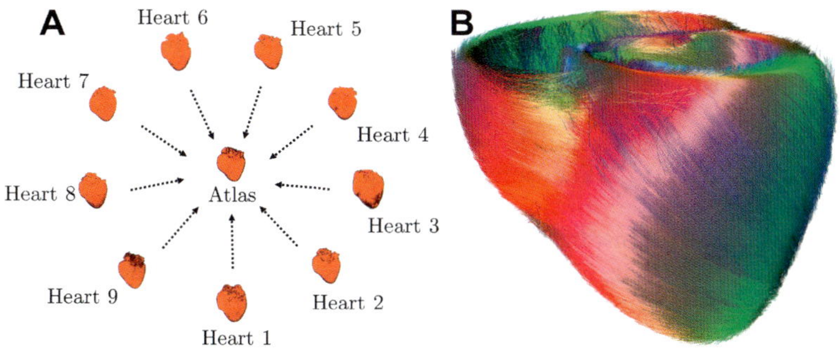

Fig. 5. Statistical atlas of cardiac fibers architecture. (*A*) A groupwise registration of the cardiac geometries to an average geometry. (*B*) Fiber tracking performed with the average DT-MRI.

- Eikonal: one static nonlinear PDE for the depolarization time derived from the previous models (Eikonal-curvature, Eikonal-diffusion) [41,42].

Solutions of the evolution PDE are computationally very demanding, because of the space scale of the electrical propagation being much smaller than the size of the ventricles, and the stability issues of the dynamic aspect. The Eikonal equation is static and the front can be observed at a larger scale, resulting in much faster computations.

For the authors' clinical applications, very fast models that can be adjusted to the data must be designed. Moreover, meaningful clinical data currently available reliably describes the propagation times, but are not suited for accurate estimation of extracellular or action potentials. For these reasons, the authors chose to base their work on the Eikonal models. Even if these models may not be able to precisely simulate the complete range of cardiac pathologies, they open up possibilities for fast parameter estimation, as well as data filtering, interpolation, and extrapolation.

An anisotropic multifront, fast marching method was developed to solve the Eikonal model equations very efficiently [43]. The Eikonal model is capable of simulating complex depolarization wavefront rotations around functional blocks. The authors base their model on the Eikonal diffusion (ED) equation. The static ED equation for the depolarization time (T_d) in the myocardium is given by

$$c_0\sqrt{D}\left(\sqrt{\nabla T_d^t \mathbf{M} \nabla T_d}\right) - (D\nabla \cdot \mathbf{M}\nabla T_d) = \tau \qquad (1)$$

where c_0 is a dimensionless constant related to the cell membrane, τ is the cell membrane time constant, and D is the square of the membrane space constant and thus related to the volumetric electrical conductivity of the tissue. The tensor quantity relating to the fiber directions is given by $\mathbf{M} = \mathbf{A}\overline{D}\mathbf{A}^t$, where A is the matrix defining the fiber directions in the global coordinate system and $\overline{D} = \mathrm{diag}(1, \lambda^2, \lambda^2)$. In this equation, λ is the anisotropic ratio of membrane space constants along and transverse to the fiber direction and is of the order 0.4 in human myocardium (see Ref. [44] for more details on the ED equation and its parameters).

Patient-specific electrophysiology

To personalize the electrophysiology model, the authors propose to estimate the cardiac cell membrane space constant (D) in the Eikonal model, which corresponds to an apparent conductivity (AC). The idea is to estimate the AC by matching the simulated propagation times of the model to clinically measured propagation times of the patient. Once this process has been achieved, a patient-specific electrophysiology model can be realized, which can help in diagnosis and therapy planning. The EP model adjustment procedure is divided into two components:

- A nominal value of the AC is estimated by minimizing the average difference between the simulated and measured depolarization times using a bisection method. This step enables the simulated and measured propagation times to be brought to the same scale.
- A multilevel approach is then taken by adaptively subdividing the entire region of the endocardium into zones where the AC on each zone is estimated using a least-squares approach and modified Brent minimization algorithm.

The authors present the application of the EP model adjustment algorithm to build a patient-specific EP model for a clinical case with left bundle branch block pathology. The patient underwent electrophysiology study in the XMR environment where an Ensite array (St. Jude Medical) is inserted into the left ventricle via a retrograde aortic approach. The baseline (normal sinus rhythm) propagation times were measured by the Ensite array and are used to adjust the Eikonal model for this particular patient (Fig. 6).

Once the EP model has been adjusted to a particular patient data, the model can then be used in its predictive capacity. Fig. 7 shows how the adjusted EP model can be used to predict a propagation map from a different pacing site. Fig. 7B presents the application of the adjusted model to predict the isochrones of propagation when paced from a postero-lateral position in the endocardium. By comparing these isochrones with those measured during pacing (Fig. 7A), it can be seen that this adjusted model can indeed be a first step toward the development of a patient specific EP model. Such models could be very useful, for example, for the planning of multisite cardiac stimulation, as used for the treatment of patients with ventricular asynchrony.

Furthermore, an additional conduction related parameter, the conduction velocity (v_{app}), can be estimated from the apparent conductivity parameter: $v_{app} = c_0\sqrt{D/\tau}$. These conduction velocity maps can aid in determining possible scars, as they show up as areas of low conduction velocity on these velocity maps. Fig. 8 shows such a resultant conduction velocity map obtained for a different clinical case after EP model adjustment. This patient had scars caused by an earlier myocardial infarction. From the figures, it can be seen from the adjusted conductivity parameter colormap, that areas of low conduction velocity (black regions on the endocardial surface) do correspond to the scar locations, as obtained by the segmentation of the late-enhancement images.

Myocardial biomechanics

Constitutive law of the myocardium

The myocardium is an active nonlinear anisotropic visco-elastic material. Its constitutive law is complex and includes an active part for contraction, controlled by the transmembrane potential propagation (which can be computed from the previous section), and a passive part representing the mechanical elasticity of the myocardium. Several constitutive laws have been proposed in the literature [45–51]. These laws are designed to precisely fit rheologic tests made on in vitro cardiac muscle.

Another approach is to model contraction from the nanomotors scale and build up a macroscopic constitutive law representing the phenomena encountered at the different scales, which is the approach followed by Bestel-Clément-Sorine [52]. A detailed study of this complex model and simulations can be found in the work of Sainte-Marie and colleagues [53] and Moireau and colleagues [54]. This model is based on the Hill-Maxwell scheme.

The electromechanical model used here was motivated by the multiscale and phenomenologic approach of Bestel-Clément-Sorine, but it is

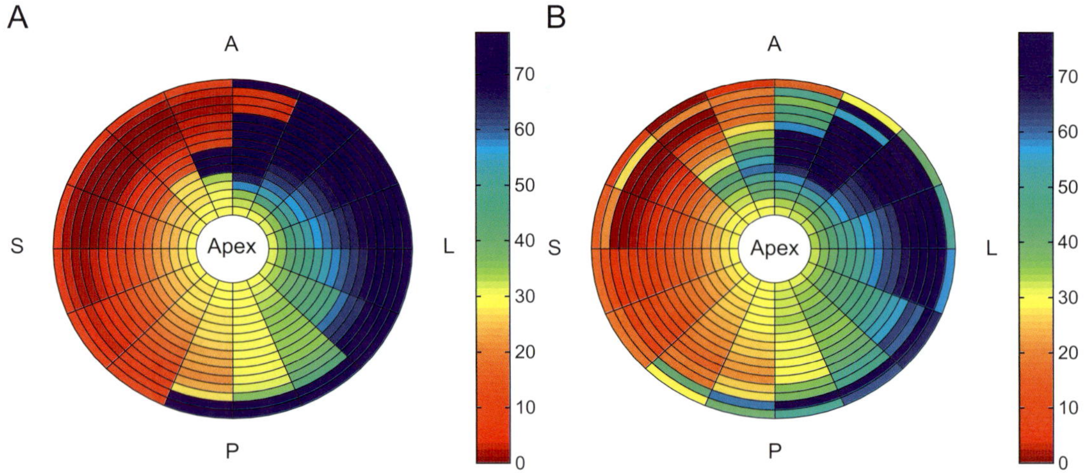

Fig. 6. Bull's-eye plots of depolarization times from a patient with left bundle branch block. (*A*) Measured isochrones using Ensite during sinus rhythm. (*B*) Simulated isochrones with the adjusted electrophysiology model.

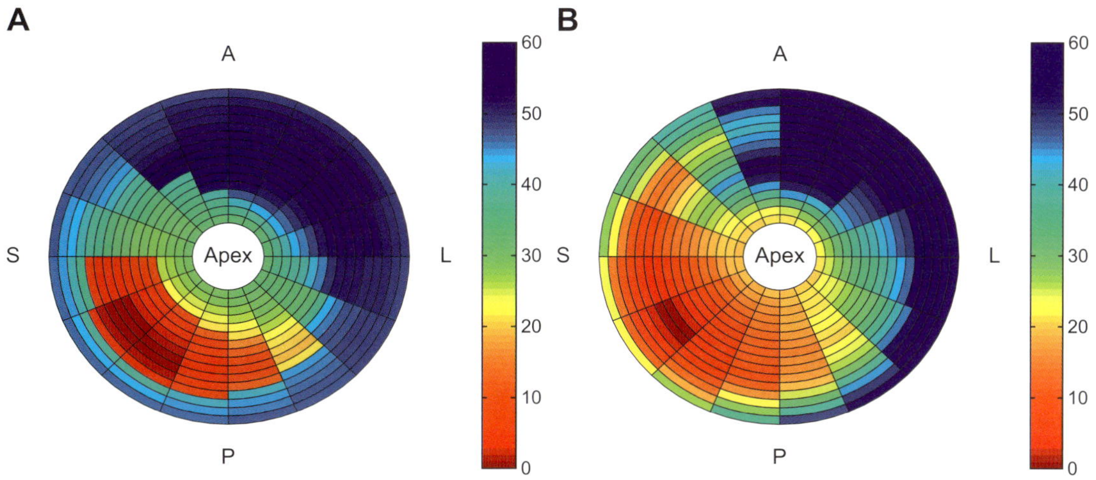

Fig. 7. Usage of the adjusted EP model to predict propagation map from a different pacing site. (*A*) Measured isochrones using Ensite during pacing. (*B*) Isochrones of depolarization predicted by the adjusted electrophysiology model.

specifically designed for cardiac image analysis and simulation. It is built to be computationally efficient and with few parameters directly related to clinical parameters, so the authors chose to simplify the constitutive law of the Bestel-Clément-Sorine approach. The simplified mechanical model has the following components:

- An active contractile element, which creates a stress tensor σ_c, controlled by the command u, depending on the depolarisation time T_d and repolarisation time T_r;
- A passive parallel element which is anisotropic linear visco-elastic and creates a stress tensor σ_p.

For the electromechanical coupling, several different laws have also been proposed [45,49]. The authors believe that it is important to keep the model simple, as relatively few clinical

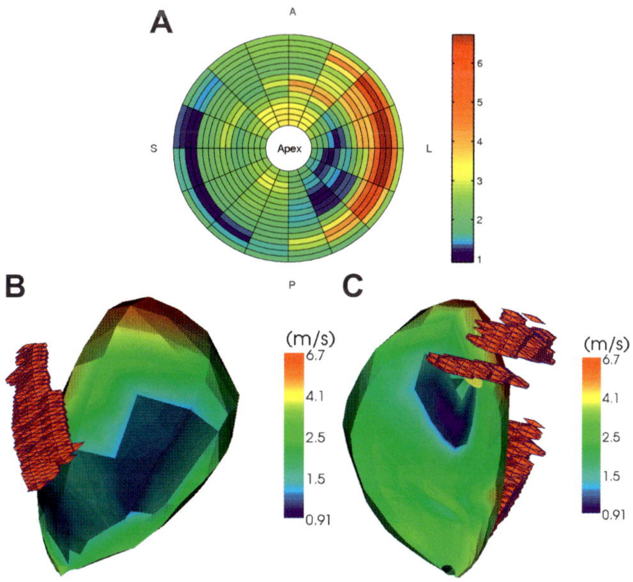

Fig. 8. (*A*) Estimated conduction velocity, where scars appear as small value regions (*blue*). (*B,C*) Areas of slow conduction (*black regions*) after EP model adjustment, compared with scar locations obtained from late-enhancement MRI image (*red wire-meshes*).

measures are available to adjust it. The contraction of a heart muscle cell (like all muscle cells) is controlled by cycling levels of calcium, which are stored in the sarcoplasmic reticulum. When depolarization occurs, the concentration of calcium increases in the cytosol and allows the adenosine diphosphate (ATP) hydrolysis, which provides energy to the molecular motors in the sarcomeres, generating the contraction of the fiber. The command u is then equal to a constant k_{ATP}, which represents the rate of the hydrolysis of the ATP. After contraction, during the depolarization, calcium moves back from the cytosol into the sarcoplasmic reticulum, and this calcium decrease leads to the relaxation of the muscle. The command u is then equal to another constant $(-\ k_{RS})$, which models the activity of the sarcoplasmic reticulum. The simplest way to model this contractile element is thus through an ordinary differential equation of the type $\dot{\sigma}_c + |u|\sigma_c = |u|_+\sigma_0$, with $\dot{\sigma}_c$ the time derivative of σ_c, σ_0 the maximum intensity of the contractionand, and $|u|_+$ the positive part of the command u, equal to u if u is greater than or equal to 0 and 0 if not. With this equation, the authors obtain the following coupling model (Equation 2 below), with T_d the depolarization time, T_r the depolarization time, HP the heart period, and $\sigma_r = \sigma_c(T_r)$.

The constants k_{ATP} and k_{RS} allow the contraction stress increase and decrease to be controlled, which is consistent with their precedent definition. A time delay between the electrical and the mechanical phenomena in this coupling can also be added. The command and the resulting contraction are represented in Fig. 9.

To numerically simulate this simplified constitutive law, the authors use the finite element method on a tetrahedral mesh to solve the discretised dynamics equation: $M\ddot{U} + C\dot{U} + KU = F_b + F_c$, with U the displacement vector, M the mass matrix, C the damping matrix for the internal viscosity part, K the stiffness matrix for the transverse anisotropic elastic part (parallel element), F_c the force vector computed from contraction (contractile element), and F_b the different external loads from the boundary conditions, detailed in the following section.

Boundary conditions: the cardiac phases

To simulate a whole cardiac cycle, the interaction of the myocardium with the blood is crucial. The cardiac cycle has four different phases (filling, isovolumetric contraction, ejection, isovolumetric relaxation), which implies different boundary conditions:

- Filling: the preload pressure is applied to the endocardium. Its intensity is equal to the pressure of the atrium. It is augmented during the P wave to represent atrial contraction. When the ventricular contraction starts, the contraction force will tend to eject blood, so when this force becomes more important than the applied pressure, the blood flow changes sign. As the blood is considered incompressible, the conservation of mass allows the computation of blood flow directly with the ventricular volume time derivative. This is used to close the atrial-ventricular valves and start the isovolumetric contraction.
- Isovolumetric contraction: the ventricular pressure computed to counterbalance the contraction force and then to keep the ventricle volume constant is applied to the vertices of the endocardium. When the ventricular pressure is more important than the arterial pressure, the ventricular-arterial valves open, and the ejection phase starts.
- Ejection: a pressure is applied to the vertices of the endocardium. Its intensity is equal to the pressure of the aorta (for the left ventricle) and the pulmonary artery (for the right ventricle). Contraction force decreases after repolarization. When the flow changes sign, the ventricular-arterial valves close, starting the isovolumetric relaxation phase.
- Isovolumetric relaxation: the ventricular pressure computed to keep the ventricular volume constant is applied to the vertices of the endocardium. When the ventricular pressure is less important than atrial pressure, the atrial-ventricular valves open, starting the filling phase.

The efficient implementation of such changing boundary conditions is an important part of

$$\begin{cases} \text{if } T_d \leq t \leq T_r: \ \sigma_c(t) = \sigma_0\left(1 - e^{k_{ATP}(T_d - t)}\right) \text{ as } \dot{\sigma}_c + k_{ATP}\sigma_c = k_{ATP}\sigma_0 \\ \text{if } T_r < t < T_d + HP: \ \sigma_c(t) = \sigma_r e^{k_{RS}(T_r - t)} \text{ as } \dot{\sigma}_c + k_{RS}\sigma_c = 0 \end{cases} \tag{2}$$

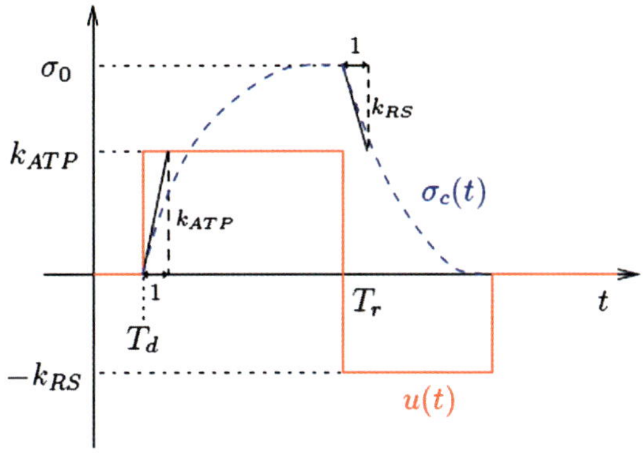

Fig. 9. Command $u(t)$ and contraction $\sigma_c(t)$ generated.

achieving fast enough mechanical simulations. In the model by Sermesant and colleagues [55], a penalty constraint was applied to the vertices of the endocardium to keep its volume constant. To achieve a balance between this constraint and the contraction, very small time steps had to be used. The authors now use the constrained optimization theory to directly compute the ventricular pressure, keeping the volume constant. The authors minimize the energy of the mechanical system of the heart $J(U) = \frac{1}{2}(U^t\tilde{K}U - U^t\tilde{F})$ under the constraints $V = V^\circ$, with V the volume in the considered ventricle (depending on U) and V° its volume at the beginning of the isovolumetric phase. $\tilde{K}$ and $\tilde{F}$ are two matrices obtained by a first integration of the dynamics equation. The pressure forces are contained in the $\tilde{F}$ matrix. At each time step, the authors compute the ventricular pressure for which the solution U of the above constrained minimization system is such that the volume is kept constant. This method can sustain much larger time steps (100 times greater than before), which allows the authors to simulate a whole heartbeat on a mesh with 50,000 elements in about 5 minutes on a standard computer. This improvement opens up possibilities in mechanical parameter adjustment and allows the behavior of the model on series of beats to be tested.

Despite its simplicity when compared with other constitutive laws proposed in the literature, this model reproduces reasonably well the global and local behavior of the myocardium. Fig. 10 shows the simulation of this model using the canine cardiac atlas for the myocardial shape and fiber structure.

In the current implementation, the atria pressures vary smoothly between two values (baseline

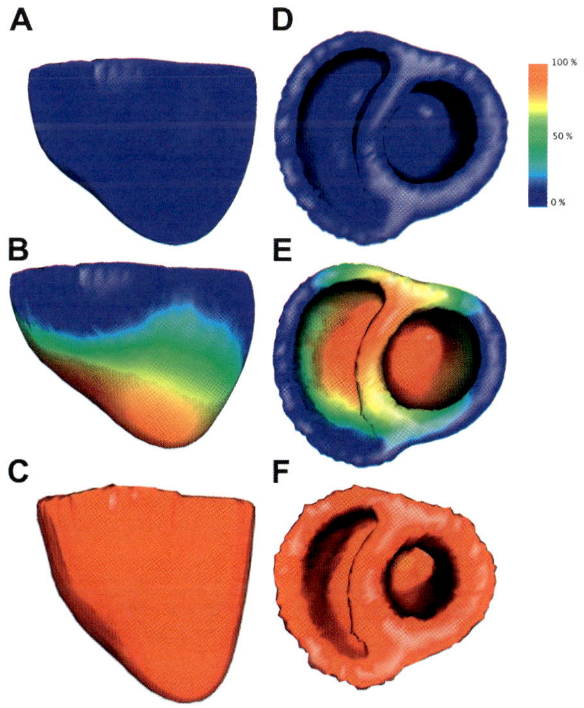

Fig. 10. Long axis and short axis views of the heart model at different phases of the heart cycle. (*A–F*) Colors represent the intensity of the contraction stress.

and atrial systolic pressure). The authors use a three-element Windkessel model to compute the arterial pressures from the arterial flow. Windkessel models are derived from electrical circuit analogies, where current and voltage represent arterial flow and pressure, respectively, and have been found to represent well (after proper adjustment of the parameters) the clinical measurements [56–58]. To hold the mesh in space, the authors simulate the fibrous structure around the valves with springs, having one extremity attached to a basal node and the other extremity attached to a fixed point. Some simulation outputs are presented in Fig. 11.

The authors can note that even with these completely independent conditions for the left and right parts of the heart, the two ventricles stay well synchronized, which shows that force development is coherent in the model. It allows calibration of the contractility parameters σ_0, k_{ATP}, and k_{RS} from the duration of the different phases, and also from the atrial and arterial pressures, before further local adjustment, using, for example, cine-MRI.

Toward patient-specific simulations

Preliminary simulations of patient heart function are already possible through this framework. Right-ventricle overload caused by congenital heart diseases, for example, can be simulated to study the effect of the abnormal myocardium anatomy and loading conditions upon the cardiac function.

To illustrate the overall framework, the authors present the adjustment of the electromechanical model to a patient with Tetralogy of Fallot. The myocardium shape is extracted from the patient image data using the presented segmentation pipeline. The biomechanical parameters are manually calibrated: maximum contraction σ_0 is obtained by comparing the simulated and real diameters of the ventricles at end-systole; contraction rate k_{ATP} and relaxation rate k_{RS} are estimated using both the dynamic images and the volume diagrams obtained from the segmentations. Because they are not accessible for this patient, electrical parameters and boundary conditions are set according to clinical observations available in the literature.

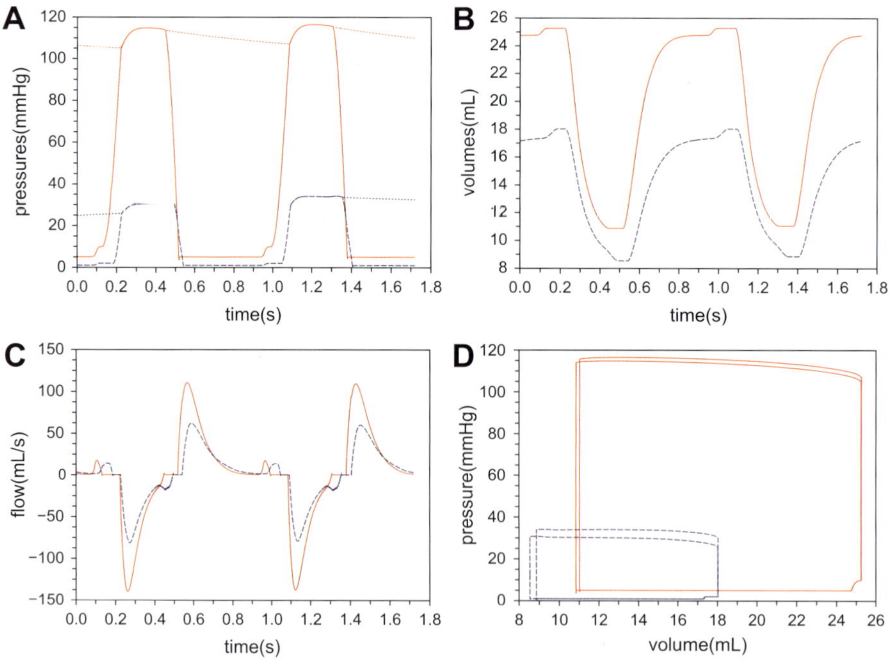

Fig. 11. (*A*) Ventricular, aorta and pulmonary artery pressures (in mm Hg). (*B*) Ventricular volumes (in mL). (*C*) Flows (in mL/mn). (*D*) Pressure-Volume cycles. The dash (and red) curves and the solid (and blue) curves represent respectively the right and the left ventricles. The dot curves in (*A*) represent the aorta and the pulmonary artery pressures.

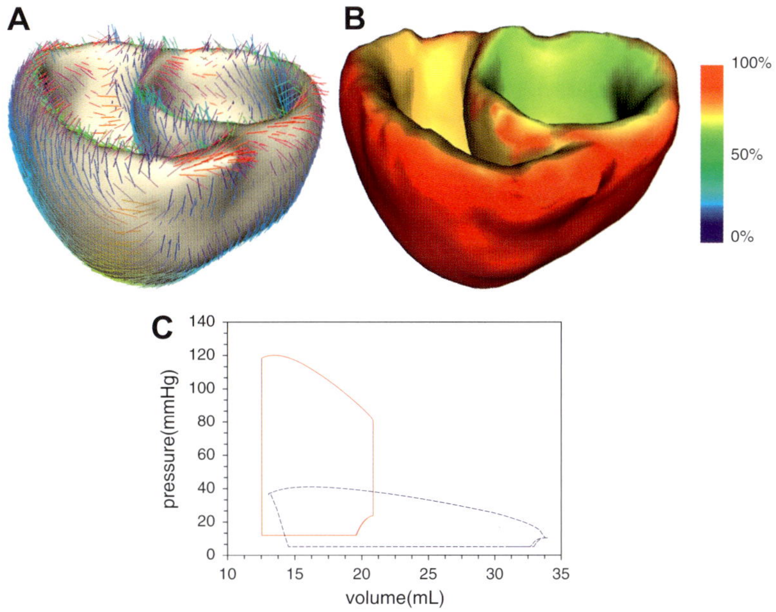

Fig. 12. (*A*) Anatomy of the right-ventricle overload patient with synthetic fiber orientations. (*B*) Contraction of the model: end-systole position; colors represent the contraction stress. (*C*) Pressure-volume loops, demonstrating right ventricle enlargement and regurgitations.

The left ventricle can be simulated successfully, as well as the regions of the right ventricle far from the outflow tract. The simulated contraction at each vertex of the mesh, the electrical propagation, and the 3D strain can be visualized in real time to assess the cardiac function (Fig. 12). Additional results on this disease-adapted work can be found on the World Wide Web (http://www-sop.inria.fr/asclepios/projects/hec/).

However, the abnormal regions of the right ventricle are still difficult to simulate because of some limitations in the model: in particular the authors' way of handling the fluid-structure interactions, which may not be suited to these pathologies. The authors introduced here a preliminary model of valve regurgitation, which is an important feature of this pathology; however, local abnormalities also have to be introduced in the model parameters to better represent the diseased behavior.

In summary, this article presents a framework toward patient-specific models of the myocardium. By integrating information about the anatomy, the electrophysiology, and the mechanics, we can explore the correlation between function and anatomy for a given patient and test different hypothesis as well as plan therapies.

To complete the personalization of the model, the parameters of the mechanical model must be adjusted locally, as was presented on the electrophysiology model. First results have been obtained on this problem, using the data assimilation framework of Sermesant and colleagues [59], but this is still very challenging. One of the additional difficulties, compared with the electrophysiology, is to precisely know the boundary conditions, such as the before-load and the after-load. In addition, the mechanical behavior depends on the electrophysiology, which is the command. Then, if errors were to occur in the electrophysiology model adjustment, this would lead to errors in the mechanical parameter adjustment. Thus, the progress made on the data acquisition and fusion will definitely play an important role in achieving a fully patient-specific heart model.

References

[1] MacLeod R, Yilmaz B, Taccardi B, et al. Direct and inverse methods for cardiac mapping using multi-electrode catheter measurements. Journal of Biomedizinische Technik 2001;46:207–9.

[2] Faris O, Evans F, Ennis D, et al. Novel technique for cardiac electromechanical mapping with magnetic resonance imaging tagging and an epicardial electrode sock. Ann Biomed Eng 2003;31(4):430–40.

[3] Masood S, Yang G, Pennell D, et al. Investigating intrinsic myocardial mechanics: the role of MR tagging, velocity phase mapping and diffusion imaging. J Magn Reson Imaging 2000;12(6):873–83.
[4] Kilner P, Yang G, Wilkes A, et al. Asymmetric redirection of flow through the heart. Nature 2000; 404:759–61.
[5] McCulloch A, Bassingthwaighte J, Hunter P, et al. Computational biology of the heart: from structure to function. Prog Biophys Mol Biol 1998;69(2–3): 151–559.
[6] Hunter P, Pullan A, Smaill B. Modeling total heart function. Annu Rev Biomed Eng 2003;5:147–77.
[7] Xia L, Huo M. Analysis of ventricular wall motion based on an electromechanical biventricular model. In: Murray A, editor. Computers in cardiology. New York: IEEE; 2003. p. 315–8.
[8] Noble D. Modeling the heart. Physiology (Bethesda) 2004;19:191–7.
[9] Nickerson D, Nash M, Nielsen P, et al. Computational multiscale modeling in the IUPS physiome project: modeling cardiac electromechanics. Systems Biology 2006;50(6):617–30.
[10] Rhode K, Sermesant M, Brogan D, et al. A system for real-time XMR guided cardiovascular intervention. IEEE Trans Med Imaging 2005;24(11):1428–40.
[11] Frangi A, Niessen W, Viergever M. Three-dimensional modeling for functional analysis of cardiac images: a review. IEEE Trans Med Imaging 2001; 1(20):2–25.
[12] Frangi A, Rueckert D. Duncan J. editors. New trends in three-dimensional cardiac image analysis. Vol. 21(9). IEEE Transactions on Medical Imaging. New York: IEEE.
[13] Montagnat J, Delingette H. 4D deformable models with temporal constraints: application to 4D cardiac image segmentation. Med Image Anal 2005;9(1): 87–100.
[14] Kaus M, von Berg J, Weese J, et al. Automated segmentation of the left ventricle in cardiac MRI. Med Image Anal 2004;8(3):245–54.
[15] Papademetris X, Sinusas A, Dione D, et al. Estimating 3D left ventricular deformation from 3D medical image sequences using biomechanical models. IEEE Trans Med Imaging 2002;21(7):786–800.
[16] Bistoquet A, Oshinski J, Skrinjar O. Left ventricular deformation recovery from cine MRI using an incompressible model. IEEE Trans Med Imaging 2007;26(9):1136–53.
[17] Linte A, Wierzbicki M, Moore J, et al. Towards subject-specific models of the dynamic heart for image-guided mitral valve surgery. In: Ayache N, Ourselin S, Maeder A, editors. Medical image computing and computer-assisted intervention. Berlin: Springer-Verlag; 2007. p. 94–101.
[18] Lorenzo-Valdes M, Sanchez-Ortiz GI, Elkington AG, et al. Segmentation of 4D cardiac MR images using a probabilistic atlas and the EM algorithm. Med Image Anal 2004;8(3):255–65.
[19] Peters J, Ecabert O, Meyer C, et al. Automatic whole heart segmentation in static magnetic resonance image volumes. In: Ayache N, Ourselin S, Maeder A, editors. Medical image computing and computer-assisted intervention. Berlin: Springer-Verlag; 2007. p. 402–10.
[20] van Assen HC, Danilouchkine MG, Frangi AF, et al. SPASM: a 3D-ASM for segmentation of sparse and arbitrarily oriented cardiac MRI data. Med Image Anal 2006;10(2):286–303.
[21] von Berg J, Lorenz C. Multi-surface cardiac modeling, segmentation, and tracking. In: Frangi A, Radeva P, Santos A, et al, editors. Functional imaging and modeling of the heart. Berlin: Springer-Verlag; 2005. p. 1–11.
[22] Sermesant M, Forest C, Pennec X, et al. Deformable biomechanical models: application to 4D cardiac image analysis. Med Image Anal 2003;7(4):475–88.
[23] Sled JG, Zijdenbos AP, Evans AC. A nonparametric method for automatic correction of intensity nonuniformity in MRI data. IEEE Trans Med Imaging 1998;17(1):87–97.
[24] Weickert J, ter Haar Romeny BM, Viergever MA. Efficient and reliable schemes for nonlinear diffusion filtering. IEEE Trans Image Process 1998;7(3): 398–410.
[25] Lorensen WE, Cline HE. Marching cubes: a high resolution 3D surface construction algorithm. In: Stone M, editor. SIGGRAPH'87: Proceedings of the 14th annual conference on Computer graphics and interactive techniques, vol. 21. New York: ACM Press; 1987. p. 163–9.
[26] Turk G, O'Brien J. Variational implicit surfaces. Technical report, Georgia Institute of Technology; 1999.
[27] Tseng W-YI, Reese TG, Weisskoff RM, et al. Cardiac diffusion tensor MRI in vivo without strain correction. Magn Reson Med 1999;42(2):393–403.
[28] Nielsen P, Grice IL, Smail B, et al. Mathematical model of geometry and fibrous structure of the heart. Am J Physiol Heart Circ Physiol 1991;260(29): H1365–78.
[29] Hsu EW, Muzikant AL, Matulevicius SA, et al. Magnetic resonance myocardial fiber-orientation mapping with direct histological correlation. Am J Physiol Heart Circ Physiol 1998;274:H1627–34.
[30] Peyrat J-M, Sermesant M, Pennec X, et al. A computational framework for the statistical analysis of cardiac diffusion tensors: Application to a small database of canine hearts. IEEE Trans Med Imaging 2007;26(11):1500–14.
[31] Streeter D. Handbook of physiology. In: Berne R, Sperelakis N, editors. The cardiovascular system: gross morphology and fiber geometry of the heart. Baltimore (MD): Williams & Wilkins; 1979.
[32] Hodgkin A, Huxley A. A quantitative description of membrane current and its application to conduction and excitation in nerve. J Physiol 1952;177:500–44.

[33] Noble D. A modification of the Hodgkin–Huxley equations applicable to Purkinje fibre action and pace-maker potentials. J Physiol 1962;160:317–52.
[34] Beeler GW, Reuter H. Reconstruction of the action potential of ventricular myocardial fibers. J Physiol 1977;268:177–210.
[35] Luo C, Rudy Y. A model of the ventricular cardiac action potential: depolarization, repolarization, and their interaction. Circ Res 1991;68:1501–26.
[36] Noble D, Varghese A, Kohl P, et al. Improved guinea-pig ventricular cell model incorporating a diadic space, I_{Kr} and I_{Ks}, and length and tension dependent processes. Can J Cardiol 1998;14:123–34.
[37] Ten Tusscher K, Noble D, Noble P, et al. A model of the human ventricular myocyte. Am J Physiol Heart Circ Physiol 2004;286(4):1573–89.
[38] FitzHugh R. Impulses and physiological states in theoretical models of nerve membrane. Biophys J 1961;1:445–66.
[39] Pollard A, Hooke N, Henriquez C. Cardiac propagation simulation. Crit Rev Biomed Eng 1992; 20(3,4):171–210.
[40] Aliev R, Panfilov A. A simple two-variable model of cardiac excitation. Chaos Solitons Fractals 1996; 7(3):293–301.
[41] Keener J, Sneyd J. Mathematical physiology. New York: Springer; 1998.
[42] Colli Franzone P, Guerri L, Rovida S. Wavefront propagation in activation model of the anisotropic cardiac tissue: asymptotic analysis and numerical simulations. J Math Biol 1990;28(2):121–76.
[43] Sermesant M, Konukoglu E, Delingette H, et al. An anisotropic multi-front fast marching method for real-time simulation of cardiac electrophysiology. In: Sachse F, Seemann G, editors. Proceedings of functional imaging and modeling of the heart. Vol 4466. Berlin: Springer-Verlag; 2007. p. 160–9.
[44] Tomlinson K. Finite element solution of an Eikonal equation for excitation wavefront propagation in ventricular myocardium, Ph.D. thesis, University of Auckland (2000).
[45] Hunter P, Smaill B. The analysis of cardiac function: a continuum approach. Prog Biophys Mol Biol 1988;52:101–64.
[46] Humphrey J, Strumpf R, Yin F. Determination of a constitutive relation for passive myocardium: I. A new functional form. J Biomech Eng 1990;112: 333–9.
[47] Guccione J, McCulloch A. Theory of heart: biomechanics, biophysics, and nonlinear dynamics of cardiac function. In: Glass L, Hunter PJ, McCulloch AD, editors. Finite element modeling of ventricular mechanics. New York: Springer-Verlag; 1991. p. 121–44.
[48] Hunter P, Nash M, Sands G. Computational biology of the heart. In: Panfilov A, Holden A, editors. Computational electromechanics of the heart. West Sussex (UK): John Wiley & Sons; 1997. p. 345–407.
[49] Nash M. Mechanics and material properties of the heart using an anatomically accurate mathematical model. Ph.D. thesis. University of Auckland; 1998.
[50] Häfner J, Sachse F, Sansour C, et al. Hyperelastic description of elastomechanic properties of the heart: A new material law and its application. Biomed Tech (Berl) 2002;47(1–2):770–3.
[51] Caillerie D, Mourad A, Raoult A. Cell-to-muscle homogenization. Application to a constitutive law for the myocardium. Mathematical Modelling and Numerical Analysis 2003;37(4):681–98.
[52] Bestel J. Clément F. Sorine M. A biomechanical model of muscle contraction. In: Niessen W, Viergever M, editors. Medical image computing and computer-assisted intervention. Vol 2208. Lecture Notes in Computer Science (LNCS). Berlin: Springer-Verlag; 2001. p.1159–61.
[53] Sainte-Marie J, Chapelle D, Cimrman R, et al. Modeling and estimation of the cardiac electromechanical activity. Comput Struct 2006;84:1743–59.
[54] Moireau P, Chapelle D, Le Tallec P. Joint state and parameter estimation for distributed mechanical systems. Computer Methods in Applied Mechanics and Engineering 2008;197:659–77.
[55] Sermesant M, Delingette H, Ayache N. An electromechanical model of the heart for image analysis and simulation. IEEE Trans Med Imaging 2006; 25(5):612–25.
[56] MacDonald A. Blood flow in the arteries. London: Edward Arnold; 1974.
[57] Stergiopulos N, Westerhof B, Westerhof N. Total arterial inertance as the fourth element of the Windkessel model. Am J Physiol 1999;276:H81–8.
[58] Muthurangu V, Atkinson D, Sermesant M, et al. Measurement of total pulmonary arterial compliance using invasive pressure monitoring and MR flow quantification during MR-guided cardiac catheterization. Am J Physiol Heart Circ Physiol 2005;289(3):1301–6.
[59] Sermesant M, Moireau P, Camara O, et al. Cardiac function estimation from MRI using a heart model and data assimilation: advances and difficulties. Med Image Anal 2006;10(4):642–56.

ELSEVIER
SAUNDERS

Heart Failure Clin 4 (2008) 303–314

HEART
FAILURE
CLINICS

Electromechanical Activation Sequence in Normal Heart

Partho P. Sengupta, MBBS, MD, DM[a,*], Fernando Tondato, MD[a], Bijoy K. Khandheria, MBBS[a], Marek Belohlavek, MD, PhD[a], Arshad Jahangir, MD[b]

[a]*Mayo Clinic, Scottsdale, AZ, USA*
[b]*Mayo Clinic, Rochester, MN, USA*

There has been extraordinary growth in the understanding of myocardial function at the molecular and genetic levels. It is rather puzzling to note that the electromechanical activation sequence, which results in the highly efficient global function of the normal heart, remain contentious and incompletely characterized, however. A report from the National Institutes of Health in 2004 drew attention to existing gaps in the understanding of the normal structure and function of a beating heart [1].

The normal electromechanical activation sequence of the left ventricle (LV) is an intricate process that involves the interaction of multiple elements, from the ultrastructural level of the myocytes and specialized conduction system to the macroscopic complex arrangement of myofibers. The complete understanding of the electromechanical activation sequence, however, is as challenging as it is fascinating. Elaborate computerized models, refined electrocardiographic systems, and the thorough analysis of the cardiac deformation sequence with high temporal resolution imaging techniques have led to substantial progress in the understanding of the heart's structure and rhythm. This review provides an in-depth experimental and theoretic exploration for understanding normal cardiac electrical propagation, electromechanical coupling, and the regional sequence of myocardial shortening and lengthening in the LV.

Intracellular conduction of electrical impulse

Cardiac myocytes are elongated structures, aligned in parallel and grouped in compact fiber bundles. The cells are electrically anisotropic, such that propagation velocity is near three times higher when the impulse propagates along the myocyte compared with conduction across the cells [2]. The term *anisotropy* (from Greek, *anisos* meaning unequal and *tropos* meaning turn) is used to describe any property or phenomenon that varies in magnitude according to the direction of measurement. A series of studies performed by Weidmann and colleagues [3] in the 1950s and 1960s demonstrated that electrical anisotropy of cardiac cells was strongly influenced by the occurrence of ionic movements between cardiomyocytes through areas of low resistance located in the intercalated disks (Fig. 1). This preferential flow of electricity makes the longitudinal propagation of the electrical stimulus happen more efficiently than in the short axis of the fiber.

The intercalated disks are made up of three types of cell junctions. The desmosome and fascia adherens are areas of strong adhesion between cells and are responsible for transmission of mechanical energy during contraction. The gap

* Corresponding author. Division of Cardiovascular Diseases, Mayo Clinic, 13400 East Shea Boulevard, Scottsdale, AZ 85259.

E-mail address: sengupta.partho@mayo.edu (P.P. Sengupta).

1551-7136/08/$ - see front matter
doi:10.1016/j.hfc.2008.02.006

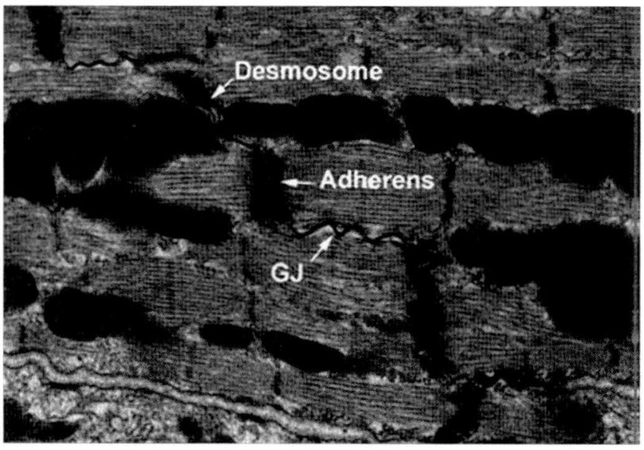

Fig. 1. Photomicrograph of intercalated disk. The line at the junction between two cells takes an irregular course, making nearly right angle step-like turns. Different parts of the intercalated disk include the transverse components (adherens) and the lateral components (GJ, gap junction). (*From* Saffitz JE. Adhesion molecules: why they are important to the electrophysiologist. J Cardiovasc Electrophysiol 2006;17:226; with permission.)

junctions are the third component of intercalated disks. These structures are transcellular channels, aggregated in the form of plaques. Gap junctions are composed of hemichannels between adjacent cells that allow the movement of ions and low molecules between the cytoplasm of the two cells involved [2]. It has been suggested that the integrity of the mechanical connections between adjacent myocytes has a strong influence on the degree to which these cells are coupled by gap junctions. Studies performed in cell culture have shown that the gap junctions are not formed until the cells are completely connected by definitive adhesion junctions and that cells with limited mechanical connections are unable to maintain normal gap junction communication [4].

The basic components of gap junctions are transmembrane protein connexins [2]. The principal connexins found in the human heart are Cx43, Cx40, and Cx45. Each gap junction is composed of two hemichannels (or connexons), which are each formed by six connexin proteins arranged in a cylindric pattern. Connexons are expressed on the surface of the cell in the intercalated disk (porous formation). During the process of cell coupling, the fusion of two hemichannels originating from each one of the cells forms low resistance channels that allow the transfer of ions between the cytoplasms of both cardiomyocytes. Mutations in genes coding connexins can result in functional and developmental abnormalities.

Factors influencing propagation of electrical impulse

The impulse propagation is influenced by active and passive properties of the myocardium, and it depends on the balance between the current generated as a result of depolarization (also called current source) and the current necessary to activate the adjacent resting portion of the tissue (known as current sink). Current source is determined by the balance between influx of sodium and calcium and efflux of potassium ions, generating a net depolarizing current. Current sink is influenced by several factors, such as the diameter and length of the cardiac myocyte and the size, number, location, and permeability of gap junctions [2,5]. Cells of the His bundle, for instance, are typically larger and longer than regular cardiomyocytes, and this feature contributes to the high propagation velocity typical of these specialized structures of the conduction system. They also have large gap junctions located mostly at the end of the fibers, with a few distributed on their sides. The His cells are aligned in series and surrounded by a large amount of collagen, which makes it easier for the stimulation to propagate in a linear fashion [6].

The arrangement of cells is also an important factor in the conductance of the stimulus. The ventricular myocardium is a laminar structure, with a characteristic three-dimensional organization. The myocytes are grouped by perimysial collagen into branching layers, which are four cells thick on average. These layers are interconnected by bridges that are one or two cells thick. Within this laminar organization, the axis of cardiac cells rotates from a right-handed helix in the endocardium to a left-handed helix in the epicardium, creating a 120° angle from the epicardium to the endocardium. In two dimensions, this complex structure can be represented by a lattice [7]. Recent studies [7–11] demonstrated how the impulse propagates in multiple branching tissues (cells crossing each other perpendicularly or the presence of bridges between layers of cardiomyocytes). Specifically, the studies showed that under physiologic conditions, the impulse propagation delays in front of each point of branching and demonstrated that the propagation safety (PS) is increased in this type of arrangement. PS is an index that correlates the charge flowing in from neighboring cells (denominator) and the charge generated by depolarization of a cell's own membrane (numerator). If the PS is greater than 1, it means that more charge is produced in the cell than is required to activate it; therefore, it incurs successful propagation. If the PS is less than 1, it means that the cell produced less charge than it received and the propagation fails [8]. This multi-branching structure can be found in distinct areas of the heart, such as the atrioventricular node, with nonlinear arrangement of cells, and the ventricular myocardium, with laminar organization of the fibers that cross or connect to each other through multiple branches or cross each other at varying angles. The tissue specialized in conduction (His-Purkinje) has a minimal amount of branching, with the cells aligned in parallel. This is one more feature of these specialized cells that enhances conduction velocity.

Sequence of ventricular activation

The patterns of wave spread observed in mouse and pig hearts are nearly identical to that in the human heart (Fig. 2) and facilitate synchronous contraction of both ventricles [12]. Durrer and colleagues [13] performed a classic study in the mid-1970s in which the sequence of electrical activation was studied in seven isolated normal human hearts from individuals who died from noncardiac causes. These investigators demonstrated that the excitatory waves initially reach the endocardial aspect of LV at three points simultaneously: (1) an area high on anterior paraseptal wall just below the mitral valve, (2) a central area in the left side of the interventricular septum, and (3) the posterior paraseptal area at approximately one third of the distance from the apex to the base. These areas quickly became confluent, and almost the entire endocardial layer of the LV was activated, with the exception of the posterobasal area, in approximately 30 milliseconds. The epicardial aspect of the LV is activated later

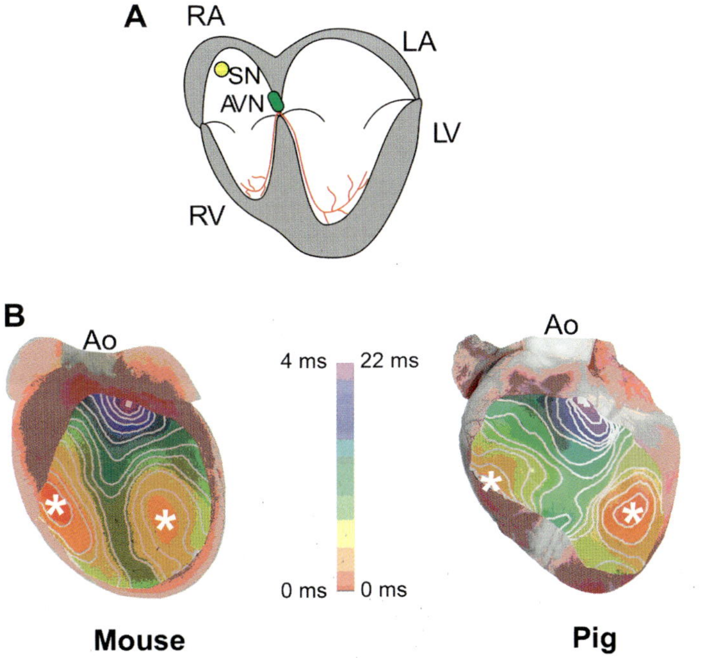

Fig. 2. Normal sequence of electrical activation in the mammalian heart. (*A*) During sinus rhythm, impulse originates from the sinoatrial node (SN, *yellow*) in the right atrium and propagates through the atrioventricular node (AVN, *green*) and the His-Purkinje system (*red*) in the LV and right ventricle (RV), respectively). (*B*) Epicardial electrical activation patterns of mouse and pig hearts are similar during normal sinus rhythm. The colored activation maps are superimposed on the digital pictures of the hearts, positioned in the same manner as in *A*. Two initial breakthroughs (*white asterisks*) appear on the LV and RV walls, after which the excitation spreads to the rest of the heart. The white lines are isochrones (0.3 milliseconds for the mouse and 1.5 milliseconds for the pig). The color scale indicates red as the earliest (0 milliseconds) and purple as the latest (4 milliseconds for the mouse and 22 milliseconds for the pig) times of activation. Ao, aorta; LA, left atrium, RA, right atrium. (*From* Noujaim SF, Berenfeld O, Kalifa J, et al. Universal scaling law of electrical turbulence in the mammalian heart. Proc Natl Acad Sci USA 2007;104:20986; with permission.)

(see Fig. 2; Fig. 3). Despite this delay, however, the activation of this outer layer starts before the propagation reaches the posterobasal area. The initial sites of activation match the distribution of the anterior and posterior divisions of the left bundle branch in the LV and the right bundle branch in the right ventricle. The delay in reaching the epicardial surface was explained by Durrer and colleagues [13] as a consequence of the slow intramural propagation of the excitation wave. The middle and epicardial layers do not have Purkinje cells, which are restricted to the inner third of the ventricular wall in humans; therefore, the conduction depends on cell-to-cell propagation, and it is influenced by anisotropy and by the angle formed between myocytes. These elements, as previously discussed, are marked by slow conduction.

The myocardial band hypothesis by Torrent-Guasp and colleagues [14,15] suggested that the electromechanical propagation followed the trajectory of the fibers, based on the principle of anisotropy. Accordingly, it was suggested that electrical activation of the muscular band starts in the right ventricle at the level of the pulmonary artery, travels across the posterobasal wall of the LV around the mitral annulus, and ends at the basal portion of the LV in the root of aorta. Although it is intuitive to expect the electrical conduction to flow preferentially from the right ventricle to the LV, following the orientation of the muscular band, this purported sequence of electromechanical activation has not been confirmed in vivo. The explanation for this discrepancy is the presence of the conduction system, which activates the myocardium through the right branch bundle and divisions of the left branch bundle. More recent studies have used electroanatomic mapping systems to confirm the sequence of LV electrical activation further. Gepstein and

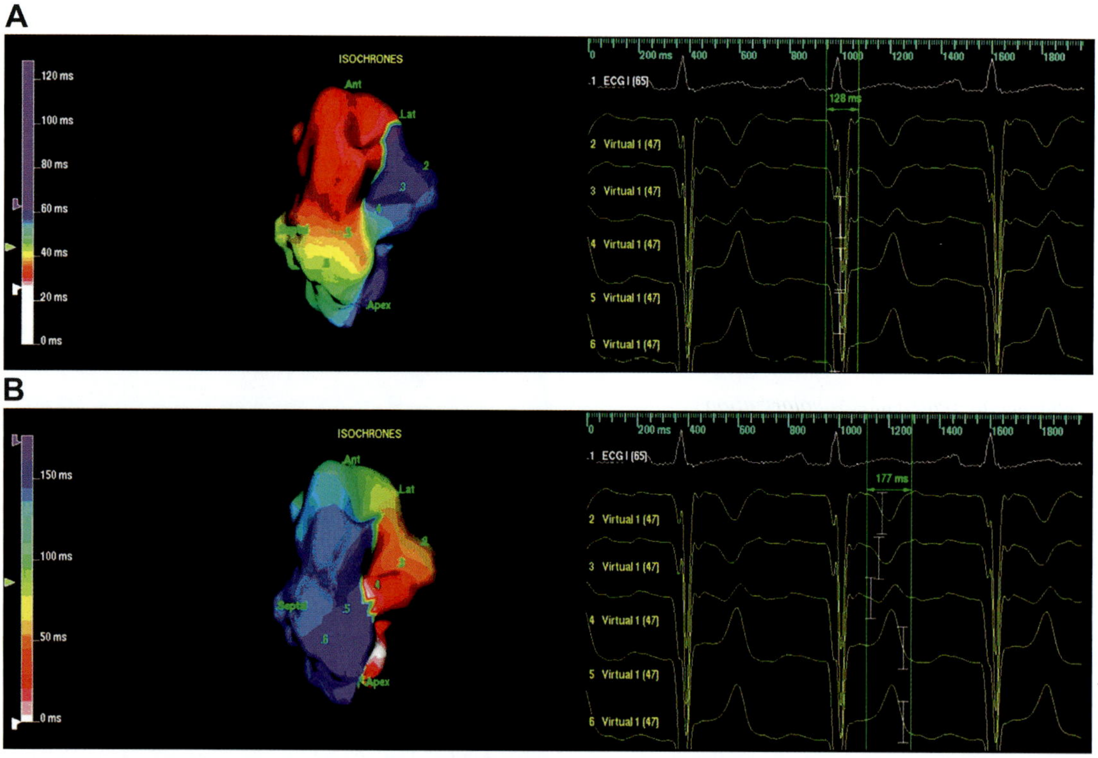

Fig. 3. Left ventricular endocardial activation sequence. Isochronal maps of the left ventricular endocardial activation sequence (left anterior oblique view) during sinus rhythm in a normal subject have been reconstructed from unipolar electrograms obtained by noncontact mapping (Ensite 3000 system; Endocardial Solutions, Inc., St. Paul, Minnesota). Activation map (*A*) and repolarization map (*B*) during T waves (positive T waves, *blue*; negative and biphasic T waves, *yellow to red*) are shown. Ant, anterior; Lat, lateral. (*From* Yue AM, Betts TR, Roberts PR, et al. Global dynamic coupling of activation and repolarization in the human ventricle. Circulation 2005;112:2596; with permission.)

colleagues [16,17] studied LV endocardial activation and repolarization patterns in 13 healthy pigs using intracardiac unipolar electrograms that were color coded and superimposed on a three-dimensional electroanatomic map of the ventricle generated with a real-time nonfluoroscopic magnetic navigation system. The earliest activation site was located in the anterosuperior septal region in all maps. Rapid conduction was noted from the earliest site of activation toward the apex. The activation then spread significantly more slowly to the rest of the endocardium, with the posterior basal wall and the atrioventricular ring being activated last. Ramanathan and colleagues [18] studied normal activation and repolarization in intact unanesthetized healthy adults under complete physiologic conditions using electrocardiographic imaging, a noninvasive cardiac electrical imaging modality that can image epicardial potentials, electrograms, and isochrones (activation sequences) using electrocardiographic measurements from many body surface locations, together with heart-torso geometry obtained from CT. The first breakthrough occurs in the right ventricular (RV) anterior-paraseptal region during early QRS and is termed *RV breakthrough*. In the LV, a broad maximum activation developed over the lateral-apical region, reflecting endocardial-to-epicardial propagation of the LV free-wall activation front, which gradually traveled toward the posterolateral base in an apex-to-base direction. The latest activation occurred in the posterior or posterolateral basal LV and the RV outflow tract.

Sequence of ventricular repolarization

Little is known about the sequence of repolarization in the human heart, because these studies are technically challenging and the results can be conflicting. Most of the information currently available is from extrapolation of animal data or studies performed in diseased human hearts. The duration of the action potential varies over different regions of the heart and between endocardial and epicardial layers, with a typically shorter duration in the latter [19]. The propagation of repolarization through the heart is still controversial. Several animal studies have suggested that the repolarization has an opposite direction-to-activation sequence. These studies were limited to epicardial mappings or to restricted areas of the heart, however. Yuan and colleagues [21] used an electroanatomic mapping system to study repolarization by constructing a three-dimensional map of human and swine hearts based on action potential duration, monophasic action potential, and end of repolarization. The authors demonstrated that the repolarization sequence followed the sequence of activation in most subjects. Taccardi and colleagues [20] confirmed these findings in a canine study. An inverse relation between local activation timing and duration of action potential was noticed; in other words, the earliest sites of activation had the longest action potential duration and the latest sites had the shortest action potential duration. This study was limited to endocardial mapping. Several other studies focused on differences in action potential duration throughout the ventricular wall. Unipolar electrograms obtained by noncontact mapping in humans showed the presence of positive T waves at the sites of earliest activation and negative T waves at the sites of latest activation [22]. Animal data have also pointed to the existence of a gradient of repolarization, with marked prolonged action potential duration in the midlayers of myocardial wall when compared with endocardial or epicardial layers [23]. These intermediate cells were called M cells [23], and their existence has been a source of controversy for many decades [24]. Ueda and colleagues [25] suggested that these cells are not a discrete group of cells with differentiated electrophysiology but that they would have what these investigators described as "M cell behavior." Studies in canine [26], swine [27], and human [28] hearts, however, reported no significant transmural gradient of electrical repolarization in the LV in vivo. Contrary to the midmyocardial location of the "M cell behavior," some studies reported that electrical repolarization in the subepicardium may occur later than in the subendocardium [27,29]. The picture is further complicated with claims that the genesis of T wave on surface electrocardiography may involve a base-to-apex gradient of repolarization [27,30]. Further studies are necessary to clarify the complexities involved in repolarization sequences of the LV observed in vivo.

Electromechanical coupling within isovolumic contraction period

After electrical activation, the time of onset of cardiac mechanical activity varies for different regions of the LV and also transmurally for a given region of the LV [27,31,32]. The heterogeneity in the timing of electromechanical coupling has recently been shown to exceed the differences in duration of the action potential of different layers of the myocardial wall (Figs. 4 and 5) [27,31,32]. The transmural propagation velocity of myofiber shortening measures 0.25 m/s and is slower than the electrical conduction velocity (0.49 m/s) [32]. Moreover, the electromechanical delay is longer in the epicardium than in the endocardium. This in vivo finding is contrary to derivations from finite element simulation [33] and in vitro studies [34]. This electromechanical delay may be partly explained by the process of myofiber prestretch. Recent experimental investigations in beating porcine hearts in situ from the authors' laboratory [35] and by others [32,36] have shown that the isovolumic contraction (IVC) phase is characterized by positive and negative waves, attributable to a physiologic asynchrony in which subendocardial shortening is accompanied by subepicardial stretching. Some stretching in the late activated regions of the subendocardium is also seen, particularly near the basal posterolateral region of the LV, which is the last area of the LV to activate. These reciprocal deformations reflect a movement that occurs

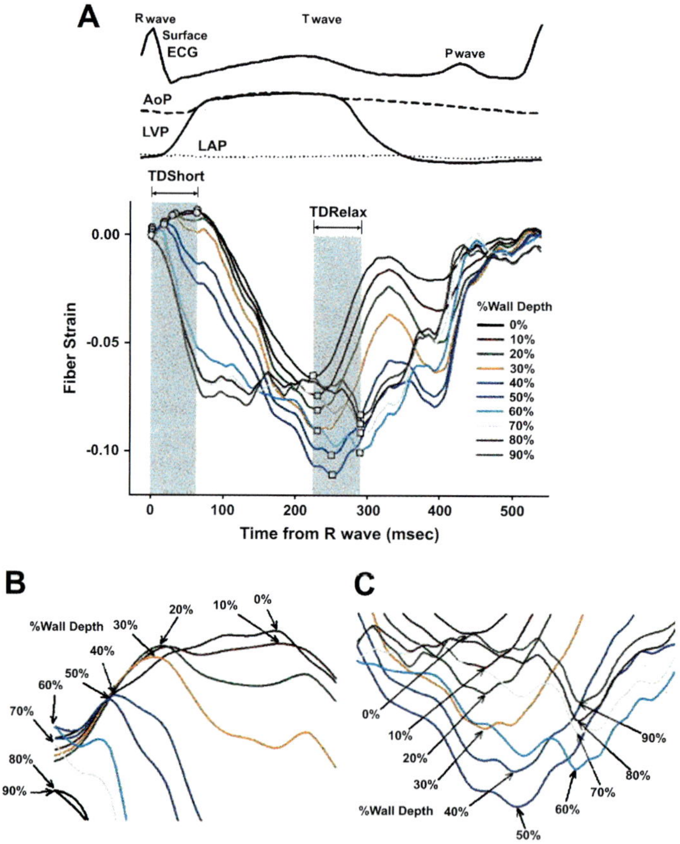

Fig. 4. Transmural heterogeneity of fiber strains. Transmural fiber strains are recorded from midanterior wall of the LV in canine hearts using transmural bead markers under biplane cineradiography. (*A*) Fiber strains during entire cardiac cycle. Different colors represent the percent wall depth from the epicardial surface. Open circles indicate onset of myofiber shortening, and open squares indicate onset of myofiber relaxation. Magnified view of transmural dispersion of myofiber shortening (TDShort) (*B*) and relaxation (TDRelax) (*C*). The onset of myofiber shortening occurs earliest at the endocardial layers and is accompanied by stretching of the epicardial layers, whereas the onset of myofiber relaxation is earliest at the epicardial layers and is accompanied by continued shortening of the subendocardial layers. There is no significant transmural gradient in electrical repolarization. AoP, central aortic pressure; ECG, electrocardiogram; LAP, left atrial pressure; LVP, left ventricular pressure. (*From* Ashikaga H, Coppola BA, Hopenfeld B, et al. Transmural dispersion of myofiber mechanics: implications for electrical heterogeneity in vivo. J Am Coll Cardiol 2007;49: 912; with permission.)

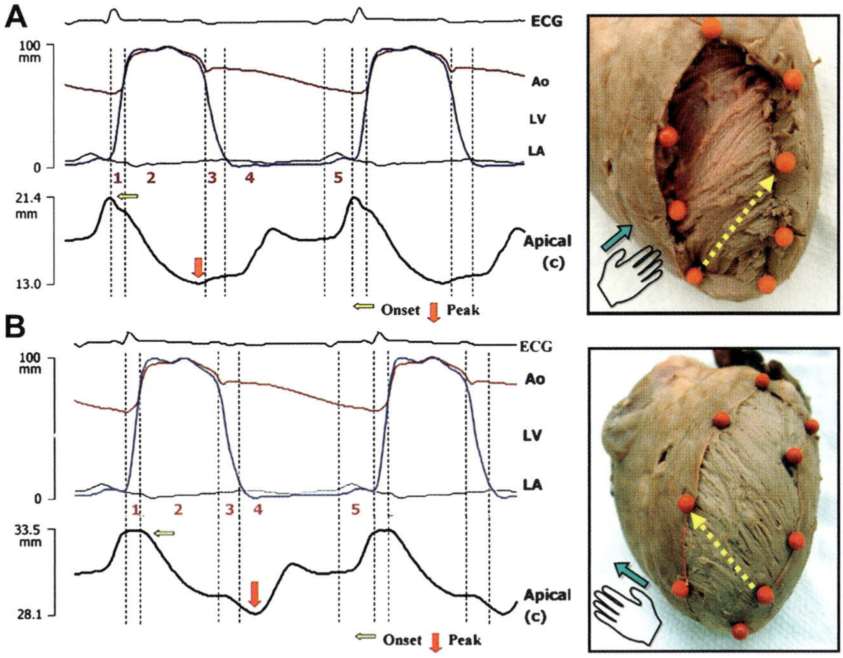

Fig. 5. Transmural sequence of deformation in anterior wall of LV near apex. Transmural strains are computed using sonomicrometry (*black tracing*). (*A*) During isovolumic contraction, shortening is initiated along the subendocardial (right-handed helical) fiber direction. (*B*) Onset of shortening in the subepicardial (left-handed helical) fiber direction is delayed and coincides with the onset of left ventricular ejection. Tissue specimens (*right*) show corresponding subendocardial and subepicardial fiber arrangements, position of sonomicrometry crystals (*orange markers*), and pairs of crystals used to determine deformation along fiber direction (*yellow arrows*). Ao, aorta (*red tracing*); ECG, electrocardiogram; LA, left atrium (*gray tracing*); LV, left ventricular (*blue tracing*); phase 1, pre-ejection; phase 2, ejection; phase 3, isovolumic relaxation; phase 4, early diastole; phase 5, late diastole. (*From* Sengupta PP, Krishnamoorthy VK, Korinek J, et al. Left ventricular form and function revisited: applied translational science to cardiovascular ultrasound imaging. J Am Soc Echocardiogr 2007;20:543; with permission.)

without a change in LV volume, (ie, shortening in one region is balanced by stretching in another region) [35]. The papillary muscles are also stretched early in systole, whereas other portions of the ventricle are contracting [37]. This has been attributed to the increasing intraventricular pressure in early systole that leads to the closing of the atrioventricular valves, increasing tension on the chordae, and, thereby, stretching of the papillary muscles [37]. Stretching of the activated myofibers during IVC has two advantages. First, it facilitates a wave of shortening to emerge in the endocardium that travels axially in an apex-to-base direction. Moreover, stretch of an activated myocyte may help to modulate the force and timing of contraction by the process of the "stretch activation response," an intrinsic length-sensing mechanism that allows muscle to adjust to the force of shortening with an autonomous regulation that reduces reliance on extrinsic regulatory systems [37–41].

The myocardial band hypothesis proposed that contraction of the posterior basal epicardial region of the LV (ie, the basal loop) would result in a rigid external cylinder [14]. The authors' observations indicate that the earliest shortening in the LV during IVC is initiated along the subendocardial myofibers in the anterior wall that are aligned in a right-handed helical direction, however [35]. The lateral and posterior basal segments of the LV that form the basal loop undergo longitudinal stretch. It has been further suggested that the basal loop would help shortening of the mitral annulus during the IVC period [14]. Nearly 90% of mitral annular shortening is directly contributed to by atrial contraction, however, and precedes the onset of systole [42]. Shortening of the mitral annulus is therefore not the result of LV myofiber contraction because the circumferential mitral annular shortening is not observed once the atrial contraction is eliminated [42].

Ejection phase

Myocardial deformation during ejection demonstrates extensive transmural tethering, such that subendocardial and subepicardial regions undergo simultaneous shortening along the fiber and cross-fiber directions during ejection (see Fig. 5) [32,35]. Subendocardial strains are higher in magnitude than subepicardial strains [27]. Within each layer, the magnitude of circumferential strains during ejection exceeds that of longitudinal strains [27]. With regard to the timing, longitudinal shortening strains for both regions show an apex-to-base gradient, such that successive shortenings are reached earlier at apex and midsegments compared with the LV base [35]. Kirn and Starc [43–45] recently mapped the contraction of the LV free wall with a high-speed digital video acquisition system and surface markers and found the presence of a continuous contraction wave traveling from the apex toward the base during LV ejection (Fig. 6). The time needed for this wave to cross the ventricle was approximately 23 milliseconds. Recent investigations using direct sonomicrometry [27], MRI tagging [46], or speckle-tracking echocardiography [47] also suggest that radial and longitudinal strains and strain rates are higher in the apex compared with the base (Fig. 7) [48].

Isovolumic relaxation and postsystolic shortening

Myofiber relaxation in vivo is primarily determined by the balance between the loading conditions and generated force within the myofiber during diastole; myofiber relaxation occurs when the afterload overcomes the generated force of the myofibers [32]. Despite the lack of a significant transmural gradient in electrical repolarization in vivo, there is a significant gradient in the onset of myofiber relaxation (see Figs. 4 and 5). Near the base, lengthening of the LV occurs along the left-handed helical subepicardial fiber direction and is accompanied by shortening and shear along the subendocardial fiber sheets (ie, right-handed fibers) [27,49]. Near the LV apex, shortening of the subepicardium (left-handed helix) continues beyond aortic valve closure and is accompanied by lengthening of the subendocardial layer (right-handed helix) near the apex (see Fig. 5) [27,50]. Delayed onset of relaxation is routinely encountered as a physiologic phenomenon in normal humans and has been referred to as postsystolic shortening [51]; experimental studies have confirmed endocardial shortening after aortic valve closure [27]. Zwanenburg and colleagues [52] timed cardiac contraction in healthy subjects with high temporal resolution MRI myocardial tagging and reported that several segments in the apical and basal segments contracted beyond aortic valve closure in diastole. The occurrence of postsystolic shortening in healthy subjects was also reported by Voigt and colleagues [51] and can be explained on the basis of the synergistic movements that occur during isovolumic relaxation (ie, lengthening of LV segment in one direction is accompanied by shortening in

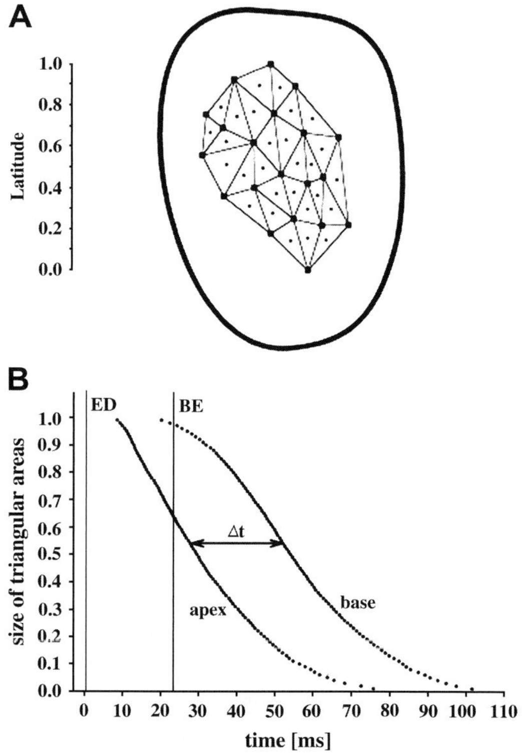

Fig. 6. Sequence of the contraction along the LV long axes. Axial sequence of LV contraction is assessed on the LV free wall of guinea pig hearts in situ using an ultrafast video system and epicardial markers by means of the latitude and the size of the areas defined by markers. The latitude of each triangular area is determined at end diastole and is normalized so that L = 0 corresponds to the position of a marker closest to the apex and L = 1 corresponds to the marker most distant from the apex. The curve for the apex precedes the curve for the base; hence, the apex achieves the same size before the regions at the base during the whole contraction. The time delay (Δt) is, on average, 23 ± 4 milliseconds. BE, beginning ejection; ED, end diastole. (*From* Kirn B, Starc V. Continuous axial contraction wave in the free wall of the guinea pig left ventricle. Comput Biol Med 2007;37:1394–7; with permission.)

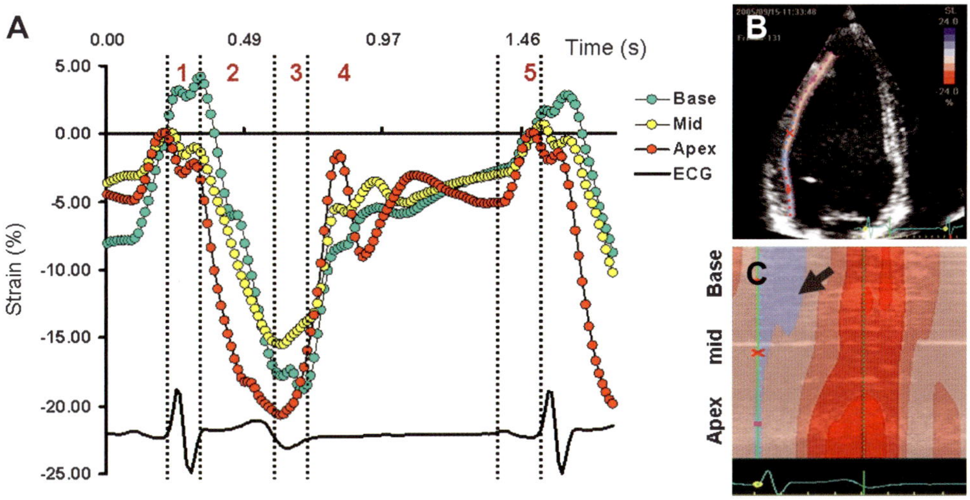

Fig. 7. Apex-to-base gradient of longitudinal deformation in the lateral wall of the LV. The sequence of longitudinal shortening has been obtained by two-dimensional speckle tracking of B-mode ultrasound images in a healthy woman. (*A*) Onset of longitudinal shortening occurs in an apical segment (*red*) of the LV and is delayed for the basal segment (*blue*) of the LV. During ejection, shortening strains at the apex are higher than those at the base. Shortening-lengthening crossover of the basal segment is delayed until the end of isovolumic relaxation. (*B*) Region of speckle tracking in the lateral wall of the LV. (*C*) Color M-mode profile of longitudinal strains obtained from basal, middle, and apical segments. Note delayed onset of longitudinal shortening in the basal segment (*arrow*). Blue indicates the presence of prestretching, whereas the apical and middle regions have already started shortening. ECG, electrocardiogram; phase 1, pre-ejection; phase 2, ejection; phase 3, isovolumic relaxation; phase 4, early diastole; phase 5, late diastole. (*From* Sengupta PP, Krishnamoorthy VK, Korinek J, et al. Left ventricular form and function revisited: applied translational science to cardiovascular ultrasound imaging. J Am Soc Echocardiogr 2007;20:546; with permission.)

the other direction). Thus, normal postsystolic contraction of the LV provides an apex-to-base and subendocardial-to-subepicardial gradient of deformation that may help in rapidly restoring the LV cavity in early diastole [27,50].

Sequence of left ventricular twist

The shortening of the right- and left-handed helical myofibers in the subendocardial and subepicardial regions of the LV is the structural basis of the wringing motion of the LV in systole, in which the apex moves counterclockwise and the base moves clockwise [1]. Rotation of the apex with respect to the base, counterclockwise in systole, is referred to as twist or torsion (twist normalized to length). Experimental and clinical explorations on LV twist have entailed the use of numerous techniques, such as implanted radioopaque markers [53], biplane cine angiography [54], sonomicrometry [55,56], optical devices [57], gyroscopic sensors [58], MRI [59–61], and echocardiography [62–64]. Recently introduced two-dimensional strain echocardiography allows rapid and accurate measurement of global and regional myocardial function, including velocity, strain and strain rate, and rotation [63]. Fig. 8 shows the time course of twist developed at the LV apex and base. During IVC, the LV apex undergoes a brief clockwise twist [57]. This correlates with the predominant mechanical activity that develops along the right-handed helical direction during IVC as a result of the shortening of the subendocardial region. During ejection, the direction of apical twist reverses, becoming counterclockwise and corresponding to the direction of the left-handed helical subepicardial myofibers. To provide a framework for interpreting LV twist during ejection, Taber and colleagues [65] proposed that an important factor influencing the twist mechanics is the moment arm of the fibers from the long axis of the LV (ie, the axis of twist). Thus, contraction of the epicardial fibers torques the apex in a counterclockwise direction and the base in a clockwise direction. Conversely, contraction of the subendocardial region torqued the LV apex and base in exactly opposite directions. Because of a larger moment arm, however, the outer epicardial layer has a mechanical advantage relative to the inner subendocardial layers.

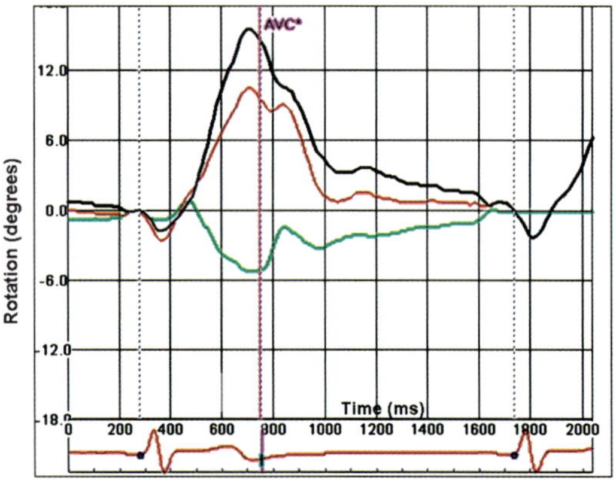

Fig. 8. Temporal sequences of LV twist during a cardiac cycle. LV rotation from apical (*red line*) and basal (*green line*) cross-sections of the LV has been obtained by speckle tracking of B-mode cardiac ultrasound images (GE Health Care, Milwaukee, Wisconsin) in a normal healthy subject. The difference between the two rotations provides an estimate of net LV twist angle (*black line*). During IVC (phase 1), the apex shows a brief clockwise rotation and the base shows a brief counterclockwise rotation. During ejection (phase 2), the direction of rotation changes to counterclockwise at the LV apex and clockwise at the LV base, respectively. Torsional recoil occurs predominantly during the phases of isovolumic relaxation (phase 3) and early diastolic filling (phase 4).

Consequently, the resulting LV twist during ejection causes rotation of the apex and base in counterclockwise and clockwise directions, respectively.

After aortic valve closure, the major extent of untwisting occurs during isovolumic relaxation. Beyar and colleagues [66] used radio-opaque markers and biplane cine angiography to follow the dynamic twist–radial shortening relation through the entire cardiac cycle and demonstrated for the first time the rapid untwisting that occurred during the early period of diastole. The fact that the major extent of the untwisting occurs before the end of isovolumic relaxation was subsequently confirmed in humans [67] and can be quantified by MRI tagging or echocardiography.

Twist of the LV base is opposite to that of the apex but is significantly lower in magnitude. During IVC, there is a brief twist in a counterclockwise direction, which is followed by clockwise twisting during ejection. The counterdirectional rotation of the LV apex with respect to the base leads to torsion of the LV, thus resulting in a wringing movement during ejection. The apex-to-base differences in the direction of twists have been explained on the basis of varying spiral myofiber architecture of the apical and basal regions and apex-to-base and transmural gradients in myosin phosphorylation [37].

In summary, the theory of electromechanical activation and LV deformation presented in this review is important for cardiac imaging techniques that intend to decipher the space-time continuum of cardiac mechanics. For example, left ventricular dysfunction, acute and chronic, irrespective of the etiology, shows specific patterns of involvement that are linked to alterations in architecture, activation sequence, and the process of electromechanical coupling. The advent of interventions like cardiac resynchronization, LV shape restoration surgery, and stem cell implantation, which intend to change the cardiac muscle scaffold and architecture, demands a careful multidisciplinary collaboration of physiologists, biomedical engineers, and clinicians. In addition, these lines of research are sufficiently complicated so as to require the cooperation of theorists and experimentalists for encouraging accurate modeling of cardiovascular function based on newer testable hypotheses concerning myocardial mechanics in health and disease.

References

[1] Buckberg GD, Weisfeldt ML, Ballester M, et al. Left ventricular form and function: scientific priorities and strategic planning for development of new views of disease. Circulation 2004;110:e333–6.

[2] Desplantez T, Dupont E, Severs NJ, et al. Gap junction channels and cardiac impulse propagation. J Membr Biol 2007;218:13–28.

[3] Weidmann S. The diffusion of radiopotassium across intercalated disks of mammalian cardiac muscle. J Physiol 1966;187:323–42.

[4] Saffitz JE. Adhesion molecules: why they are important to the electrophysiologist. J Cardiovasc Electrophysiol 2006;17:225–9.

[5] Wang Y, Rudy Y. Action potential propagation in inhomogeneous cardiac tissue: safety factor considerations and ionic mechanism. Am J Physiol Heart Circ Physiol 2000;278:H1019–29.

[6] Reckova M, Rosengarten C, deAlmeida A, et al. Hemodynamics is a key epigenetic factor in development of the cardiac conduction system. Circ Res 2003;93:77–85.

[7] Hooks DA, Trew ML, Caldwell BJ, et al. Laminar arrangement of ventricular myocytes influences electrical behavior of the heart. Circ Res 2007;101: e103–12.

[8] Shaw RM, Rudy Y. Ionic mechanisms of propagation in cardiac tissue. Roles of the sodium and L-type calcium currents during reduced excitability

and decreased gap junction coupling. Circ Res 1997; 81:727–41.
[9] Kucera JP, Kleber AG, Rohr S. Slow conduction in cardiac tissue, II: effects of branching tissue geometry. Circ Res 1998;83:795–805.
[10] Kucera JP, Rudy Y. Mechanistic insights into very slow conduction in branching cardiac tissue: a model study. Circ Res 2001;89:799–806.
[11] Rohr S. Role of gap junctions in the propagation of the cardiac action potential. Cardiovasc Res 2004; 62:309–22.
[12] Noujaim SF, Berenfeld O, Kalifa J, et al. Universal scaling law of electrical turbulence in the mammalian heart. Proc Natl Acad Sci U S A 2007;104: 20985–9.
[13] Durrer D, van Dam RT, Freud GE, et al. Total excitation of the isolated human heart. Circulation 1970;41:899–912.
[14] Torrent-Guasp F, Ballester M, Buckberg GD, et al. Spatial orientation of the ventricular muscle band: physiologic contribution and surgical implications. J Thorac Cardiovasc Surg 2001;122:389–92.
[15] Ballester-Rodes M, Flotats A, Torrent-Guasp F, et al. The sequence of regional ventricular motion. Eur J Cardiothorac Surg 2006;29(Suppl 1):S139–44.
[16] Gepstein L, Hayam G, Ben-Haim SA. Activation-repolarization coupling in the normal swine endocardium. Circulation 1997;96:4036–43.
[17] Gepstein L, Hayam G, Ben-Haim SA. A novel method for nonfluoroscopic catheter-based electroanatomical mapping of the heart. In vitro and in vivo accuracy results. Circulation 1997;95:1611–22.
[18] Ramanathan C, Jia P, Ghanem R, et al. Activation and repolarization of the normal human heart under complete physiological conditions. Proc Natl Acad Sci U S A 2006;103:6309–14.
[19] Conrath CE, Opthof T. Ventricular repolarization: an overview of (patho)physiology, sympathetic effects and genetic aspects. Prog Biophys Mol Biol 2006;92:269–307.
[20] Taccardi B, Punske BB, Sachse F, et al. Intramural activation and repolarization sequences in canine ventricles. Experimental and simulation studies. J Electrocardiol 2005;38:131–7.
[21] Yuan S, Kongstad O, Hertervig E, et al. Global repolarization sequence of the ventricular endocardium: monophasic action potential mapping in swine and humans. Pacing Clin Electrophysiol 2001;24(10):1479–88.
[22] Yue AM, Betts TR, Roberts PR, et al. Global dynamic coupling of activation and repolarization in the human ventricle. Circulation 2005;112:2592–601.
[23] Antzelevitch C. Cellular basis for the repolarization waves of the ECG. Ann N Y Acad Sci 2006;1080: 268–81.
[24] Anyukhovsky EP, Sosunov EA, Gainullin RZ, et al. The controversial M cell. J Cardiovasc Electrophysiol 1999;10:244–60.
[25] Ueda N, Zipes DP, Wu J. Functional and transmural modulation of M cell behavior in canine ventricular wall. Am J Physiol Heart Circ Physiol 2004;287: H2569–75.
[26] Janse MJ, Sosunov EA, Coronel R, et al. Repolarization gradients in the canine left ventricle before and after induction of short-term cardiac memory. Circulation 2005;112:1711–8.
[27] Sengupta PP, Khandheria BK, Korinek J, et al. Apex-to-base dispersion in regional timing of left ventricular shortening and lengthening. J Am Coll Cardiol 2006;47:163–72.
[28] Taggart P, Sutton P, Opthof T, et al. Electrotonic cancellation of transmural electrical gradients in the left ventricle in man. Prog Biophys Mol Biol 2003;82:243–54.
[29] Franz MR, Bargheer K, Rafflenbeul W, et al. Monophasic action potential mapping in human subjects with normal electrocardiograms: direct evidence for the genesis of the T wave. Circulation 1987;75: 379–86.
[30] Opthof T. In vivo dispersion in repolarization and arrhythmias in the human heart. Am J Physiol Heart Circ Physiol 2006;290:H77–8.
[31] Prinzen FW, Augustijn CH, Allessie MA, et al. The time sequence of electrical and mechanical activation during spontaneous beating and ectopic stimulation. Eur Heart J 1992;13:535–43.
[32] Ashikaga H, Coppola BA, Hopenfeld B, et al. Transmural dispersion of myofiber mechanics: implications for electrical heterogeneity in vivo. J Am Coll Cardiol 2007;49:909–16.
[33] Guccione JM, Costa KD, McCulloch AD. Finite element stress analysis of left ventricular mechanics in the beating dog heart. J Biomech 1995;28: 1167–77.
[34] Cordeiro JM, Greene L, Heilmann C, et al. Transmural heterogeneity of calcium activity and mechanical function in the canine left ventricle. Am J Physiol Heart Circ Physiol 2004;286:H1471–9.
[35] Sengupta PP, Khandheria BK, Korinek J, et al. Biphasic tissue Doppler waveforms during isovolumic phases are associated with asynchronous deformation of subendocardial and subepicardial layers. J Appl Physiol 2005;99:1104–11.
[36] Goetz WA, Lansac E, Lim HS, et al. Left ventricular endocardial longitudinal and transverse changes during isovolumic contraction and relaxation: a challenge. Am J Physiol Heart Circ Physiol 2005;289: H196–201.
[37] Davis JS, Hassanzadeh S, Winitsky S, et al. The overall pattern of cardiac contraction depends on a spatial gradient of myosin regulatory light chain phosphorylation. Cell 2001;107:631–41.
[38] Stelzer JE, Brickson SL, Locher MR, et al. Role of myosin heavy chain composition in the stretch activation response of rat myocardium. J Physiol 2007; 579:161–73.

[39] Stelzer JE, Patel JR, Walker JW, et al. Differential roles of cardiac myosin-binding protein C and cardiac troponin I in the myofibrillar force responses to protein kinase A phosphorylation. Circ Res 2007; 101:503–11.
[40] Stelzer JE, Dunning SB, Moss RL. Ablation of cardiac myosin-binding protein-C accelerates stretch activation in murine skinned myocardium. Circ Res 2006;98:1212–8.
[41] Stelzer JE, Larsson L, Fitzsimons DP, et al. Activation dependence of stretch activation in mouse skinned myocardium: implications for ventricular function. J Gen Physiol 2006;127:95–107.
[42] Glasson JR, Komeda M, Daughters GT, et al. Most ovine mitral annular three-dimensional size reduction occurs before ventricular systole and is abolished with ventricular pacing. Circulation 1997;96:II-115–22 [discussion: II-123].
[43] Kirn B, Starc V. Continuous axial contraction wave in the free wall of the guinea pig left ventricle. Comput Biol Med 2007;37:1394–7.
[44] Kirn B, Starc V. Contraction wave in axial direction in free wall of guinea pig left ventricle. Am J Physiol Heart Circ Physiol 2004;287:H755–9.
[45] Kirn B, Starc V. The video technique developed for measuring epicardial strains on guinea pig's left ventricle. J Biomech 2005;38:169–73.
[46] Bogaert J, Rademakers FE. Regional nonuniformity of normal adult human left ventricle. Am J Physiol Heart Circ Physiol 2001;280:H610–20.
[47] Korinek J, Wang J, Sengupta PP, et al. Two-dimensional strain—a Doppler-independent ultrasound method for quantitation of regional deformation: validation in vitro and in vivo. J Am Soc Echocardiogr 2005;18:1247–53.
[48] Sukmawan R, Watanabe N, Toyota E, et al. Application of novel echocardiographic two-dimensional tracking system to define regional heterogeneity of radial and longitudinal myocardial strain and strain-rate. Circulation 2005;112:2561.
[49] Ashikaga H, Criscione JC, Omens JH, et al. Transmural left ventricular mechanics underlying torsional recoil during relaxation. Am J Physiol Heart Circ Physiol 2004;286:H640–7.
[50] Buckberg GD, Castella M, Gharib M, et al. Active myocyte shortening during the 'isovolumetric relaxation' phase of diastole is responsible for ventricular suction; 'systolic ventricular filling.' Eur J Cardiothorac Surg 2006;29(Suppl 1):S98–106.
[51] Voigt JU, Lindenmeier G, Exner B, et al. Incidence and characteristics of segmental postsystolic longitudinal shortening in normal, acutely ischemic, and scarred myocardium. J Am Soc Echocardiogr 2003;16:415–23.
[52] Zwanenburg JJ, Gotte MJ, Kuijer JP, et al. Timing of cardiac contraction in humans mapped by high-temporal-resolution MRI tagging: early onset and late peak of shortening in lateral wall. Am J Physiol Heart Circ Physiol 2004;286:H1872–80.
[53] Arts T, Hunter WC, Douglas AS, et al. Macroscopic three-dimensional motion patterns of the left ventricle. Adv Exp Med Biol 1993;346:383–92.
[54] Hansen DE, Daughters GT 2nd, Alderman EL, et al. Torsional deformation of the left ventricular midwall in human hearts with intramyocardial markers: regional heterogeneity and sensitivity to the inotropic effects of abrupt rate changes. Circ Res 1988;62:941–52.
[55] Bell SP, Nyland L, Tischler MD, et al. Alterations in the determinants of diastolic suction during pacing tachycardia. Circ Res 2000;87:235–40.
[56] Gorman JH 3rd, Gupta KB, Streicher JT, et al. Dynamic three-dimensional imaging of the mitral valve and left ventricle by rapid sonomicrometry array localization. J Thorac Cardiovasc Surg 1996;112:712–26.
[57] Gibbons Kroeker CA, Ter Keurs HE, Knudtson ML, et al. An optical device to measure the dynamics of apex rotation of the left ventricle. Am J Physiol 1993;265:H1444–9.
[58] Marcelli E, Plicchi G, Cercenelli L, et al. First experimental evaluation of cardiac apex rotation with an epicardial coriolis force sensor. ASAIO J 2005;51: 696–701.
[59] Buchalter MB, Weiss JL, Rogers WJ, et al. Noninvasive quantification of left ventricular rotational deformation in normal humans using magnetic resonance imaging myocardial tagging. Circulation 1990;81:1236–44.
[60] Buchalter MB, Rademakers FE, Weiss JL, et al. Rotational deformation of the canine left ventricle measured by magnetic resonance tagging: effects of catecholamines, ischaemia, and pacing. Cardiovasc Res 1994;28:629–35.
[61] Henson RE, Song SK, Pastorek JS, et al. Left ventricular torsion is equal in mice and humans. Am J Physiol Heart Circ Physiol 2000;278:H1117–23.
[62] Kim HK, Sohn DW, Lee SE, et al. Assessment of left ventricular rotation and torsion with two-dimensional speckle tracking echocardiography. J Am Soc Echocardiogr 2007;20:45–53.
[63] Notomi Y, Lysyansky P, Setser RM, et al. Measurement of ventricular torsion by two-dimensional ultrasound speckle tracking imaging. J Am Coll Cardiol 2005;45:2034–41.
[64] Helle-Valle T, Crosby J, Edvardsen T, et al. New noninvasive method for assessment of left ventricular rotation: speckle tracking echocardiography. Circulation 2005;112:3149–56.
[65] Taber LA, Yang M, Podszus WW. Mechanics of ventricular torsion. J Biomech 1996;29:745–52.
[66] Beyar R, Yin FC, Hausknecht M, et al. Dependence of left ventricular twist-radial shortening relations on cardiac cycle phase. Am J Physiol 1989;257: H1119–26.
[67] Knudtson ML, Galbraith PD, Hildebrand KL, et al. Dynamics of left ventricular apex rotation during angioplasty: a sensitive index of ischemic dysfunction. Circulation 1997;96:801–8.

ELSEVIER
SAUNDERS

Heart Failure Clin 4 (2008) 315–324

HEART
FAILURE
CLINICS

Twist and Untwist Mechanics of the Left Ventricle

Partho P. Sengupta, MBBS, MD, DM[a,*],
Bijoy K. Khandheria, MBBS[a],
Jagat Narula, MD, PhD[b]

[a]*Mayo Clinic, Scottsdale, AZ, USA*
[b]*University of California, Irvine, CA, USA*

The twisting motion of the left ventricle about its long axis results from the contraction of the obliquely oriented epicardial and endocardial fibers. Cardiothoracic surgeons intuitively check this twisting movement as a sign of healthy left ventricular (LV) function. Lower [1] studied LV torsion in the late seventeenth century. He described the twisting motion of the left ventricle as "the wringing of a linen cloth to squeeze out the water." Over the past 3 centuries, experimental and clinical explorations on LV twist have entailed the use of numerous techniques such as implanted radiopaque markers [2], biplane cineangiography [3], sonomicrometry [4,5], optical devices [6], gyroscopic sensors [7], MRI [8–10], and echocardiography [11–14]. Furthermore, the rapid pace of technologic advancements has resulted in the development of innovative techniques in which LV twist is readily computed from grayscale cardiac ultrasound images obtained at the bedside.

Significance of left ventricular torsion

Torsion helps bring a uniform distribution of LV fiber stress and fiber shortening across the wall [15]. It has been demonstrated in a mathematic model that normal torsion causes sarcomere shortening of 0.20 μm in the epicardium and 0.48 μm in the endocardium [16]. Elimination of the torsion, however, decreases epicardial shortening (0.10 μm) and increases endocardial shortening (0.55 μm). Thus, disappearance of torsion would increase endocardial stress and strain and increase oxygen demand, thereby reducing the efficiency of LV systolic function. In the subepicardium, torsion aids contraction in the principal fiber direction [17]. In the midwall, LV torsion enhances shortening in the circumferential direction [17]. In the subendocardium, torsion causes fiber rearrangement such that subendocardial fibers are sheared toward the left ventricle cavity for LV wall thickening while the left ventricle base is pulled toward the apex, shortening the longitudinal axis of the left ventricle. Torsion also provides a key association between systole and diastole. Twisting and shearing of the subendocardial fibers deforms the matrix and results in storage of potential energy during systole, then abruptly releases with sudden untwisting during isovolumic relaxation, generating intraventricular pressure gradients for LV diastolic filling [4].

Definitions for characterizing left ventricular twist deformation

The term *rotation* refers to the rotation of a short-axis section of the left ventricle as viewed from the apical end and is defined as the angle between radial lines connecting the center of mass of that specific cross-sectional plain to a specific point in the myocardial wall at end diastole and at any other time during systole [10]. Rotation is measured in degrees or radians. In solid mechanics, torsion is defined as the twisting of an object

* Corresponding author. Division of Cardiovascular Diseases, Mayo Clinic, 13400 East Shea Boulevard Scottsdale, AZ 85259.
E-mail address: sengupta.partho@mayo.edu (P.P. Sengupta).

1551-7136/08/$ - see front matter
doi:10.1016/j.hfc.2008.03.001

due to an applied torque. In circular sections, the resultant shearing stress is perpendicular to the radius. Therefore, the terms *twist* and *torsion* refer to the same mechanical phenomenon. LV twist or torsion represents the base-to-apex gradient in the rotation angle along the longitudinal axis of the left ventricle, expressed in degrees per centimeter or radians per meter [18]. The absolute apex-to-base difference in LV rotation (also in degrees or radians) is stated as the net LV twist angle or net LV torsion angle (Fig. 1) [18]. Some investigators have also expressed torsion as the axial gradient in the rotation angle multiplied by the average of the outer radii in apical and basal cross-sectional planes, thereby representing the shear deformation angle on the epicardial surface (in degrees or radians) [19].

Link between myofiber geometry and twist mechanics

Cardiac myocytes are arranged in axial tracts that branch and interconnect to form a three-dimensional network. These fibers resemble vortices that emanate from the left ventricle apex and spiral upward to the left ventricle base in counter-directional helices (Fig. 2). In a right-handed helix, if the thumb of an open hand points to the longitudinal axis of the ascent, the fingers orient along the ascending strand of the helix, and vice versa for the left-handed helix. The subendocardial fibers ascend in the form of a right-handed helix, whereas the subepicardial fibers spiral in the form of a left-handed helix. From the endocardium to the epicardium, the helix angle, therefore, changes continuously, typically ranging from +85° at the subendocardium to −85° at the subepicardium [20–23]. In the midwall, the fibers are perpendicular to the long axis, forming a sort of "equator of the heart."

To provide a framework for interpreting LV twist, Taber and colleagues [24] proposed a model of helical layer architecture on a one-layer cylinder composed of obliquely aligned muscle fibers embedded in an isotropic matrix. The contraction of the epicardial fibers rotates the apex in a counterclockwise direction and the base in a clockwise direction. The contraction of the subendocardial region, however, rotates the left ventricle apex and base in exactly the opposite directions.

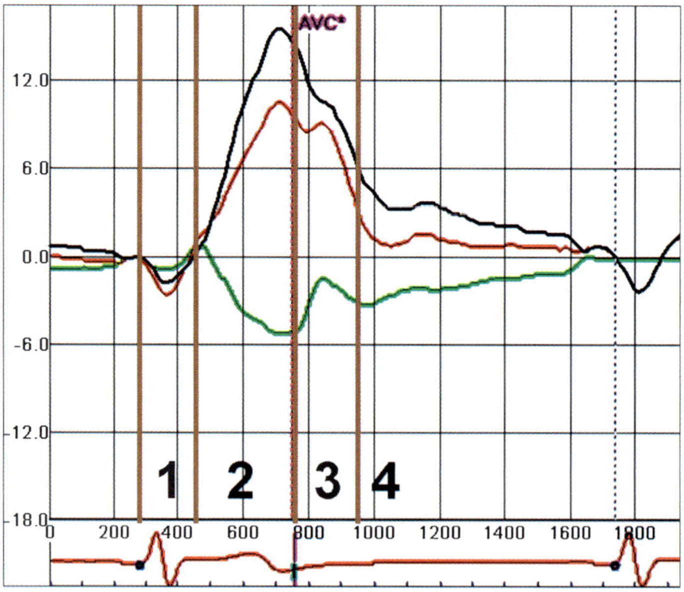

Fig. 1. Temporal sequences of LV twist during a cardiac cycle. LV rotation from apical (*red line*) and basal (*green line*) cross sections of the left ventricle were obtained by speckle tracking of B-mode cardiac ultrasound images (GE Health Care, Milwaukee, Wisconsin) in a normal healthy subject. The difference between the two rotations provides an estimate of net LV twist angle (*black line*). During isovolumic contraction (phase 1), the apex shows a brief clockwise rotation and the base shows a brief counterclockwise rotation. During ejection (phase 2), the direction of rotation changes to counterclockwise at the left ventricle apex and clockwise at the left ventricle base. Torsional recoil occurs predominantly during isovolumic relaxation (phase 3) and early diastolic filling (phase 4). AVC*, aortic valve closure.

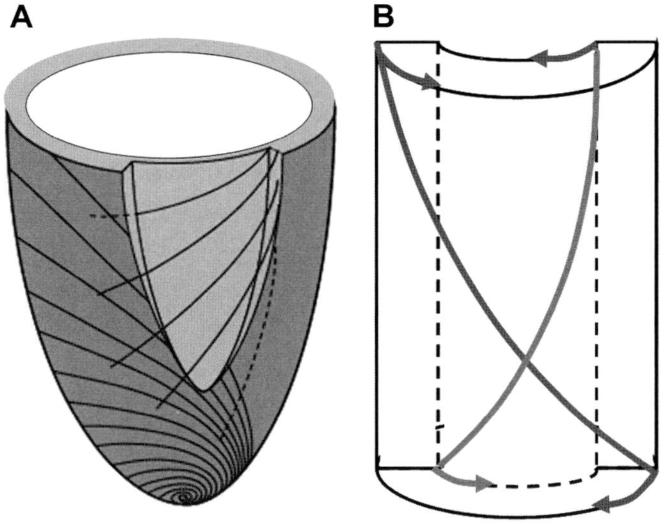

Fig. 2. Myofiber architecture of the left ventricle and a model for understanding LV twist dynamics. (*A*) Myofiber orientation in the left ventricle changes smoothly from a left-handed helix in the subepicardium to a right-handed helix in the subendocardium. (*B*) Myofiber model proposed by Ingels and colleagues [17] shows the subendocardial fiber wrapped in a right-handed helix and a subepicardial fiber wrapped in a left-handed helix. Arrows depict the circumferential components of force that result from force development in each fiber. The subepicardial fibers have a larger arm of moment than the subendocardial fibers.

When both layers contract simultaneously, a larger radius of rotation for the outer epicardial layer results in epicardial fibers having a mechanical advantage in dominating the overall direction of rotation [24].

Sequence of left ventricular twist

Figs. 2–4 link the spatial and temporal sequence of LV twist with mechanical events during different phases of the cardiac cycle.

Pre-ejection phase

During pre-ejection, the left ventricle apex shows brief clockwise rotation [17,25]. This brief clockwise rotation is related to a brief asynchrony in myocardial deformation. In a normally conducting heart, the subendocardium at the apex is the first to be electrically stimulated [23]. Cardiac muscle shortening is initiated in the subendocardial fiber direction [23]. Because the left ventricle volume does not change, there is a counterbalancing stretch in the direction of the subepicardial fibers that are aligned in the direction of the left ventricle outflow tract. It has been speculated that this stretch primes the heart for an optimal force development during ejection, a phenomenon that has been referred to as stretch activation [26]. The ideal isovolumic contraction phase is one in which the blood that has been received during diastole, even as it is being received, is redirected toward the outflow track without loss of much energy. This rheologic sequence has been demonstrated to occur through the formation of a vortex across the anterior mitral leaflet [27]. The transient clockwise rotation of the apex thus represents stretch and recoil that results from the momentum of the redirected blood stream toward the left ventricle outflow.

The description of LV apical rotation during the phase of isovolumic contraction has varied depending on the technique used. Studies that have measured LV apical rotation using cineangiographic markers [17], sonomicrometry [11,14], rotational devices [6,14], and echocardiography [11,14] have recorded an initial clockwise motion of the left ventricle apex and a counterclockwise motion of the left ventricle base during isovolumic contraction, whereas studies with magnetic resonance tagging have reported that the left ventricle base and apex rotate in a counterclockwise direction during isovolumic contraction [10,28]. The reason for this discrepancy remains unclear, although some investigators have attributed this observation to the lower temporal resolution of magnetic resonance tagging [11,14].

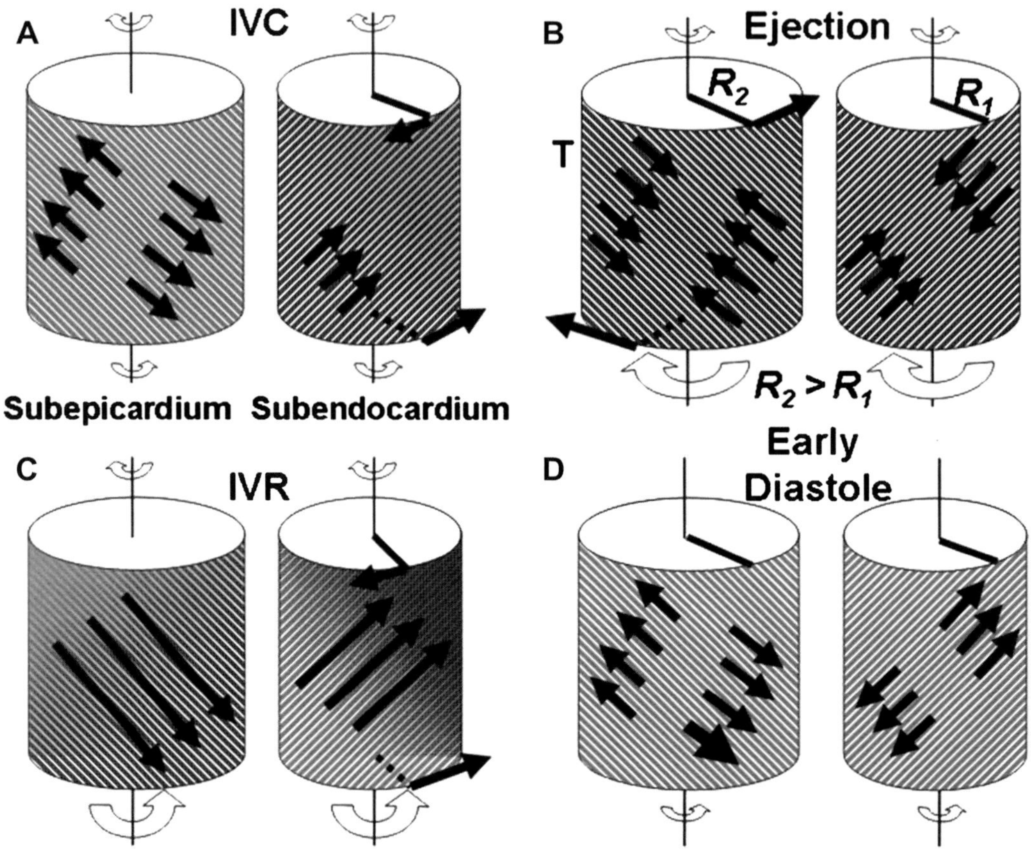

Fig. 3. Sequence of twist mechanics explained in a cylindric myofiber model. Electric and mechanical activation are initiated in the apical subendocardial region. (*A*) During isovolumic contraction (IVC), the subendocardial myofibers (right-handed helix) shorten with stretching of the subepicardial myofibers (left-handed helix), producing a brief clockwise rotation of the left ventricle apex and counterclockwise rotation of the left ventricle base. (*B*) During ejection, the subendocardial and subepicardial layers shorten simultaneously, with shortening strains near the apex exceeding those of the base. The larger arm of moment of the subepicardial fibers dominates the direction of twist, causing rotation of the apex and the base to be in a counterclockwise and clockwise direction, respectively. (*C*) During isovolumic relaxation (IVR), the subepicardium lengthens from the base toward the apex, and the subendocardium from the apex toward the base. (*D*) The subsequent period of diastole is characterized by relaxation in both layers, with minimum untwisting. R_1, radius of subendocardium; R_2, radius of subepidcardium.

Ejection phase

The transmural spread of electrical activation results in sequential subendocardial-to-subepicardial fiber shortening [23,29]. The myocardium shortens along the entire transmural course, resulting in longitudinal and circumferential shortening of the left ventricle. The onset of ejection coincides with the contraction of the subepicardial fibers [30]. During ejection, even though the subendocardial forces exceed subepicardial forces, the larger radius of subepicardial region produces higher torque to dominate the direction of rotation. The large subepicardial torque is coupled transmurally to the midwall and subendocardium and results in global counterclockwise LV rotation near the apex and clockwise rotation near the left ventricle base during ejection.

Isovolumic relaxation and diastolic filling

The torsional recoil during isovolumic relaxation and early diastole releases the potential energy stored in the deformed matrix of the subendocardium [4,31,32]. This process is facilitated by the presence of two mechanical gradients: axial and transmural. The apical subendocardium is the first to relax. While the subendocardium is relaxing, the subepicardium persists in its contraction [30]. This ongoing shortening has been

<table>
<tr><th>Phase</th><th>Subendocardium</th><th>Subepicardium</th><th>Apical Rotation</th><th></th><th>LV Cavitary Flow</th></tr>
<tr><td>Baseline</td><td>Relaxed</td><td>Relaxed</td><td>None</td><td>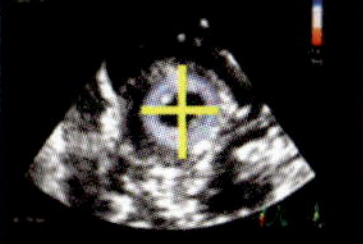</td><td>Concluding flow from atrial contraction</td></tr>
<tr><td>Isovolumic Contraction</td><td>Rapid apex to base electro-mechanical activation and initiation of shortening</td><td>Reciprocal stretching</td><td>Minimal clockwise twist (along subendocardial fiber direction)</td><td>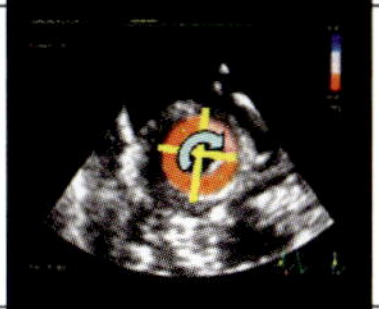</td><td>Apex-to-base flow redirection without change in volume, flow acceleration accentuates vortex</td></tr>
<tr><td rowspan="2">Ejection</td><td>Apex-to-base contraction continues</td><td>Shortening starts and continues during ejection</td><td rowspan="2">Counter-clockwise twist (along subepicardial fiber direction)</td><td rowspan="2">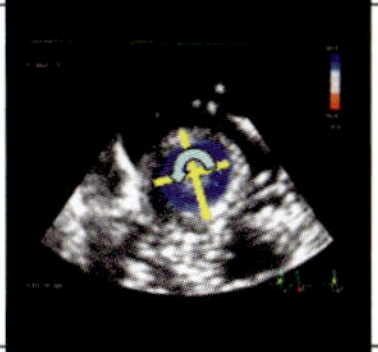</td><td rowspan="2">Continued flow acceleration into aorta, flow from LV base redirected towards outflow</td></tr>
<tr><td colspan="2">Higher shortening strains at apex compared to base; descent of LV base</td></tr>
<tr><td rowspan="2">Isovolumic and early Relaxation</td><td>Relaxation starts at apex and extends to base</td><td>Relaxation starts at base and extends to apex, apex still contracting</td><td rowspan="2">Clockwise untwisting (recoil and release of strain energy stored in deformed matrix)</td><td rowspan="2">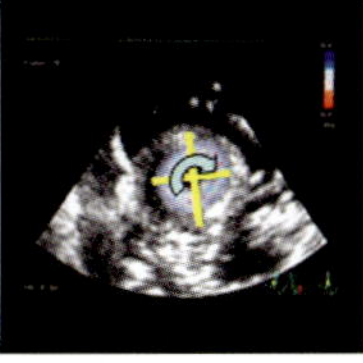</td><td rowspan="2">Base-to-apex flow reversal, LV volume remains unchanged till the onset of early diastole</td></tr>
<tr><td colspan="2">Subendocardial apex enlarges to initiate suction, subepicardial base relaxes to allow recoil. LV base ascends</td></tr>
</table>

Fig. 4. LV transmural mechanics, rotation, and intracavitary flow sequences during various phases of the cardiac cycle. (*Modified from* Narula J, Vannan MA, DeMaria AN. Of that waltz in my heart. J Am Coll Cardiol 2007;49:918.)

defined as postsystolic shortening of the myocardium. In the context of the opposing helices, it is easy to imagine that a relaxing subendocardium (right-handed helix) is facilitated by the contracting subepicardium (left-handed helix) to untwist and create a suction gradient toward the apex for efficient filling. The presence of simultaneous shortening and lengthening vectors of deformation within the left ventricle wall allows diastolic restoration to be initiated without changes in the left ventricle volume.

In contrast to the left ventricle apex, rotation of the left ventricle base is significantly lower in magnitude and opposite in direction. During isovolumic contraction, there is a brief counterclockwise rotation that is followed by clockwise rotation during ejection and counterclockwise rotation during isovolumic relaxation and early diastolic filling.

Variables affecting left ventricular twist

Age

LV twist increases gradually from infancy to adulthood [33]. This progressive change has been attributed to the maturation of the helical myofiber architecture of the left ventricle wall [33]. Subsequently, with increasing age in adult life, subendocardial function may gradually attenuate and LV twist increases further due to unopposed increase in LV apical rotation [34,35]. Age-related degenerative changes reduce the elastic resilience of the myocardial wall and, therefore, the velocity of untwisting in early diastole progressively reduces [35].

Load

LV preload and afterload alter the extent of twist [36–38]. Twist is greater with higher preload. For example, higher end-diastolic volumes of the left ventricle, with end-systolic volume held constant, produces higher LV twist. Similarly, afterload affects twist; that is, twist decreases at higher end-systolic volumes when end-diastolic volumes are held constant. The effect of preload on twist is about two thirds as great as that of afterload.

Contractility

Increasing contractility increases LV twist. For example, positive inotropic interventions such as dobutamine infusion and paired pacing greatly increase LV twist [9,37,39,40], whereas negative inotropic interventions markedly reduce twist [9]. In the intact circulation, changes in contractility are often accompanied by changes in loading conditions for increasing the twist mechanics of the left ventricle. For example, LV systolic twist and untwisting can almost double with short-term exercise due to augmented rotation of apical and basal levels [41], storing additional potential energy that is released for improving diastolic suction [42,43]. Long-term exercise training may, however, reduce the LV twist at rest. Soccer players demonstrate lower LV twist values and untwisting velocities than nontrained individuals [44]. It has been postulated that reduced LV twist in soccer players may represent increased torsional reserves that are used in increased-demand situations such as high-intensity sports. Indeed, a higher resting LV twist value, as seen with advancing age, is associated with attenuation of torsional reserves at peak exercise [45].

Imaging techniques for measuring left ventricular rotation

MRI

For several years, MRI examination was considered the reference standard for noninvasive assessment of cardiac biomechanics. The two most common MRI methods to measure myocardial motion are tagging and phase contrast velocity mapping [46]. Border and tag detection can be performed manually or semiautomatically; however, semiautomatic techniques generally require some extent of manual correction, and both techniques are usually time-consuming. Tissue phase mapping, however, directly encodes the velocity of myocardial motion into the magnetic resonance signal and offers high spatial resolution of the functional information (1–3 mm) [28]. Because both methods in MRI are based on multiple breath-held two-dimensional measurements, the temporal resolution is limited by the length of the breath-hold period to 30 to 80 milliseconds. This limitation has been addressed by the development of a respiratory-gated free-breathing method for tissue phase mapping that allows measurement with a temporal resolution comparable to tissue Doppler imaging.

Echocardiography

Echocardiography has wide availability and is therefore a more feasible technique for bedside assessment of LV twist, including use in patients who have a pacemaker, an internal cardioverter-defibrillator, or both. Applications for measuring twist using echocardiography were initially applied semiqualitatively by studying the rotational motion of papillary muscles [47]. Subsequently, there were attempts to decipher the rotational mechanics using tissue Doppler imaging [13]; however, the angle dependency of Doppler has remained a major limitation. Another echocardiographic method for motion estimation that has gained recent acceptance is based on two-dimensional tracking of unique speckle patterns created by the constructive and destructive interference of ultrasound beams within tissue [11,12,14]. These speckles are cross-correlated and tracked on a frame-by-frame basis. Because the tracking is fundamentally based on gray-scale B-mode images, it is independent of cardiac translation and angle dependency. The accuracy of speckle-tracking imaging has been validated against sonomicrometry and tagged MRI [12,14]; however, the quality of tracking depends on the image quality and is vulnerable to dropouts of ultrasound data and reverberations. Moreover, clinical studies with speckle-tracking echocardiography have reported wide variability in the values for resting LV systolic torsion [48]. This variability may be related to the incongruent locations of the left ventricle apical and basal cross-sectional planes, errors related to through-plane motion, and variable transmural depth of the region of interest for measuring LV rotation in each cross-sectional view. Methods for improving reproducibility of measurements should be addressed in future investigations.

Clinical applications

Diastolic dysfunction

Assessment of twist and peak untwisting rates were previously proposed to accurately reflect LV relaxation [49]. Two recent studies, however, have shown that LV twist may remain preserved in patients who have diastolic dysfunction in the presence of normal ejection fraction [50,51]. The onset of LV untwisting and the magnitude of peak untwisting velocities, however, showed variability in the two studies, remaining normal [50] or becoming reduced and significantly delayed [51]. More studies are required for understanding the variability of this observation.

Coronary artery disease

LV apical rotation and torsion may be variably affected in patients who have coronary artery disease, depending on the transmural extent of myocardial ischemia. Observations from experimental studies have previously reported greater than normal apical rotation with subendocardial ischemia and less than normal apical rotation with transmural ischemia [9,52]. Thus, patients who have subendocardial ischemia have normal LV torsion due to relative sparing of subepicardial function that determines LV torsion. For example, in a study of patients undergoing angioplasty, Knudtson and colleagues [53] demonstrated reduction in apical LV rotation with transient ischemia resulting from balloon occlusion of the left anterior descending coronary artery. Alternately, alteration of LV torsion was not reported in patients who had subendocardial ischemia provoked by dobutamine infusion [54].

LV twist is severely depressed in patients who have LV anterior wall infarction with reduced LV ejection fraction [55]. In contrast, systolic twist is maintained in patients who have anterior wall myocardial infarction with relatively preserved LV systolic function [55,56]. LV systolic torsion was directly related to the extent of infarction. Patients who had multiregional involvement had significantly less LV systolic torsion compared with those who had infarcts confined to a single vascular territory [54].

Valvular heart diseases

In aortic valve stenosis, coronary flow diminishes in the subendocardial region relative to the subepicardial region. LV twist is therefore significantly increased, although diastolic apical untwisting is prolonged compared with normal subjects [57–59]. The delay in apical untwisting is associated with diastolic dysfunction and elevated LV end-diastolic filling pressures [57,58]. After aortic valve replacement, LV twist normalizes. The level of recovery, however, depends on underlying coronary artery disease [60].

Changes in LV twist have also been studied in patients who have mitral regurgitation [61–63]. It has been suggested that chronic mitral regurgitation reduces systolic LV twist due to a decreased "leverage" of the epicardial fibers relative to the endocardial muscle fibers. Although increased preload tends to increase systolic twist [36], chronic mitral regurgitation is associated with complex LV adaptive remodeling and eccentric hypertrophy. The effect of chronic mitral regurgitation on twist likely depends on the extent of subclinical LV systolic dysfunction. Peak untwisting velocity in mitral regurgitation remains normal but correlates negatively with end-systolic dimension and regurgitant volume, suggesting that peak untwisting velocity, like peak systolic twist, depends on the stage of the disease [64].

Congenital heart diseases

Bedside assessment of LV strain and twist deformation may provide important insights into mechanical adaptive responses of the right and left ventricles in congenital heart diseases. For example, in the normal heart, the right and left ventricles are coupled for twisting in the same direction [65]; however, in patients who have transposition of the great arteries, the morphologic right ventricle supports the systemic circulation. It has been recently shown that the systemic right ventricular contraction in these patients resembles that of the normal left ventricle, without the ventricular twist [66]. The global performance of the systemic ventricle depends more on the circumferential than the longitudinal free wall contraction and may represent an adaptive response to the systemic load [67]. Becuase twist contributes to energy-efficient ejection, reduced twist might represent a potential for myocardial dysfunction [66].

Dilated and hypertrophic cardiomyopathy

In dilated cardiomyopathy, the amplitude of peak LV systolic twist is impaired in proportion to the global LV function [68]. This reduction in LV twist is accounted by marked attenuation of LV apical rotation, whereas basal rotation may be spared. After the initial part of the systole, the rotation diverges into one of two patterns: continuation of identical rotation at all levels for the remainder of systole or a divergence of rotation so that the apex and base rotate in opposite directions [69,70]. In contrast to dilated cardiomyopathy, patients who have hypertrophic cardiomyopathy show relatively preserved net LV twist [71], although the apex-to-base progression of the LV twist sequence is altered. Despite a preserved LV twist magnitude, patients who have hypertrophic cardiomyopathy have reduced efficiency in generating untwisting. At rest, peak untwisting velocities are only marginally reduced compared with normal subjects; however, these differences become more dramatic with exercise in patients showing much lower untwisting velocities compared with normal subjects [42].

Constrictive pericarditis versus restrictive cardiomyopathy

The marked endocardial dysfunction with relative sparing of epicardial function leads to abnormal longitudinal mechanics with relative sparing of circumferential and twist mechanics in restrictive cardiomyopathy [72]. In constrictive pericarditis, however, marked epicardial dysfunction leads to predominant impairment of circumferential shortening [73] and twist mechanics [72] while relatively sparing subendocardial longitudinal mechanics. Similarly, congentital defects of pericardium cause a lack of LV twist while maintaining LV regional myocardial function [74], suggesting that normal pericardial layers may have important roles in modulating LV rotational mechanics.

In summary, a growing body of evidence suggests that assessment of LV rotation and twist is feasible in clinical settings. Evolving applications in three-dimensional echocardiography will enable more accurate quantification of LV rotational deformation in three dimensions and in real time. Randomized and blinded studies in larger and diverse patient populations are needed to better define their eventual role in clinical practice.

References

[1] Lower R. Tractatus de Corde. London: Oxford University Press; 1669.

[2] Arts T, Hunter WC, Douglas AS, et al. Macroscopic three-dimensional motion patterns of the left ventricle. Adv Exp Med Biol 1993;346:383–92.

[3] Hansen DE, Daughters GT 2nd, Alderman EL, et al. Torsional deformation of the left ventricular midwall in human hearts with intramyocardial markers: regional heterogeneity and sensitivity to the inotropic effects of abrupt rate changes. Circ Res 1988; 62:941–52.

[4] Bell SP, Nyland L, Tischler MD, et al. Alterations in the determinants of diastolic suction during pacing tachycardia. Circ Res 2000;87:235–40.

[5] Gorman JH 3rd, Gupta KB, Streicher JT, et al. Dynamic three-dimensional imaging of the mitral valve and left ventricle by rapid sonomicrometry array localization. J Thorac Cardiovasc Surg 1996;112: 712–26.

[6] Gibbons Kroeker CA, Ter Keurs HE, Knudtson ML, et al. An optical device to measure the dynamics of apex rotation of the left ventricle. Am J Physiol 1993;265:H1444–9.

[7] Marcelli E, Plicchi G, Cercenelli L, et al. First experimental evaluation of cardiac apex rotation with an epicardial coriolis force sensor. ASAIO J 2005;51: 696–701.

[8] Buchalter MB, Weiss JL, Rogers WJ, et al. Noninvasive quantification of left ventricular rotational deformation in normal humans using magnetic resonance imaging myocardial tagging. Circulation 1990;81:1236–44.

[9] Buchalter MB, Rademakers FE, Weiss JL, et al. Rotational deformation of the canine left ventricle measured by magnetic resonance tagging: effects of catecholamines, ischaemia, and pacing. Cardiovasc Res 1994;28:629–35.

[10] Lorenz CH, Pastorek JS, Bundy JM. Delineation of normal human left ventricular twist throughout systole by tagged cine magnetic resonance imaging. J Cardiovasc Magn Reson 2000;2:97–108.

[11] Kim HK, Sohn DW, Lee SE, et al. Assessment of left ventricular rotation and torsion with two-dimensional speckle tracking echocardiography. J Am Soc Echocardiogr 2007;20:45–53.

[12] Notomi Y, Lysyansky P, Setser RM, et al. Measurement of ventricular torsion by two-dimensional ultrasound speckle tracking imaging. J Am Coll Cardiol 2005;45:2034–41.

[13] Notomi Y, Setser RM, Shiota T, et al. Assessment of left ventricular torsional deformation by Doppler tissue imaging: validation study with tagged magnetic resonance imaging. Circulation 2005;111: 1141–7.

[14] Helle-Valle T, Crosby J, Edvardsen T, et al. New noninvasive method for assessment of left ventricular rotation: speckle tracking echocardiography. Circulation 2005;112:3149–56.

[15] Arts T, Veenstra PC, Reneman RS. Epicardial deformation and left ventricular wall mechanisms during ejection in the dog. Am J Physiol 1982;243: H379–90.

[16] Beyar R, Sideman S. Left ventricular mechanics related to the local distribution of oxygen demand throughout the wall. Circ Res 1986;58:664–77.

[17] Ingels NB Jr, Hansen DE, Daughters GT 2nd, et al. Relation between longitudinal, circumferential, and oblique shortening and torsional deformation in the left ventricle of the transplanted human heart. Circ Res 1989;64:915–27.

[18] Henson RE, Song SK, Pastorek JS, et al. Left ventricular torsion is equal in mice and humans. Am J Physiol Heart Circ Physiol 2000;278:H1117–23.

[19] Delhaas T, Kotte J, van der Toorn A, et al. Increase in left ventricular torsion-to-shortening ratio in children with valvular aortic stenosis. Magn Reson Med 2004;51:135–9.

[20] Streeter DD, Ramon C. Muscle pathway geometry in the heart wall. J Biomech Eng 1983;105: 367–73.

[21] Nielsen PM, Le Grice IJ, Smaill BH, et al. Mathematical model of geometry and fibrous structure of the heart. Am J Physiol 1991;260:H1365–78.

[22] Chen J, Liu W, Zhang H, et al. Regional ventricular wall thickening reflects changes in cardiac fiber and sheet structure during contraction: quantification with diffusion tensor MRI. Am J Physiol Heart Circ Physiol 2005;289:H1898–907.

[23] Sengupta PP, Khandheria BK, Korinek J, et al. Biphasic tissue Doppler waveforms during isovolumic phases are associated with asynchronous deformation of subendocardial and subepicardial layers. J Appl Physiol 2005;99:1104–11.

[24] Taber LA, Yang M, Podszus WW. Mechanics of ventricular torsion. J Biomech 1996;29:745–52.

[25] Narula J, Vannan MA, DeMaria AN. Of that waltz in my heart. J Am Coll Cardiol 2007;49:917–20.

[26] Stelzer JE, Moss RL. Contributions of stretch activation to length-dependent contraction in murine myocardium. J Gen Physiol 2006;128:461–71.

[27] Sengupta PP, Khandheria BK, Korinek J, et al. Left ventricular isovolumic flow sequence during sinus and paced rhythms: new insights from use of high-resolution Doppler and ultrasonic digital particle imaging velocimetry. J Am Coll Cardiol 2007;49: 899–908.

[28] Jung B, Markl M, Foll D, et al. Investigating myocardial motion by MRI using tissue phase mapping. Eur J Cardiothorac Surg 2006;29(Suppl 1): S150–7.

[29] Ashikaga H, Coppola BA, Hopenfeld B, et al. Transmural dispersion of myofiber mechanics: implications for electrical heterogeneity in vivo. J Am Coll Cardiol 2007;49:909–16.

[30] Sengupta PP, Khandheria BK, Korinek J, et al. Apex-to-base dispersion in regional timing of left ventricular shortening and lengthening. J Am Coll Cardiol 2006;47:163–72.

[31] Rademakers FE, Buchalter MB, Rogers WJ, et al. Dissociation between left ventricular untwisting and filling. Accentuation by catecholamines. Circulation 1992;85:1572–81.

[32] Ashikaga H, Criscione JC, Omens JH, et al. Transmural left ventricular mechanics underlying torsional recoil during relaxation. Am J Physiol Heart Circ Physiol 2004;286:H640–7.

[33] Notomi Y, Srinath G, Shiota T, et al. Maturational and adaptive modulation of left ventricular torsional biomechanics: Doppler tissue imaging observation from infancy to adulthood. Circulation 2006;113: 2534–41.

[34] Lumens J, Delhaas T, Arts T, et al. Impaired subendocardial contractile myofiber function in asymptomatic aged humans, as detected using MRI. Am J Physiol Heart Circ Physiol 2006;291:H1573–9.

[35] Takeuchi M, Nakai H, Kokumai M, et al. Age-related changes in left ventricular twist assessed by two-dimensional speckle-tracking imaging. J Am Soc Echocardiogr 2006;19:1077–84.

[36] Dong SJ, Hees PS, Huang WM, et al. Independent effects of preload, afterload, and contractility on left ventricular torsion. Am J Physiol 1999;277: H1053–60.

[37] Hansen DE, Daughters GT 2nd, Alderman EL, et al. Effect of volume loading, pressure loading, and inotropic stimulation on left ventricular torsion in humans. Circulation 1991;83:1315–26.

[38] MacGowan GA, Burkhoff D, Rogers WJ, et al. Effects of afterload on regional left ventricular torsion. Cardiovasc Res 1996;31:917–25.

[39] Gibbons Kroeker CA, Tyberg JV, Beyar R. Effects of load manipulations, heart rate, and contractility on left ventricular apical rotation. An experimental study in anesthetized dogs. Circulation 1995;92: 130–41.

[40] Moon MR, Ingels NB Jr, Daughters GT 2nd, et al. Alterations in left ventricular twist mechanics with inotropic stimulation and volume loading in human subjects. Circulation 1994;89:142–50.

[41] Neilan TG, Ton-Nu TT, Jassal DS, et al. Myocardial adaptation to short-term high-intensity exercise in highly trained athletes. J Am Soc Echocardiogr 2006;19:1280–5.

[42] Notomi Y, Martin-Miklovic MG, Oryszak SJ, et al. Enhanced ventricular untwisting during exercise: a mechanistic manifestation of elastic recoil described by Doppler tissue imaging. Circulation 2006;113:2524–33.

[43] Notomi Y, Popovic ZB, Yamada H, et al. Ventricular untwisting: a temporal link between left ventricular relaxation and suction. Am J Physiol Heart Circ Physiol 2008;294:H505–13.

[44] Zocalo Y, Bia D, Armentano RL, et al. Assessment of training-dependent changes in the left ventricle torsion dynamics of professional soccer players using speckle-tracking echocardiography. Conf Proc IEEE Eng Med Biol Soc 2007;1:2709–12.

[45] Burns AT, La Gerche A, Macisaac AI, et al. Augmentation of left ventricular torsion with exercise is attenuated with age. J Am Soc Echocardiogr 2008;21(4):315–20.

[46] Epstein FH. MRI of left ventricular function. J Nucl Cardiol 2007;14:729–44.

[47] Rothfeld JM, LeWinter MM, Tischler MD. Left ventricular systolic torsion and early diastolic filling by echocardiography in normal humans. Am J Cardiol 1998;81:1465–9.

[48] Weyman AE. The year in echocardiography. J Am Coll Cardiol 2007;49:1212–9.

[49] Dong SJ, Hees PS, Siu CO, et al. MRI assessment of LV relaxation by untwisting rate: a new isovolumic phase measure of tau. Am J Physiol Heart Circ Physiol 2001;281:H2002–9.

[50] Wang J, Khoury DS, Yue Y, et al. Left ventricular untwisting rate by speckle tracking echocardiography. Circulation 2007;116:2580–6.

[51] Takeuchi M, Borden WB, Nakai H, et al. Reduced and delayed untwisting of the left ventricle in

patients with hypertension and left ventricular hypertrophy: a study using two-dimensional speckle tracking imaging. Eur Heart J 2007;28:2756–62.

[52] Kroeker CA, Tyberg JV, Beyar R. Effects of ischemia on left ventricular apex rotation. An experimental study in anesthetized dogs. Circulation 1995;92:3539–48.

[53] Knudtson ML, Galbraith PD, Hildebrand KL, et al. Dynamics of left ventricular apex rotation during angioplasty: a sensitive index of ischemic dysfunction. Circulation 1997;96:801–8.

[54] Bansal M, Leano RL, Marwick TH. Clinical assessment of left ventricular systolic torsion: effects of myocardial infarction and ischemia. J Am Soc Echocardiogr 2008, in press.

[55] Takeuchi M, Nishikage T, Nakai H, et al. The assessment of left ventricular twist in anterior wall myocardial infarction using two-dimensional speckle tracking imaging. J Am Soc Echocardiogr 2007;20:36–44.

[56] Garot J, Pascal O, Diebold B, et al. Alterations of systolic left ventricular twist after acute myocardial infarction. Am J Physiol Heart Circ Physiol 2002;282:H357–62.

[57] Nagel E, Stuber M, Burkhard B, et al. Cardiac rotation and relaxation in patients with aortic valve stenosis. Eur Heart J 2000;21:582–9.

[58] Stuber M, Scheidegger MB, Fischer SE, et al. Alterations in the local myocardial motion pattern in patients suffering from pressure overload due to aortic stenosis. Circulation 1999;100:361–8.

[59] Van Der Toorn A, Barenbrug P, Snoep G, et al. Transmural gradients of cardiac myofiber shortening in aortic valve stenosis patients using MRI tagging. Am J Physiol Heart Circ Physiol 2002;283:H1609–15.

[60] Biederman RW, Doyle M, Yamrozik J, et al. Physiologic compensation is supranormal in compensated aortic stenosis: does it return to normal after aortic valve replacement or is it blunted by coexistent coronary artery disease? An intramyocardial magnetic resonance imaging study. Circulation 2005;112:I429–36.

[61] Tibayan FA, Yun KL, Fann JI, et al. Torsion dynamics in the evolution from acute to chronic mitral regurgitation. J Heart Valve Dis 2002;11:39–46 [discussion: 46].

[62] Tibayan FA, Lai DT, Timek TA, et al. Alterations in left ventricular curvature and principal strains in dilated cardiomyopathy with functional mitral regurgitation. J Heart Valve Dis 2003;12:292–9.

[63] Tibayan FA, Rodriguez F, Langer F, et al. Alterations in left ventricular torsion and diastolic recoil after myocardial infarction with and without chronic ischemic mitral regurgitation. Circulation 2004;110:II109–14.

[64] Borg AN, Harrison JL, Argyle RA, et al. Left ventricular torsion in primary chronic mitral regurgitation. Heart 2008, in press.

[65] Haber I, Metaxas DN, Geva T, et al. Three-dimensional systolic kinematics of the right ventricle. Am J Physiol Heart Circ Physiol 2005;289:H1826–33.

[66] Pettersen E, Lindberg H, Smith HJ, et al. Left ventricular function in patients with transposition of the great arteries operated with atrial switch. Pediatr Cardiol 2008, in press.

[67] Pettersen E, Helle-Valle T, Edvardsen T, et al. Contraction pattern of the systemic right ventricle shift from longitudinal to circumferential shortening and absent global ventricular torsion. J Am Coll Cardiol 2007;49:2450–6.

[68] Kanzaki H, Nakatani S, Yamada N, et al. Impaired systolic torsion in dilated cardiomyopathy: reversal of apical rotation at mid-systole characterized with magnetic resonance tagging method. Basic Res Cardiol 2006;101:465–70.

[69] Setser RM, Kasper JM, Lieber ML, et al. Persistent abnormal left ventricular systolic torsion in dilated cardiomyopathy after partial left ventriculectomy. J Thorac Cardiovasc Surg 2003;126:48–55.

[70] Setser RM, Smedira NG, Lieber ML, et al. Left ventricular torsional mechanics after left ventricular reconstruction surgery for ischemic cardiomyopathy. J Thorac Cardiovasc Surg 2007;134:888–96.

[71] Young AA, Kramer CM, Ferrari VA, et al. Three-dimensional left ventricular deformation in hypertrophic cardiomyopathy. Circulation 1994;90:854–67.

[72] Sengupta PP, Krishnamoorthy VK, Abhayaratna W, et al. Disparate patterns of left ventricular mechanics differentiate constrictive pericarditis from restrictive cardiomyopathy. J Am Coll Cardiol Img 2008;1:29–38.

[73] Sekino E, Suzuki S, Momokawa T, et al. Left ventricular function studies in constrictive pericarditis. Jpn J Surg 1978;8:186–91.

[74] Tanaka H, Oishi Y, Mizuguchi Y, et al. Contribution of the pericardium to left ventricular torsion and regional myocardial function in patients with total absence of the left pericardium. J Am Soc Echocardiogr 2008;21:268–74.

Heart Failure Clin 4 (2008) 325–332

Following the Flow in Chambers

Partho P. Sengupta, MBBS, MD, DM*, Robert Burke, MD,
Bijoy K. Khandheria, MBBS,
Marek Belohlavek, MD, PhD

Mayo Clinic, Scottsdale, AZ, USA

The form and function of the heart creates time varying and spatially complex pulsatile flow patterns that are optimal for minimizing energy dissipation. One of the most intriguing features of these intracardiac flow patterns is the formation of intracavitary vortex rings. Historically, Leonardo da Vinci was the first to use flow visualization as a tool for discovery and exploration, and he masterfully followed this principle in his studies of heart valves [1]. He observed the development of vortices within the sinus of Valsalva and attempted to uncover a function to fit a known form. He described that the structure of the vortex was in perfect agreement with the curved geometry of the aortic sinus and therefore suitable for providing a closure mechanism for the aortic valve. Four centuries later, experimental and clinical explorations on cardiac flow have entailed the use of physical or computational models and imaging techniques such as echocardiography and magnetic resonance imaging to provide unique insights into the efficient suction and ejection performance of a beating heart.

Experimental insights into the significance of vortex ring formation

Using physical and numerical models, investigators have attempted to explore the significance of vortex formation by focusing on the analysis of particular aspects of the problem; therefore, these models are characterized by specific simplifying assumptions. Bellhouse [2] conducted experimental studies on the left ventricular (LV) diastolic vortex in the context of cardiac physiology in the early 1970s and proposed that vortical motion might assist in valve closure. Taylor and Yamaguchi [3] suggested that the presence of LV diastolic vortical flow may help in the ensuing process of ejection by conversion of vortex kinetic energy into kinetic energy of outflow with aortic valve opening. According to that view, vortices within the ventricle would act as energy-preserving flow structures. Indeed, Bolger and coworkers [4] recently estimated that $16 \pm 8\%$ of the kinetic energy of diastolic mitral flow would be conserved to the end of diastole and carried over into the next beat.

Investigators have suggested that the asymmetric geometry of the LV and the orientation of its valves may favor vortex formation and automatic redirection of blood from the LV inflow to the outflow. In an experimental model, Pedrizetti and Domenichini [5] showed that asymmetric circulation in the LV largely develops owing to the physiologic eccentricity of the mitral orifice. When the mitral orifice is oriented more centrally, energy dissipation increases because the flow pattern at the end of filling is not favorable for ejection, and fluid elements are subjected to more strain for redirection toward the exit. In contrast, when the mitral orifice is highly eccentric, the entering flow collides with the ventricular wall, enhancing the dissipative interaction with the boundary layer. This interaction promotes natural swirling of blood flow inside the LV and serves as an efficient physiologic adaptation to facilitate the ejection of blood.

* Corresponding author.
E-mail address: sengupta.partho@mayo.edu (P.P. Sengupta).

1551-7136/08/$ - see front matter
doi:10.1016/j.hfc.2008.02.005

The formation of vortices also aids ventricular filling. In the initial phase of LV filling, the local acceleration gradient favors forward flow, corresponding to the upstroke (acceleration phase) of the early diastolic filling wave (E-wave) [6]. During the E-wave downstroke (deceleration phase), the convective forces are augmented, resulting in flow reversal. This change leads to disruption of the boundary between oncoming blood and endocardial walls, or "flow separation," and to the formation of a toroidal vortex. The vortical swirl inside the LV cavity ascends and strikes the undersurface of the mitral valve causing transient approximation of the mitral leaflets. Furthermore, the vortical swirl breaks down into smaller eddies, and this process is continued during diastasis until the vortices are reduced to micron-sized eddies (Kolmogorov "microscale"), when they dissipate under the action of viscous forces [7], a process also known as the vortical cascade mechanism. Persistent ongoing interaction of diastolic vortices with the endocardial wall ensures a continuous presence of lateral pressure for effecting ongoing expansion of the endocardial surface and assists in attaining higher LV end-diastolic volumes [6,8].

Bot and colleagues [9] studied the relations between vortex size and speed of flow for clarifying whether LV diastolic inflow volume and the LV size have a role in vortex ring formation. An important parameter discerned in their equations was the relative injection length, that is, the ratio of the length of the injected bolus and the radius of the orifice (L/R). It was estimated that the highest value in humans, $L/R = 15$, would produce a dense vortex ring (relative thickness, 0.77). Gharib and colleagues recently described the use of a similar dimensionless numerical index for characterizing vortex ring formation [10]. This index, called the "vortex formation time," is a measure of the length-to-diameter ratio (L/D) of the ejected fluid column. A vortex ring will continue to grow larger during the process of fluid transport until a vortex formation time $T = 4$ is reached. After this point, the vortex ring is unable to grow larger because of energetic constraints, and ejected fluid subsequently forms a trailing jet behind the vortex ring. These fluid principles also apply to the function of the LV. Normal flow across the mitral valve in early diastole is completed within a vortex formation time of $3.3 < T < 5.5$, a range consistent with the optimal range of vortex formation time found in the in vitro vortex formation studies [10].

Direct in vivo observations

Cardiac MRI

Cardiac MRI techniques have been developed for direct quantitative assessment of intracardiac blood flow (Fig. 1). A variety of cardiac MR techniques have been developed to measure blood flow in clinical practice, including time of flight and phase flow imaging methods [11]. The most common flow assessment technique available in commercial scanners is phase contrast velocity mapping, which is based on detection of the acquired phase shift of proton spins moving along a magnetic field gradient [11,12]. In this technique, stationary protons acquire zero phase shifts [13]. Applying bipolar gradients with equal magnitude and opposite directions creates a linear relation between the motion of proton spins along the gradient and the net phase shift in each voxel of the image. As a result, temporally and spatially resolved flow maps can be reconstructed on the basis of phase shift measurements. For the purpose of imaging with cardiac MR, the protons in question reside in the hydrogen in water, obviating the need for a blood pool contrast agent. This technique has been well validated and is reproducible in clinical and research settings [12,14].

Direct measurement of LV intracavitary vortices requires a volumetric technique, which provides three-dimensional flow information. Using cardiac MR phase contrast velocity mapping, the development of vortices within the human LV was initially described by Kim and coworkers [15]. Specifically, they elucidated the formation of an anterior vortex within the LV that developed immediately after the peak of early mitral inflow (after the onset of middiastolic anterior leaflet closure) and reappeared at the time of final mitral valve closure. This initial study described a complex pattern in which two different velocities were found in the vortex—one central and one peripheral. The occurrence of a late diastolic vortex ring was confirmed in subsequent investigations [16]. Bolger and colleagues recently showed that direct flow entering with the atrial contraction shows the least change in velocity and follows the shortest route from inflow to ejection [4]. The atrial wave also appears to boost the mitral vortical flow velocity and, in doing so, accelerates blood flow toward the LV outflow tract. Retained flow, on the other hand, spends more than a single beat within the body of the ventricle and contributes to the delayed ejection

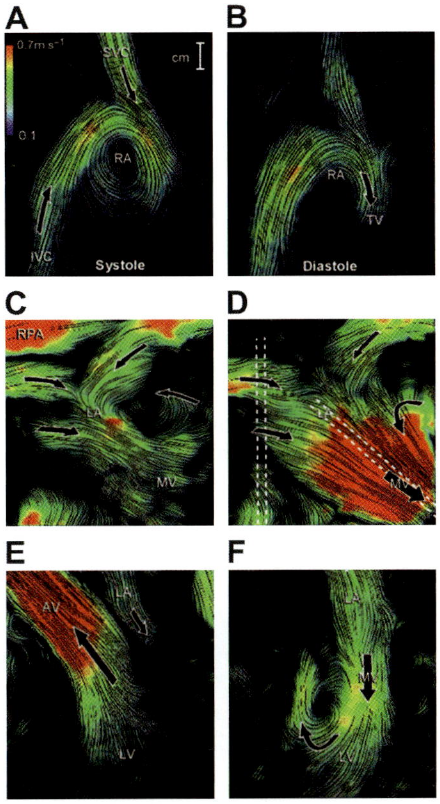

Fig. 1. Intracardiac flow sequence in a beating heart. Colored streamlines computed from MR velocity acquisitions show local speed as indicated by the color scale. (*A*) The right atrial flow has been viewed in ventricular systole in a sagittal plane from the subject's right side. Blood entering from superior and inferior caval veins rotates and forms a well-defined vortex in the expanding chamber. (*B*) In early ventricular diastole, blood is redirected through the open tricuspid valve. (*C*) In the left atrium in ventricular systole, blood enters from the upper and lower pulmonary veins on each side, indicated by arrows in this coronal plane viewed from the front (lower veins lie out of the plane posteriorly). Rotating streams of blood flow are redirected toward the mitral valve. (*D*) In early ventricular diastole, there is further inflow from veins while blood passes through the open mitral valve to the LV. Vertical and oblique dotted lines indicate planes orthogonal to this panel, represented by panels A, B, E, and F. (*E*) In the LV in systole, streamlines pass from the LV through the aortic valve. (*F*) In early diastole, flow from the left atrium is redirected from the inflow to the outflow through the formation of a large anterior vortex. In panels E and F only, the color scale is modified to reach red at 1 ms^{-1}. AV, aortic valve; IVC, inferior vena cava; LA, left atrium; MV, mitral valve; RA, right atrium; RPA, right pulmonary artery; SVC, superior vena cava; TV, tricuspid valve. (*From* Kilner PJ, Yang GZ, Wilkes AJ, et al. Asymmetric redirection of flow through the heart. Nature 2000;404:759; with permission.)

volume for the subsequent beat and, as expected, takes a longer path through the LV before ejection.

Cardiac MR studies have confirmed the existence of vortical swirl in other chambers of the human heart. In the right atrium, flows through the superior and inferior caval veins were shown to swirl into a vortex that emptied into the inlet of the tricuspid valve. The blood flow through the tricuspid valve surged into the right ventricle, giving rise to recirculating flows beneath the leaflets, the dominant direction being toward the outflow region [6,14]. The change in direction between inflow and outflow is less acute than in the left ventricle.

In the left atrium, two temporally discrete left atrial vortices have been identified, with the axis of rotation being approximately crescent shaped and parallel to the mitral annular plane [17]. Vortical flow in the left atrium begins to develop immediately before ventricular systole and increases in magnitude during systole. The vortex disappears with the onset of early diastole, during which flow from all four pulmonary veins propagates rapidly through the left atrium and the mitral valve for rapid LV filling. A second left atrial vortex develops during middiastole and disappears at the time of atrial contraction. Transient reversal of flow into the pulmonary veins can be recorded during this phase [17].

Cardiac MR has also been used for deciphering flow in the aorta (Fig. 2). Following ejection, vortices can be identified in the coronary sinuses of Valsalva [18]. The central jet continues in the main aortic arch. An initial jet of blood streams toward the anterior right wall of the ascending aorta and is reflected posterolaterally toward the inner curvature, creating opposing helices, a right-handed helix along the left wall and a left-handed helix along the right wall [19]. Furthermore, retrograde flow occurs along the inner curvature between the location of the two helices [19]. Looking down the aorta from its origin, rapid systolic forward blood flow follows a right-handed helix of approximately 360 degrees from the ascending aorta to the descending aorta [20]. Except in young individuals, blood flow is not continuously forward during all of systole but instead reverses in mid and late systole and goes forward again in diastole. Blood flows from the aortic valve to the middescending aorta in rapid systole in young individuals (<50 years) and in two-to-three beats in older individuals [20].

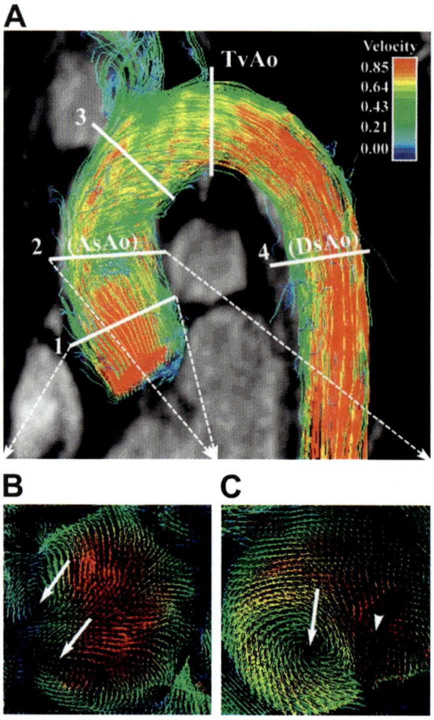

Fig. 2. Pattern of blood flow in the thoracic aorta discerned by MR phase contrast velocity mapping. Streamlines in a healthy volunteer are shown at 15% of the cardiac cycle. (*A*) A right-handed helix can be seen on the surface of the streamlines, as well as a slowing of velocities at the aortic arch. Velocities in all images are measured in meters per second. (*B*) Cross-sectional plane with velocity vectors placed orthonormal to the aorta at plane 1 shows two opposing helices, one clockwise and one counterclockwise along the posterior wall of the aorta (*arrows*). (*C*) At plane 2, the right-handed helix to the left (*arrow*) is larger than the left-handed helix on the right (*arrowhead*). All planes are viewed from a perspective distal to the plane, with the inner curvature at the bottom of the image. For example, the larger vortex (*arrow*) would be graded as occurring at a 9 o'clock angle, rotating in a counterclockwise direction, encompassing 50% of the aortic lumen, and with its center 50% of the way between the center of the lumen and the vessel wall. AsAo, ascending aorta; DsAo, descending aorta; TvAo, transverse aorta. (*From* Hope TA, Markl M, Wigstrom L, et al. Comparison of flow patterns in ascending aortic aneurysms and volunteers using four-dimensional magnetic resonance velocity mapping. J Magn Reson Imaging 2007;26:1473; with permission.)

Echocardiography

Doppler echocardiography remains a cornerstone application for understanding blood flow patterns in clinical practice. Doppler imaging has been used in experimental and clinical settings for deciphering intracavitary vortex ring formation [21–25]. One of the specific advantages of Doppler imaging is the high temporal resolution, which helps to decipher the flow during the brief pre-ejection and post-ejection isovolumic intervals of the cardiac cycle (Fig. 3). Conventionally, the timing of mitral valve closure divides the pre-ejection period into two composite intervals [25]. The interval from the onset of the Q-wave on surface electrocardiography to mitral valve closure is referred to as "electromechanical delay," whereas isovolumic contraction is the period that follows mitral valve closure and is characterized by a rapid rise in LV pressure before opening of the aortic valve. During sinus rhythm, initial Doppler velocities in the pre-ejection period are directed from

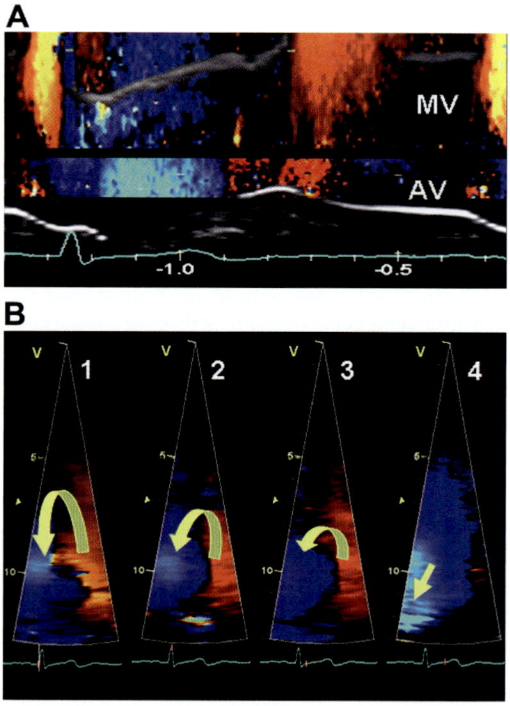

Fig. 3. Left ventricular intracavitary flow sequence by high-resolution Doppler imaging. (*A*) Anatomic M-mode across the mitral valve (MV) and aortic valve (AV) delineates the timing of onset and closure of mitral and aortic leaflet. (*B*) Frames 1–4 show the dynamic flow across the submitral region obtained with the use of high frame rate flow Doppler during the isovolumic contraction phase. Note the counterdirectional flow moving toward the LV cavity in the submitral region (red) and then toward the LV outflow tract (blue, *arrows*). Biphasic flow signals in the LV represent counterdirectional motions of a vortex formation.

the apex toward the LV base [25]. After the mitral leaflets close, during the phase of isovolumic contraction, the direction of flow in the submitral region reverses briefly toward the apex before accelerating again in the apex-to-base direction, which further continues into the period of ejection. During isovolumic relaxation, the flow is transiently bidirectional. An initial flow in the base-to-apex direction is followed by a brief reversed flow in the apex-to-base direction. Vortex formation during early and late diastolic filling appears in the form of antegrade and retrograde bidirectional velocities in the inflow and outflow compartments of the LV. These bidirectional flow signals occur earlier and are higher, at the level of the deflected anterior mitral leaflet tip when compared with more apical levels [23,25].

Color Doppler imaging has limitations in measuring absolute fluid velocities (average uncertainty $\pm$ 10 cm/s) [24]. As an alternative to the Doppler technique, contrast echocardiography has been used for semiqualitative assessment of intracardiac flows [25,26]. The LV cavity is opacified with contrast microbubbles, and the movement of contrast bubbles is tracked from one frame to the other by using high temporal resolution imaging. In an M-mode display, the flow paths of contrast bubbles appear as streaks in the dark blood pool (Fig. 4). Both the speed and direction of blood flow influence the shape and length of these streaks. In a two-dimensional display, the contrast motion can be tracked from one frame to the other in real time using a computational technique called "echo particle imaging velocimetry" (Echo PIV) [25,27–30]. Displacement of the particles in the second image relative to the position of the particles in the first image is a measure of the motion of the fluid. Pairs of sequential frames are cross-correlated for generating instantaneous flow vectors. Echo PIV has shown good agreement with optical PIV for in vitro models of pulsatile flow [27].

Echo PIV has been recently used for deciphering blood flow and vortex ring formation during the isovolumic intervals [25]. The initial pre-ejection period is characterized with movement of contrast bubbles from the apical region toward the outflow, whereas the contrast bubbles moving from the submitral region form a large vortex from the inflow toward the outflow (see Fig. 4). The vortex ring formation continues after mitral valve closure as the flow is seen to accelerate toward the LV outflow during isovolumic contraction. Following ejection, the isovolumic relaxation is characterized with reversal of flow in a base-to-apex direction. The brisk reversal of flow collides with the LV wall and transiently rolls upward toward the LV base before the opening of mitral leaflets. The intracavitary flow sequences during the isovolumic intervals are temporally matched with transient asynchronous movements of the subendocardial and subepicardial regions of the LV. It has been suggested that although the intrinsic LV and mitral valve geometries are important contributors to asymmetric flow redirection [14], the apex-to-base differences in electromechanical forces at the onset of systole and diastole are critical for further continuation and stabilization of flow reversal [25].

Aberrant flow patterns in diseased states

Flow patterns inside the LV can be predicted to change in a diseased state. For example, mathematical models have predicted that the presence of global LV dysfunction, such as in dilated cardiomyopathy, would result in the wake vortex detaching from the mitral valve at later times, resulting in increased intensity and reduced propagation velocity and longer stagnation near the apex [31]. From a pathophysiologic point of view, this fluid stagnation may result in the formation of apical thrombi. These observations have been confirmed in clinical studies [32]. In patients with a dilated LV, the inflow is seen to be directed toward the free wall, giving rise to a well-developed circular flow pattern turning back toward the septum and an outflow tract that persists through the diastole [33].

Intracavitary flows are also altered in the presence of regional myocardial dysfunction. For example, in coronary artery disease, infarcted segments of the LV can show complex blood flow vortex formation not identified in healthy ventricles [34]. Beppu and colleagues [35] demonstrated the existence of recirculation flow in the basal LV during coronary ligation in dog hearts using contrast echocardiography. This recirculation vortex differs from the vortices that form at the tips of the mitral valve. Recirculation vortex is largely observed during diastasis, as opposed to the vortices at the mitral tips, which are stronger during the rapid filling phases. Abnormal recirculation flows suggestive of stasis have also been identified in humans by Doppler echocardiography and have been reported to be superior to conventional clinical and two-dimensional echocardiographic assessment for estimating the

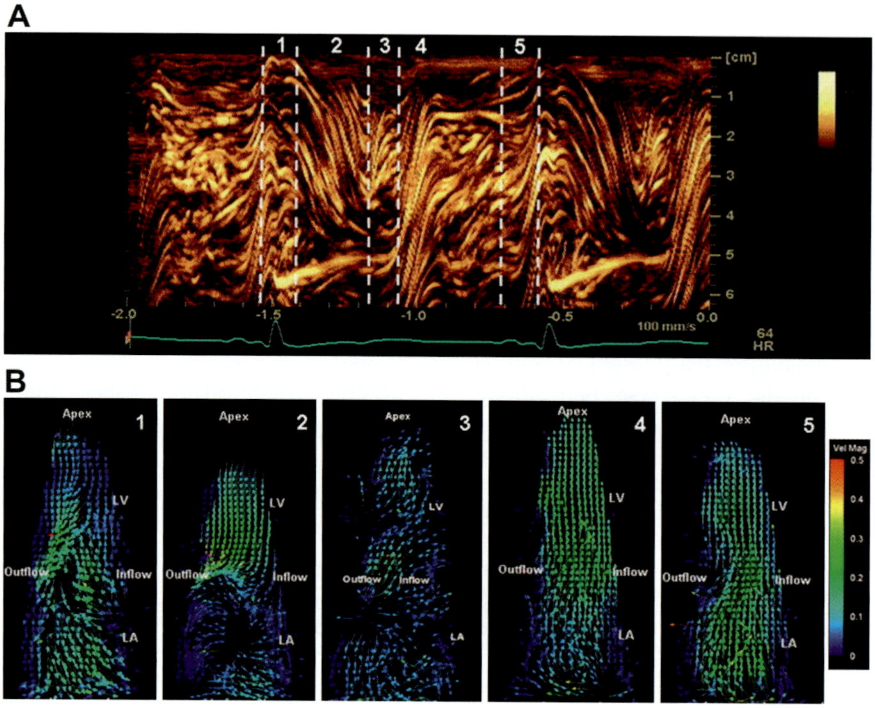

Fig. 4. Left ventricular flow during phases of the cardiac cycle. (*A*) Anatomic M-mode characteristics of LV intracavitary flow have been obtained along the long axis of the LV cavity during contrast infusion. (*B*) Time-related changes in two-dimensional intracardiac flow have been obtained by using high temporal resolution imaging at 200 frames/s and echocontrast particle imaging velocimetry. High frame rates allow tracking of bubbles sufficiently to determine the two-dimensional component of local vectors of blood motion before bubbles move out of the scan plane. For each phase, the local ensemble-averaged axis-normal velocity magnitude is superimposed on the vector field. LA, left atrium; 1, pre-ejection period enclosing isovolumic contraction; 2, ejection; 3, isovolumic relaxation; 4, early diastole; 5, late diastole. (*From* Sengupta PP, Krishnamoorthy VK, Korinek J, et al. Left ventricular form and function revisited: applied translational science to cardiovascular ultrasound imaging. J Am Soc Echocardiogr 2007;20:548; with permission.)

risk of LV thrombosis after myocardial infarction [32].

LV intracavitary diastolic flow may be useful for differentiating normal from pseudonormal patterns of LV filling. Ishizu and colleagues studied 29 patients with a pseudonormalized pattern and 26 normal controls using contrast echocardiography [26]. Although in both groups vortices were observed at the ridge of the mitral valve during acceleration of the E-wave, the mean radius of the vortices was greater in the pseudonormalized filling group than in the control group.

Flow visualization has also been used for understanding the mechanism of outflow tract obstruction in patients with hypertrophic cardiomyopathy [36]. In the normal LV, large anterior vortex formation helps maintain the mitral leaflets closer to the posterior wall of the LV while simultaneously prepositioning the upcoming systolic outflow stream close to the septum, thereby minimizing the flow forces acting on the mitral valve. In contrast, in hypertrophic cardiomyopathy, anterior displacement of the papillary muscles moves the entire mitral apparatus into the outflow tract. It also reverses the direction of the diastolic vortex, which now promotes the initiation of systolic anterior motion of the mitral leaflets by displacing the closing mitral leaflets anteriorly and by positioning the systolic outflow stream close to the posterior wall. These events lead to the creation of drag forces as the systolic flow impacts the posterior side of the mitral leaflets, initiating systolic anterior motion of the mitral valve [36].

Blood flow patterns in arterial disease can be investigated with the use of cardiac MR imaging and echocardiography. Carotid atheromatous disease is associated with a reduction in the prevalence of systolic spiral flow pattern in the aortic arch [37]. Loss of spiral flow in the abdominal aorta has also been associated with increasing severity of renal artery stenosis and more rapid deterioration of renal function [38]. It has been proposed that spiral blood flow structure may protect the arterial wall from damage by reducing laterally directed forces, just like a bullet from a rifle has directional stability conferred by the spiral configuration within the gun barrel [39,40]. The role of flow visualization as a tool for allowing the prediction of vascular health and atherosclerotic disease progression requires systematic assessment in future investigations.

In summary, this article illustrates how functional assessment of the cardiovascular system is possible by observing intracardiac and intravascular flow structure. In vivo techniques such as MRI and Echo PIV offer promise as tools for the routine assessment of flow and the computation of new integrative markers of cardiovascular function.

References

[1] Gharib M, Kremers D, Koochesfahani MM, et al. Leonardo's vision of flow visualization. Experiments in Fluids 2002;33:219–23.

[2] Bellhouse BJ. Fluid mechanics of model aortic and mitral valves. Proc R Soc Med 1970;63:996.

[3] Taylor TW, Yamaguchi T. Flow patterns in three-dimensional left ventricular systolic and diastolic flows determined from computational fluid dynamics. Biorheology 1995;32:61–71.

[4] Bolger AF, Heiberg E, Karlsson M, et al. Transit of blood flow through the human left ventricle mapped by cardiovascular magnetic resonance. J Cardiovasc Magn Reson 2007;9:741–7.

[5] Pedrizzetti G, Domenichini F. Nature optimizes the swirling flow in the human left ventricle. Phys Rev Lett 2005;95:108101–4.

[6] Pasipoularides A, Shu M, Shah A, et al. RV instantaneous intraventricular diastolic pressure and velocity distributions in normal and volume overload awake dog disease models. Am J Physiol Heart Circ Physiol 2003;285:H1956–65.

[7] Mukdadi OM, Kim HB, Hertzberg J, et al. Numerical modeling of microbubble backscatter to optimize ultrasound particle image velocimetry imaging: initial studies. Ultrasonics 2004;42:1111–21.

[8] Pasipoularides A, Shu M, Shah A, et al. Diastolic right ventricular filling vortex in normal and volume overload states. Am J Physiol Heart Circ Physiol 2003;284:H1064–72.

[9] Bot H, Verburg J, Delemarre BJ, et al. Determinants of the occurrence of vortex rings in the left ventricle during diastole. J Biomech 1990;23:607–15.

[10] Gharib M, Rambod E, Kheradvar A, et al. Optimal vortex formation as an index of cardiac health. Proc Natl Acad Sci U S A 2006;103:6305–8.

[11] Chai P, Mohiaddin R. How we perform cardiovascular magnetic resonance flow assessment using phase-contrast velocity mapping. J Cardiovasc Magn Reson 2005;7:705–16.

[12] Yang GZ, Merrifield R, Masood S, et al. Flow and myocardial interaction: an imaging perspective. Philos Trans R Soc Lond B Biol Sci 2007;362:1329–41.

[13] Mohiaddin RH, Pennell DJ. MR blood flow measurement: clinical application in the heart and circulation. Cardiol Clin 1998;16:161–87.

[14] Kilner PJ, Yang GZ, Wilkes AJ, et al. Asymmetric redirection of flow through the heart. Nature 2000;404:759–61.

[15] Kim WY, Walker PG, Pedersen EM, et al. Left ventricular blood flow patterns in normal subjects: a quantitative analysis by three-dimensional magnetic resonance velocity mapping. J Am Coll Cardiol 1995;26:224–38.

[16] Walker PG, Cranney GB, Grimes RY, et al. Three-dimensional reconstruction of the flow in a human left heart by using magnetic resonance phase velocity encoding. Ann Biomed Eng 1996;24:139–47.

[17] Fyrenius A, Wigstrom L, Ebbers T, et al. Three-dimensional flow in the human left atrium. Heart 2001;86:448–55.

[18] Markl M, Draney MT, Miller DC, et al. Time-resolved three-dimensional magnetic resonance velocity mapping of aortic flow in healthy volunteers and patients after valve-sparing aortic root replacement. J Thorac Cardiovasc Surg 2005;130:456–63.

[19] Hope TA, Markl M, Wigstrom L, et al. Comparison of flow patterns in ascending aortic aneurysms and volunteers using four-dimensional magnetic resonance velocity mapping. J Magn Reson Imaging 2007;26:1471–9.

[20] Bogren HG, Buonocore MH. 4D magnetic resonance velocity mapping of blood flow patterns in the aorta in young vs. elderly normal subjects. J Magn Reson Imaging 1999;10:861–9.

[21] Steen T, Steen S. Filling of a model left ventricle studied by colour M mode Doppler. Cardiovasc Res 1994;28:1821–7.

[22] Kim WY, Bisgaard T, Nielsen SL, et al. Two-dimensional mitral flow velocity profiles in pig models using epicardial Doppler echocardiography. J Am Coll Cardiol 1994;24:532–45.

[23] Rodevand O, Bjornerheim R, Edvardsen T, et al. Diastolic flow pattern in the normal left ventricle. J Am Soc Echocardiogr 1999;12:500–7.

[24] Cooke J, Hertzberg J, Boardman M, et al. Characterizing vortex ring behavior during ventricular filling with Doppler echocardiography: an in vitro study. Ann Biomed Eng 2004;32:245–56.

[25] Sengupta PP, Khandheria BK, Korinek J, et al. Left ventricular isovolumic flow sequence during sinus and paced rhythms: new insights from use of

high-resolution Doppler and ultrasonic digital particle imaging velocimetry. J Am Coll Cardiol 2007;49: 899–908.

[26] Ishizu T, Seo Y, Ishimitsu T, et al. The wake of a large vortex is associated with intraventricular filling delay in impaired left ventricles with a pseudonormalized transmitral flow pattern. Echocardiography 2006;23:369–75.

[27] Drost T, Zimmer T, Kim HB, et al. Study of in vitro mitral valve filling flow. Biomed Sci Instrum 2004; 40:350–6.

[28] Mukdadi O, Shandas R. Ultrasound wave propagation in tissue and scattering from microbubbles for echo particle image velocimetry technique. Biomed Sci Instrum 2004;40:364–70.

[29] Zheng H, Mukdadi O, Hertzberg J, et al. Advantages in using multi-frequency driving ultrasound for optimizing echo particle image velocimetry techniques. Biomed Sci Instrum 2004;40:371–6.

[30] Zheng H, Mukdadi O, Kim H, et al. Advantages in using multifrequency excitation of contrast microbubbles for enhancing echo particle image velocimetry techniques: initial numerical studies using rectangular and triangular waves. Ultrasound Med Biol 2005;31:99–108.

[31] Baccani B, Domenichini F, Pedrizzetti G, et al. Fluid dynamics of the left ventricular filling in dilated cardiomyopathy. J Biomech 2002;35:665–71.

[32] Van Dantzig JM, Delemarre BJ, Bot H, et al. Doppler left ventricular flow pattern versus conventional predictors of left ventricular thrombus after acute myocardial infarction. J Am Coll Cardiol 1995;25: 1341–6.

[33] Mohiaddin RH. Flow patterns in the dilated ischemic left ventricle studied by MR imaging with velocity vector mapping. J Magn Reson Imaging 1995;5:493–8.

[34] Taylor TW, Suga H, Goto Y, et al. The effects of cardiac infarction on realistic three-dimensional left ventricular blood ejection. J Biomech Eng 1996;118:106–10.

[35] Beppu S, Izumi S, Miyatake K, et al. Abnormal blood pathways in left ventricular cavity in acute myocardial infarction: experimental observations with special reference to regional wall motion abnormality and hemostasis. Circulation 1988;78: 157–64.

[36] Lefebvre XP, He S, Levine RA, et al. Systolic anterior motion of the mitral valve in hypertrophic cardiomyopathy: an in vitro pulsatile flow study. J Heart Valve Dis 1995;4:422–38.

[37] Houston JG, Gandy SJ, Sheppard DG, et al. Two-dimensional flow quantitative MRI of aortic arch blood flow patterns: effect of age, sex, and presence of carotid atheromatous disease on prevalence of spiral blood flow. J Magn Reson Imaging 2003;18: 169–74.

[38] Houston JG, Gandy SJ, Milne W, et al. Spiral laminar flow in the abdominal aorta: a predictor of renal impairment deterioration in patients with renal artery stenosis? Nephrol Dial Transplant 2004;19: 1786–91.

[39] Stonebridge PA, Brophy CM. Spiral laminar flow in arteries? Lancet 1991;338:1360–1.

[40] Stonebridge PA, Hoskins PR, Allan PL, et al. Spiral laminar flow in vivo. Clin Sci (Lond) 1996;91:17–21.

ELSEVIER
SAUNDERS

Heart Failure Clin 4 (2008) 333–345

HEART
FAILURE
CLINICS

Development of Strategies for Guiding Cardiac Resynchronization Therapy

Leonard M. Rademakers, MD[a], Bart W.L. de Boeck, MD[b], Jos G. Maessen, MD, PhD[a], Frits W. Prinzen, PhD[a,*]

[a]Cardiovascular Research Institute Maastricht, Maastricht, The Netherlands
[b]University Medical Centre, Utrecht, The Netherlands

In approximately one third of patients who have heart failure, ventricular conduction disturbances are found, most commonly manifested as left bundle-branch block (LBBB). Patients who have heart failure and LBBB have a higher mortality rate than those without LBBB. For such patients, cardiac resynchronization therapy (CRT) has emerged as an important therapy, in addition to optimized pharmacologic treatment [1].

Approximately 7 years after its formal introduction in clinical practice, CRT can be regarded as having survived its childhood diseases and is now is in its adolescence. Indeed, there are signs that there is still growing potential for CRT; however, conversely, CRT has some behavioral problems, such as the approximately one third of nonresponders. Proper growth to adulthood requires better understanding of the mechanisms of CRT and of the various relevant diagnostic and monitoring tools.

In this article, the authors review the following:

1. Dyssynchrony and resynchronization
2. Better selection of CRT candidates: mechanical dyssynchrony
3. Better therapy application: site of stimulation, optimization of atrioventricular (AV) delay and interventricular (VV)-interval
4. New growth areas: narrow QRS complex, prevention of heart failure

Dyssynchrony and resynchronization

Leftbundle-branch block and dyssynchrony?

In healthy subjects, the left ventricle (LV) is activated almost synchronously, predominantly through the rapid conduction system, and this is followed by synchronous and coordinated contraction [2]. Patients who have LBBB and other conduction abnormalities have a markedly altered ventricular activation sequence, however. In LBBB, the septum and right ventricle (RV) are activated early, whereas the LV lateral wall is activated late. Fig. 1 shows data on mechanical consequences of asynchronous activation from a canine heart in which LBBB was induced. The early activated septum also contracts early, thereby prestretching the still quiescent LV lateral wall. This prestretch, in turn, leads to increased lateral wall strain later in systole (see Fig. 1) [3,4]. Consequences of these abnormal contraction patterns are delayed increase of LV pressure, uncoordinated papillary muscle contraction, prolonged relaxation, and mitral valve regurgitation (MR) [5]. This discoordinate contraction results in a 10% to 20% decline in indices of systolic (eg, cardiac output, maximal rate of LV pressure rise [LV$dP/dt_{max}$]) and diastolic (eg, maximal rate of LV pressure fall [LV$dP/dt_{min}$], peak filling rate, τ) function and a decline in efficiency (Fig. 2), as reviewed in the article by Prinzen and Peschar [6]. These acute detrimental mechanical consequences seem to be

* Corresponding author. Department of Physiology, Cardiovascular Research Institute Maastricht, Universiteitssingel 50, NL-6229 ER Maastricht, The Netherlands.

E-mail address: frits.prinzen@fys.unimaas.nl (F.W. Prinzen).

1551-7136/08/$ - see front matter
doi:10.1016/j.hfc.2008.02.008

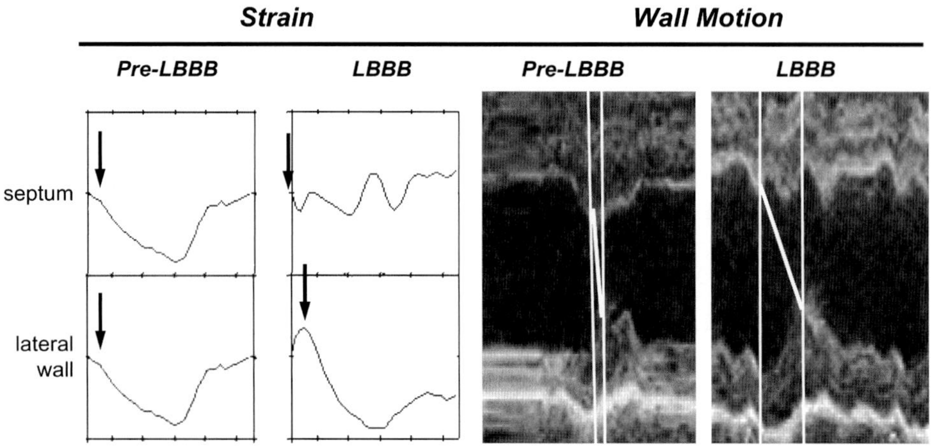

Fig. 1. (*Left panel*) Typical example of myocardial circumferential shortening tracings of the septum and LV lateral wall in a canine heart before and after induction of LBBB. Arrows indicate the time of onset of myocardial shortening. (*Right panel*) M-mode echocardiographic images illustrate the paradoxical septal motion after LBBB and the septal-to-posterior wall motion delay (SPWMD). Thin vertical white lines indicate the moment of maximal inward movement of the septum and LV lateral wall. Thick white lines indicate SPWMD.

amplified in the long run because of structural [4], contractile, and electrical remodeling [5], part of which shows regional differences within the LV wall, presumably attributable to the local differences in workload [4,5]. These remodeling processes may predispose to development of heart failure over time. Clear evidence for a relation between abnormal conduction and heart failure also comes from several studies in patients with RV pacing [7].

Mechanisms of cardiac resynchronization therapy and acute hemodynamics studies

Resynchronization of ventricular activation and contraction can be achieved in two ways (Fig. 3). The most common approach for CRT is to stimulate the RV and LV (almost) simultaneously, resulting in two activation wave fronts, merging approximately halfway down the LV wall. Such resynchronization can also be obtained by pacing the LV lateral wall using an AV delay that allows the wave front emerging from the intrinsic activation, originating from the right bundle branch, to merge with the wave front originating from the LV pacing lead [8,9].

In 1994, Cazeau and colleagues [10] were the first to apply CRT ("multisite pacing") to a patient who had heart failure and conduction disturbances and demonstrated a significant improvement in the clinical status after 6 weeks of pacing. This experience paved the way for hemodynamic studies,

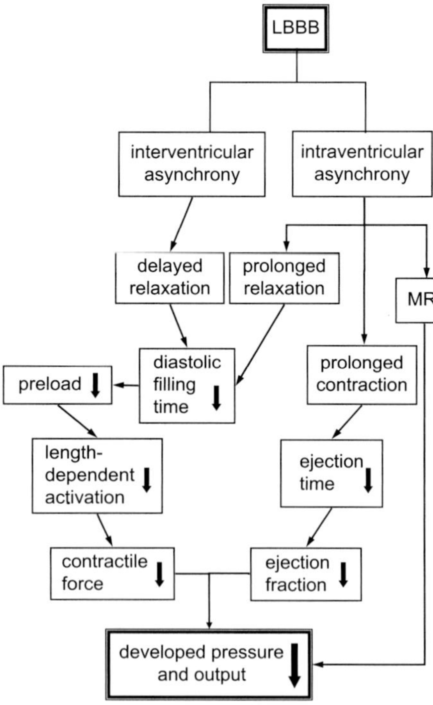

Fig. 2. Schematic relation between the various consequences of asynchronous activation of the ventricles attributable to LBBB and the deterioration of pump function over time.

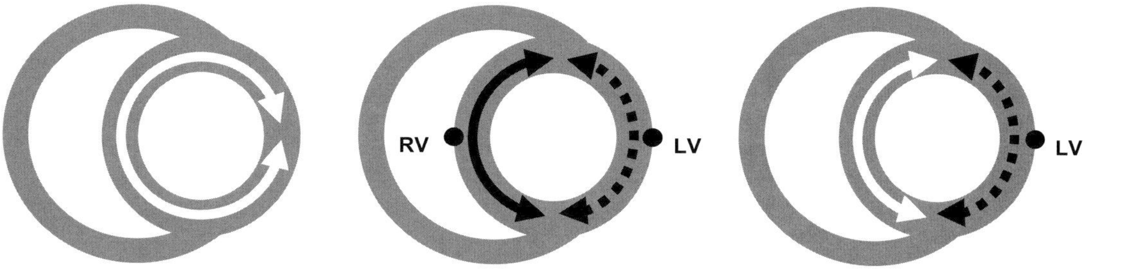

Fig. 3. Schematic LV activation through intrinsic activation from the right bundle branch (as is seen in LBBB; *left*), biventricular pacing (*middle*), and fusion of the LV pacing activation wave front with intrinsic activation through the right bundle branch (*right*). Black dots indicate pacing location.

further proving the benefit of CRT [9,11]. CRT essentially corrects the disturbances induced by LBBB, as displayed in Fig. 2. Consequently, CRT improves pump function, as indicated by increased $LVdP/dt_{max}$, pulse pressure, LV stroke work, and cardiac index [9,11], and decreases pulmonary–capillary wedge pressure [12]. These improvements occur almost instantaneously and without increasing myocardial energy consumption [13]. CRT also shortens the isovolumic contraction and relaxation times, resulting in an increased filling time [14].

Various mechanistic studies evaluated the long-term effects of CRT. In canine (nonfailing) hearts, Vernooy and colleagues [15] showed that on induction of LBBB, $LVdP/dt_{max}$ decreased to 79% of the pre-LBBB value. $LVdP/dt_{max}$ recovered to 89% and 95% of pre-LBBB values with acute CRT and after 8 weeks of CRT, respectively. Also, in patients, it has been shown that the benefit for LV pump function is maintained in the long run [16], if not improved further [17]. Furthermore, CRT leads to a reduction in LV end-systolic and end-diastolic volumes and LV wall mass in addition to a reduction in asymmetric hypertrophy in the canine LBBB model [15] (Fig. 4) and in human patients [17–19]. Thus, improved ventricular pump function and geometry over time indicate that CRT is able to reverse pathologic ventricular remodeling. Yu and colleagues [17] demonstrated that on cessation of CRT, the process of maladaptive remodeling (ie, gradual decrease in LV pump function and increase in LV volumes) returns.

Clinical trials

Currently, approximately 4000 patients who have heart failure have been included in major single- or double-blind randomized controlled trials of CRT [20–26].

Inclusion criteria for these trials were presence of impaired functional status (New York Heart Association [NYHA] functional class III or IV congestive heart failure), normal sinus rhythm, QRS duration of at least 120 or 150 milliseconds on surface electrocardiography (ECG) with interventricular conduction disturbances, and an impaired LV function (left ventricular ejection fraction [LVEF] <35%). Mostly, end points reflected functional status or LV reverse remodeling; however, the Comparison of Medical Therapy, Pacing, and Defibrillation in Heart Failure (COMPANION) trial [25] and Cardiac Resynchronization-Heart Failure (CARE-HF) trial [26] also showed a reduction in mortality by CRT. Data from selected randomized trials are summarized in Table 1.

Points of concern for selection: nonresponders and mechanical dyssynchrony

Despite the uniform success of clinical trials, a significant proportion of apparently suitable patients do not respond to CRT. Studies that used functional status as the determinant of response (ie, improvement in NYHA functional class) reported nonresponse rates of 20% to 30% [27,28]. In contrast, when using LV reverse remodeling as an end point (ie, a decrease in left ventricular end systolic volume [LVESV] or an increase in LVEF), the rate of nonresponse was 40% to 50% [29,30]. The former relates to subjective patient-experienced improvement, whereas the latter is a more objective criterion. In the Multicenter InSync Randomized Clinical Evaluation (MIRACLE) trial [22], approximately 30% of patients in the control group (ie, device implanted but inactive) improved at least one NYHA functional class, showing that factors like inclusion and extra care in a clinical trial, in addition to

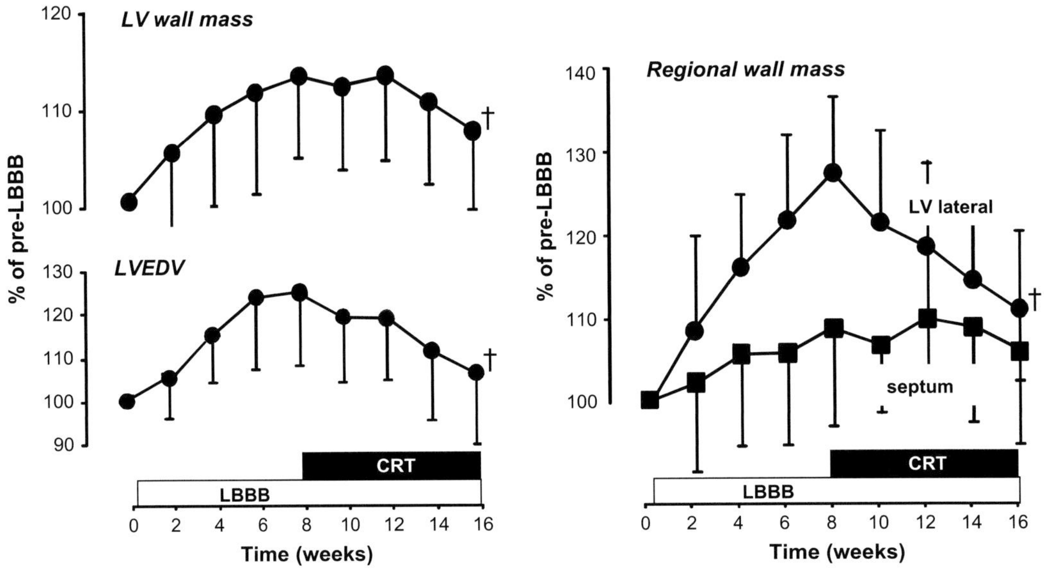

Fig. 4. Relative changes in left ventricle end-diastolic volume (LVEDV; *left panel, top*) and total LV wall mass (*left panel, bottom*) and change (*right panel*) in septal (*squares*) and LV lateral (*circles*) wall mass. †$P < .05$ at 16 weeks versus 8 weeks. Values are presented as mean ± SD. (*Modified from* Vernooy K, Cornelussen RN, Verbeek XA, et al. Cardiac resynchronization therapy cures dyssynchronopathy in canine left bundle-branch block hearts. Eur Heart J 2007;28: 2153; with permission.)

the placebo effect regarding device implantation, have important consequences for the patients' perceived fitness. The 40% to 50% of nonresponders, as observed by echocardiography, may thus better reflect the lack of a clear (patho)physiologic benefit in almost half of the patients who receive CRT and indicates that considerable efforts are needed to increase the efficiency of CRT in health care.

Electrical or mechanical dyssynchrony

In all large multicenter CRT trials, a widened QRS complex (ranging from >120 to >150 milliseconds) was an important inclusion criterion. Later studies (not clinical trials) suggested an additional role for "mechanical dyssynchrony" in predicting response to CRT. Arguments were that prediction of the success of CRT did not correlate perfectly with QRS width and that the hemodynamic and clinical benefits of CRT were not related to narrowing of the QRS complex [22]. Recently, however, mechanical dyssynchrony has been criticized because it did not improve the prediction of response to CRT in multicenter trials [31–33]. The authors discuss these disappointing findings in the next sections.

Measuring mechanical dyssynchrony

Over the past decade, various techniques and approaches have been used to determine mechanical dyssynchrony. An extensive review of imaging techniques is not within the scope of this article and can be found elsewhere [34]. In short, measures of mechanical dyssynchrony may be based on timing of valve opening or on displacement, velocity, or deformation (strain) of tissue. The relation between the latter three mechanical variables is displayed in Fig. 5.

Interventricular dyssynchrony

Interventricular dyssynchrony can be measured by pulsed-wave Doppler echocardiography, assessing the difference in left and right ventricular pre-ejection intervals, measured from QRS onset to the beginning of aortic and pulmonary Doppler flow velocity curves. An aortic-pulmonary pre-ejection interval of more than 40 milliseconds is regarded as a significant delay [34].

Measures relying on displacement of tissue

These methods measure displacement of tissue with respect to a certain reference point. The septal-to-posterior wall motion delay (SPWMD) is measured using conventional

Table 1
Randomized controlled trials of cardiac resynchronization therapy

Study	Enrollment (publication) dates	N	Length of FU (months)	End points: 6-MWT	Peak VO_2	NYHA fc	QOL	LV remodeling	Hospitalization for CHF	All-cause mortality
PATH-CHF [20]	1995–1998 (2002)	41	3	1[a]	1	2[a]	2[a]		2[a]	2
MUSTIC-SR [21]	1998–1999 (2001)	58	3	1	2[a]	2[a]	2[a]	2[a]	2	2
MIRACLE [22]	1998–2000 (2002)	453	6	1[a]	2	1[a]	1[a]	2[a]	2[a]	2
COMPANION [25]	2000–2002 (2004)	1520	15						1[a,b]	1[a,b], 2
CARE-HF [26]	2001–2003 (2004)	813	29			2[a]	2[a]	2[a]	2[a]	1[a]

Indicated are the primary (1) and secondary end points (2) and whether these end points were met.

Abbreviations: CHF, congestive heart failure; FU, follow-up; MUSTIC-SR, Multisite Stimulation in Cardiomyopathy—Sinus Rhythm; 6-MWT, 6-minute walk test; NYHA fc, New York Heart Association functional class; PATH-CH, Pacing Therapies for Congestive Heart Failure; QOL, quality of life; VO_2, oxygen uptake.

[a] Statistically significant improvement.

[b] Composite of time to first all-cause mortality or admission.

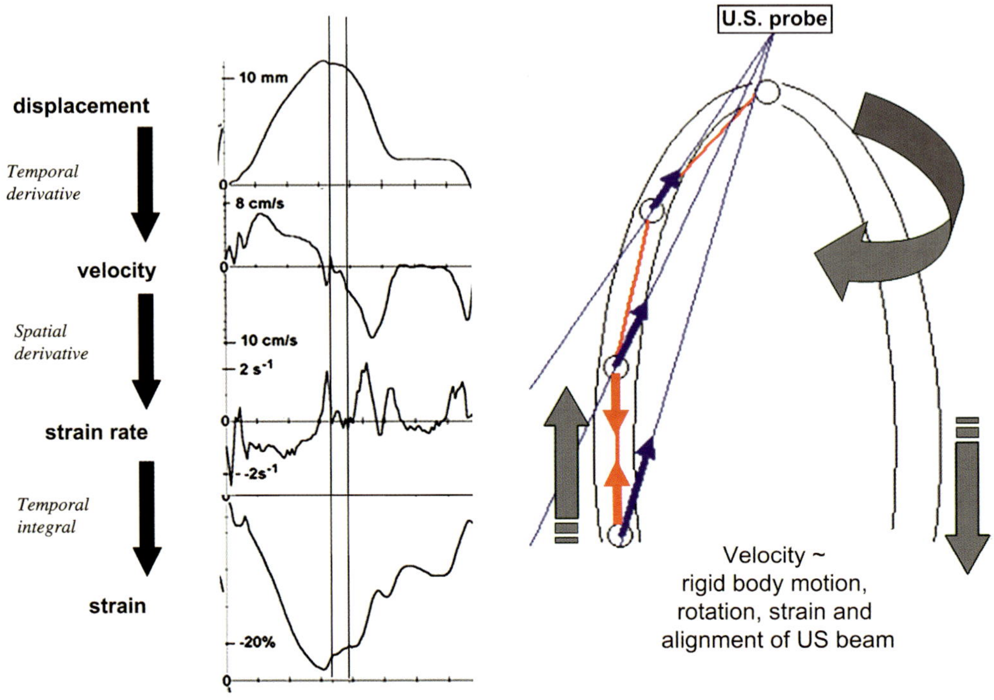

Fig. 5. Principles of measurement of myocardial displacement, velocity, strain rate, and strain using ultrasound (US) techniques. Tissue Doppler imaging (TDI) measures velocities of the tissue with respect to the US probe (*blue lines*). Local velocity depends on rigid body motion of the ventricle and on rotation (*gray arrows*) and shortening (*red arrows*), whereas only the latter reflects local mechanical behavior of the tissue. (*Data from* Stoylen A. Basic ultrasound for clinicians. Trondheim (Norway): Norwegian University of Science and Technology; 2006. Available at: http://folk.-ntnu.no/stoylen/strainrate/Ultrasound/index.html#section_index.)

M-mode echocardiography and is defined as the delay between the maximal inward movement of the septum and the LV lateral wall (see Fig. 1, right panel). An SPWMD greater than 130 milliseconds has been shown to predict the clinical and echocardiographic response to CRT [29].

Novel three-dimensional (3D) echocardiography technology allows us to measure endocardial wall motion in many LV wall segments. From this motion, regional ejection fraction is derived, as calculated using a central cavitary reference point [34]. The regional differences in peak endocardial wall motion are then used to describe ventricular dyssynchrony.

Tissue tracking (TT) measures the displacement of segments of myocardium with respect to the ultrasound transducer. Dyssynchrony is assessed by determining the location and the number of wall segments with delayed longitudinal displacement (ie, after aortic valve closure) and by measuring the magnitude of the time delay for each segment [34].

Measures relying on tissue velocity of tissue

Tissue Doppler imaging (TDI) measures the velocity of myocardial displacement and, consequently, results in noisier signals than displacement measurements (see Fig. 5; Fig. 6). Commonly measured parameters include the time from end-diastole to onset or peak systolic velocity. Regional differences in these times are the most commonly used indicators of mechanical dyssynchrony. Examples are the septal-to-lateral wall delay in peak systolic velocity and the standard deviation of the time to peak systolic velocity for 12 LV wall segments (Ts-SD-12) [34].

TDI has theoretic and technical limitations (Fig. 5), some of which were demonstrated in a recent study [33]. TDI measures velocity in the direction of the ultrasound beam rather than along the muscle fibers. Fig. 5 shows that local velocity (blue arrows) is a function of many factors, with only one of them being local shortening. It can be seen that TDI can make significant errors in estimating local myocardial behavior when

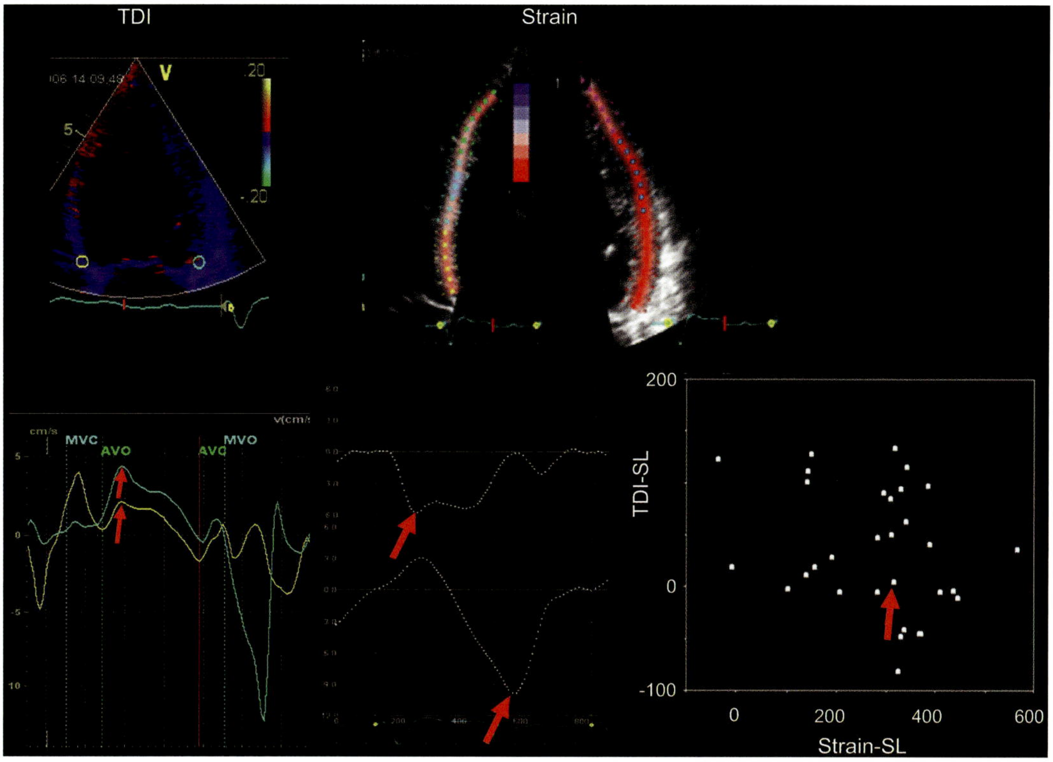

Fig. 6. TDI and strain registrations in a candidate for CRT. The left part of the figure shows that the time of peak velocity was similar in the septum (*yellow*) and LV posterior wall (*blue*). The middle panel shows strain signals, as obtained by speckle-tracking analysis in the same patient. Peak shortening is clearly dyssynchronous. The right panel shows the poor relation between dyssynchrony as measured by strain (*horizontal axis*) and velocity (*vertical axis*). The red arrows point to peak velocity (*right panel*), peak shortening (*middle panel*), and the data point related to the presented patient (*right panel*). AVO, aorta valve opening; MVC, mitral valve closure; MVO, mitral valve opening; Strain-SL, peak 2-dimensional longitudinal strain; TDI-SL, TDI-derived septal-to-lateral delays of peak velocities.

wall segments are not aligned with the ultrasound beam [33]. Velocity tracings can also change considerably by even slight changes in the position of the sample volume, thereby also changing the timing of peak velocities (see Fig. 5) [33]. Because of the complex signals and the flexible criteria, even experienced observers disagreed on the choice of a peak in the velocity tracing in most of 18 TDI measurements [33].

Although these problems seem to be well dealt with in single-center studies, the PROSPECT multicenter trial showed disappointing predictions of CRT success by echocardiographic indices of mechanical dyssynchrony. Preliminary results indicate that although some indices of dyssynchrony did correlate with CRT response, their sensitivity and specificity were fairly poor. As a consequence, it was concluded that no single measure of mechanical dyssynchrony could be recommended to improve patient selection further beyond the current guidelines [32]. Additionally, marked inter- and intraobserver variability was noticed, indicating that methodology to determine mechanical dyssynchrony needs further elaboration.

Measures relying on strain

Strain represents the extent of deformation of a tissue segment over time and is expressed as the percentage of segmental shortening or lengthening in relation to its original dimension. Thus, strain describes the mechanical performance of a specific myocardial region. As shown in Figs. 1 and 5, strain signals are easier to analyze than velocity signals because they contain less peaks and are less noisy.

The first measurements on strain-based indices of "mechanical dyssynchrony" with imaging techniques were performed using MRI tagging [35]. Tags are temporarily applied changes in the magnetic field, creating planes of saturation, leading to a family of lines usually imposed at end diastole. These lines stick to the myocardium and move during subsequent phases of the cardiac cycle. Strain is calculated by measuring the difference in displacement between adjacent sites (see red arrows in Fig. 5). Various indices of mechanical dyssynchrony have been calculated from strain information [36]. MRI tagging is regarded as the "gold standard" for strain imaging, but it is expensive and time-consuming. Therefore, it is primarily a research tool.

Strain can also be determined by postprocessing of TDI velocities on two adjacent regions to strain rate and, subsequently, strain (see Fig. 5). Doing so, Breithardt and colleagues [37] showed that in describing dyssynchrony and its changes attributable to CRT, the calculated strain yielded more reliable information than tissue Doppler velocities. Strain analysis from TDI is problematic, however, because all errors of TDI, as mentioned previously, make subtraction of two such signals cumbersome, time-consuming, and operator dependent [34].

A novel approach to quantify myocardial strain from echocardiographic data is speckle tracking [38]. The gray-scale echo image consists of a speckled pattern. Speckle-tracking software tracks the frame-to-frame movement of these acoustic markers throughout the myocardium, similar to the analysis of MRI tagging. De Boeck and colleagues [33] showed that dyssynchrony based on speckle-tracking strains provides a more reliable prediction of CRT response than TDI. Fig. 6 shows an example of a patient in whom nearly synchronous TDI velocities coincide with highly dyssynchronous strains.

Strategies to improve response to cardiac resynchronization therapy further using mechanical information

Deformations in dyssynchronous hearts are complex; in comparison with regionally ischemic hearts, for example, they show considerably larger regional differences and multiphasic signals. Accordingly, only techniques providing comprehensive and reliable data on deformation can be expected to provide a good estimation of mechanical dyssynchrony. The best way to characterize the mechanical behavior of the asynchronous heart seems to be by using strain analysis. With the availability of novel strain measuring techniques (eg, speckle tracking, velocity vector imaging), such characterization may improve over the following years.

Mechanical dyssynchrony inherently relates to time differences in, for example, onset or peak strain. Such differences may only partially reflect the loss of ventricular pump function, however. A more comprehensive impression may be achieved from indices describing discoordination (ie, amount or distribution of stretch and shortening within the LV wall). Examples of such indices are the CURE index [39] and the recently presented internal stretch fraction (ISF). With respect to the latter index, preliminary data indicate that distinction between CRT responders (defined as reduction in LVESV $>15\%$) and nonresponders can be made using ISF but not by using timing differences in onset and peak shortening, as measured by MRI tagging [40]. Therefore, in the near future, studies need to explore to what extent discoordination and dyssynchrony provide additive information on the prediction of the response of a patient to CRT.

Points for better therapy application: site of stimulation and atrioventricular and interventricular intervals

Site of stimulation

Initially, LV pacing leads for CRT were placed on the epicardium surgically [10], but these approaches were largely abandoned because of morbidity from surgery. In 1998, Daubert and colleagues [41] introduced a transvenous approach for LV lead placement using the branches of the coronary sinus. Since that time, most LV leads have been placed transvenously. From a mechanistic point of view, optimal pacing sites are those that render the maximal reduction in total electrical activation time. Optimal transvenous lead positioning is limited by venous anatomy, accessibility of the vein, lead stability, pacing threshold, and phrenic nerve stimulation, however.

Several studies show that a (postero)lateral lead position is a good location and an anterior lead position is a poor location. Optimal pacing sites seem to depend on the patient, however. In nonischemic CRT candidates, Ansalone and colleagues [42] used echocardiography to show that the last activated site was the lateral wall in 35%, the anterior wall in 26%, the posterior wall in 23%, and the inferior or septal region in 16% of patients. Murphy and colleagues [43] showed that the largest LV remodeling occurred when the LV lead was positioned at the site of latest mechanical activation. Dekker and colleagues

[44] investigated acute hemodynamic effects of various predefined epicardial pacing locations in patients receiving CRT using pressure-volume loops. They demonstrated that optimal lead position varies among patients and that suboptimal lead positioning may even deteriorate the acute hemodynamic response.

If transvenous leads cannot be properly positioned, there are at least two options: the transatrial septal approach and the epicardial approach. The atrial transseptal approach is successfully applied by other centers when lead placement in the coronary veins is not possible [45,46]

If access can be achieved, epicardial LV lead implantation is easy and well controllable, and may thus enhance individually tailored LV lead positioning. Another benefit is the avoidance of the vascular system, which may reduce the risk for venous complications, such as perforations or dissections of the coronary sinus. In the recent past, minimally invasive techniques have been developed to avoid the attendant morbidity from full sternotomy surgery. Joshi and colleagues [47] reported follow-up data of 84 patients undergoing robot-assisted epicardial lead placement after thoracotomy. In all patients, the site of latest mechanical activation (assessed by TDI before surgery) could be reached. They reported a higher clinical response rate when compared with coronary sinus approaches. Zenati and colleagues [48] described a minimally invasive surgical approach for epicardial lead implantation requiring only a limited subxiphoid incision. Sosa and colleagues [49] described an even less invasive subxiphoid technique to access the pericardium using a blunted epidural (17-gauge) needle advanced toward the cardiac area under fluoroscopic guidance. The technique proved to be safe, easy to perform, and reproducible. In the future, this approach may be modified to allow introduction of pacing leads. Lead placement in this way may also be combined with epicardial mapping strategies to determine the optimal LV pacing site [50]. An alternative approach is to position the LV lead at the LV endocardium, which is approached with a lead through the atrial septum and the mitral valve. This has been successfully used by two groups, and hemodynamic benefit seems to be at least as high as using the transvenous approach [46]. Finally, several groups report successful addition of a second LV lead if the first one did not result in a good response to CRT [51]. These studies are, however, small and require further validation.

Device programming

Another way to optimize CRT is to program the best AV delay and VV interval. These parameters can be programmed after implantation of the device, and thus can be adapted later on when necessary.

Several techniques, such as transmitral Doppler flow, tissue tracking, LV$dP/dt_{max}$, and digital photoplethysmography (Finapres Medical Systems, Amsterdam, The Netherlands), have been described for this optimization, as recently reviewed elsewhere [52]. It is remarkable how different the results of these optimization procedures are. Some studies show little effect, whereas other studies find considerable benefit of sequential over simultaneous biventricular pacing. Also, RV and LV pre-excitation are reported to be optimal in case of sequential biventricular pacing. These differences are poorly understood and seem to necessitate determining all possible combinations of the two delays during hemodynamic measurements, which seems to be too time-consuming for routine application.

Recently, Vernooy and colleagues [53] published a novel concept for finding the optimal combination of AV delay and VV interval. Important is the notion that although AV delay is a determinant of filling in conventional pacing therapy, in CRT, AV delay also determines the degree of synchronization. As shown in Fig. 7, at short AV delays, both ventricles are activated by RV and LV stimulation. On prolongation of the AV delay, intrinsic activation from the right bundle branch starts to dominate, thus reducing the degree of synchronization and hemodynamic benefit. In the Pacing Therapies for Congestive Heart Failure (PATH-CHF) study [54], the best hemodynamic effects were achieved at AV delays less than half of the PR interval. Therefore, AV delay and VV interval both influence the degree of resynchronization. To simplify optimal programming, the effective VV interval (VV_{eff}) can be calculated. This VV_{eff} is the time between LV stimulation and RV activation, wherein the latter can be caused by intrinsic activation or by RV stimulation, whichever occurs first. It was shown that the time of intrinsic RV activation can be easily measured by means of surface ECG. Using this concept, it was also shown experimentally that the same hemodynamic effect can be obtained by different combinations of AV delay and VV interval yet lead to the same hemodynamic effect (Fig. 8) [53].

These data indicate that a conceptual rather than empiric approach facilitates optimization of device programming, especially because many

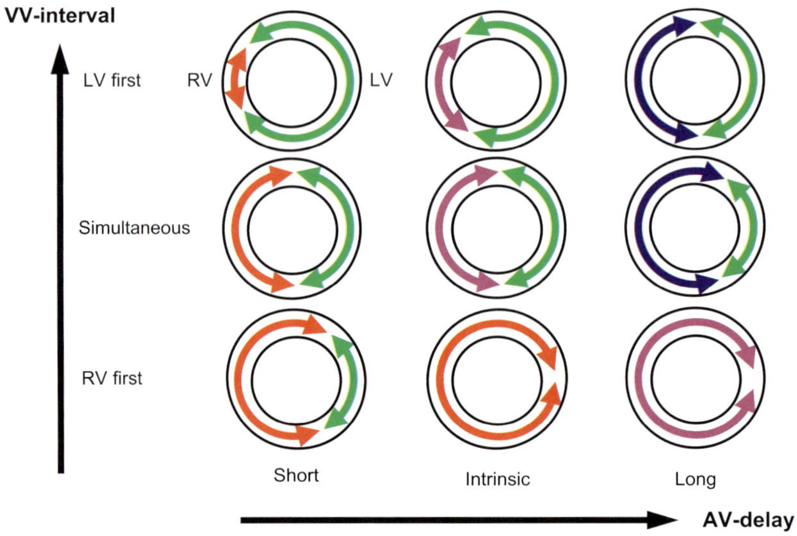

Fig. 7. Schematic LV electrical activation at various AV delays and VV intervals. Arrows indicate conduction paths induced by intrinsic activation (*blue*), RV pacing (*red*), combination of intrinsic activation and RV pacing (*purple*), and LV pacing (*green*). For explanation, see text. At longer AV delays, the LV lateral wall still can be activated by LV pacing, because activation of the LV lateral wall is delayed as a result of slow myocardial conduction. Also note that the same synchrony of activation can be achieved by multiple combinations of AV delay and VV interval. (*Modified from* Vernooy K, Verbeek XA, Cornelussen RN, et al. Calculation of effective VV interval facilitates optimization of AV delay and VV interval in cardiac resynchronization therapy. Heart Rhythm 2007;4:76; with permission.)

parameters used for device optimization are subject to considerable variability.

New growth areas: prevention of heart failure, narrow QRS complex

Prevention of heart failure

Studies in animals and human patients showed that asynchronous activation reduces pump function even in the absence of heart failure. Similarly, a study in canine hearts showed that biventricular pacing reverses the negative hemodynamic effects and the ventricular remodeling attributable to isolated LBBB in the absence of heart failure (see Fig. 2) [15]. Therefore, it seems reasonable to suppose that all patients with asynchronous activation (eg, RV pacing, LBBB) would benefit from resynchronization, irrespective of heart failure classification. In patients who do not have heart failure, CRT may be regarded as a prophylactic therapy, preventing progression to (more severe) heart failure. The MIRACLE Implantable Cardioverter-Defibrillator (ICD) II trial [55] compared the benefit of CRT in patients with NYHA class II and an indication for an ICD. Although patients with CRT did not show significant clinical improvement

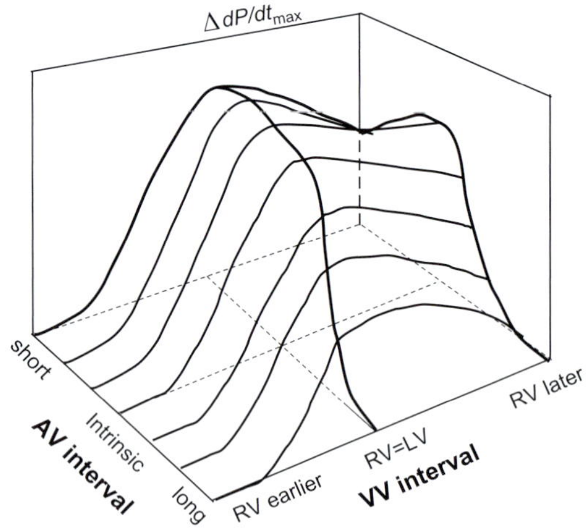

Fig. 8. Schematic changes in LV$dP/dt_{max}$ during biventricular pacing at various combinations of AV delay and VV interval in the canine heart with LBBB. (*Data from* Vernooy K, Verbeek XA, Cornelussen RN, et al. Calculation of effective VV interval facilitates optimization of AV delay and VV interval in cardiac resynchronization therapy. Heart Rhythm 2007;4:75–82.)

(6-minute walk test and quality-of-life score) compared with those without CRT, their LVEF, LV remodeling indices (LV diastolic and systolic volumes), and composite clinical response improved significantly over 6 months. Also, Bleeker and colleagues [56] found similar reverse remodeling in class II patients as compared with class III and IV patients. These data are supported by a large sample size study with 12 months of follow-up [57]. More studies in patients who have milder degrees of heart failure are required to substantiate the idea that CRT can be used to prevent the development of heart failure. Of course, it remains to be seen whether such prevention is worth covering the costs of the devices.

Cardiac resynchronization therapy in narrow QRS complex?

The great success of CRT in patients with a wide QRS complex has led some investigators to extend CRT to patients with a narrow QRS complex, especially in case of mechanical dyssynchrony. The physiologic explanation for a benefit in this category of patients is not clear, however; a benefit could only be explained by the presence of considerable electromechanical dissociation. After all, in the presence of synchronous electrical activation, considerable mechanical dyssynchrony can only be achieved when there are extensive regional differences in the electromechanical interval (at least ~100 milliseconds). Such large electromechanical dissociation has never been demonstrated convincingly, however. As recently pointed out by Kass [58], the mechanical dyssynchrony in the presence of narrow QRS complexes may be related to regional differences in contractile force rather than to different timing. Because regional differences in contractile force are likely not amenable for pacing therapy, it may not be surprising that the recent RethinQ study [31] showed no benefit of CRT. This multicenter, prospective, randomized controlled trial evaluated the efficacy of CRT in patients with a narrow QRS complex (< 130 milliseconds) and evidence of mechanical dyssynchrony on echocardiography. As compared with a control group, 6 months of CRT did not improve peak oxygen consumption or echocardiographic parameters (eg, LVESV, LVEF).

This negative finding may not completely exclude a beneficial effect of CRT in patients with a narrow QRS complex and heart failure. Bleasdale and colleagues [59] showed that irrespective of QRS width, in patients with increased pulmonary capillary wedge pressure (> 15 mm Hg), LV pre-excitation results in better filling of the LV, and thus, through the Frank-Starling effect, better pump function. This mechanism is referred to as ventricular interaction. This alternative and potentially additive effect of LV-based stimulation clearly deserves further investigation, especially in long-term studies.

In summary, this article illustrates the highly interesting possibilities of CRT yet also discusses several problems for optimal implementation. After a period of rapid growth of the number of implants and enthusiasm on the part of many cardiologists, it is now time for a more critical view of the real potential. The authors have presented possible strategies to improve CRT further by designing and using better measurements of mechanical dyssynchrony or discoordination, leading to better patient selection. In addition, application of CRT can be improved by developing techniques to reach the optimal pacing site(s) easier and algorithms for easier programming of optimal AV delay and VV interval. Also, application of CRT in patients with less severe heart failure deserves further attention. Finally, the mechanism of ventricular interaction may open new fields of application of LV-based pacing in patients who have heart failure, even with a narrow QRS complex. Some of these aspects can only be developed if basic mechanisms of CRT are understood better.

References

[1] McAlister FA, Ezekowitz J, Hooton N, et al. Cardiac resynchronization therapy for patients with left ventricular systolic dysfunction: a systematic review. JAMA 2007;297:2502–14.

[2] Clayton PD, Bulawa WF, Klausner SC, et al. The characteristic sequence for the onset of contraction in the normal human left ventricle. Circulation 1979;59:671–9.

[3] Grines CL, Bashore TM, Boudoulas H, et al. Functional abnormalities in isolated left bundle branch block. The effect of interventricular asynchrony. Circulation 1989;79:845–53.

[4] Vernooy K, Verbeek XA, Peschar M, et al. Left bundle branch block induces ventricular remodelling and functional septal hypoperfusion. Eur Heart J 2005;26:91–8.

[5] Spragg DD, Kass DA. Pathobiology of left ventricular dyssynchrony and resynchronization. Prog Cardiovasc Dis 2006;49:26–41.

[6] Prinzen FW, Peschar M. Relation between the pacing induced sequence of activation and left

ventricular pump function in animals. Pacing Clin Electrophysiol 2002;25:484–98.
[7] Sweeney MO, Prinzen FW. A new paradigm for physiologic ventricular pacing. J Am Coll Cardiol 2006;47:282–8.
[8] Verbeek XA, Vernooy K, Peschar M, et al. Intraventricular resynchronization for optimal left ventricular function during pacing in experimental left bundle branch block. J Am Coll Cardiol 2003; 42:558–67.
[9] Auricchio A, Stellbrink C, Block M, et al. Effect of pacing chamber and atrioventricular delay on acute systolic function of paced patients with congestive heart failure. The Pacing Therapies for Congestive Heart Failure Study Group. The Guidant Congestive Heart Failure Research Group. Circulation 1999;99:2993–3001.
[10] Cazeau S, Ritter P, Bakdach S, et al. Four chamber pacing in dilated cardiomyopathy. Pacing Clin Electrophysiol 1994;17:1974–9.
[11] Kass DA, Chen CH, Curry C, et al. Improved left ventricular mechanics from acute VDD pacing in patients with dilated cardiomyopathy and ventricular conduction delay. Circulation 1999;99: 1567–73.
[12] Blanc JJ, Etienne Y, Gilard M, et al. Evaluation of different ventricular pacing sites in patients with severe heart failure: results of an acute hemodynamic study. Circulation 1997;96:3273–7.
[13] Nelson GS, Berger RD, Fetics BJ, et al. Left ventricular or biventricular pacing improves cardiac function at diminished energy cost in patients with dilated cardiomyopathy and left bundle-branch block. Circulation 2000;102:3053–9.
[14] Zhou Q, Henein M, Coats A, et al. Different effects of abnormal activation and myocardial disease on left ventricular ejection and filling times. Heart 2000;84:272 6.
[15] Vernooy K, Cornelussen RN, Verbeek XA, et al. Cardiac resynchronization therapy cures dyssynchronopathy in canine left bundle-branch block hearts. Eur Heart J 2007;28:2148–55.
[16] Nelson GS, Curry CW, Wyman BT, et al. Predictors of systolic augmentation from left ventricular preexcitation in patients with dilated cardiomyopathy and intraventricular conduction delay. Circulation 2000;101:2703–9.
[17] Yu CM, Chau E, Sanderson JE, et al. Tissue Doppler echocardiographic evidence of reverse remodeling and improved synchronicity by simultaneously delaying regional contraction after biventricular pacing therapy in heart failure. Circulation 2002;105:438–45.
[18] St John Sutton MG, Plappert T, Abraham WT, et al. Effect of cardiac resynchronization therapy on left ventricular size and function in chronic heart failure. Circulation 2003;107:1985–90.
[19] Zhang Q, Fung JW, Auricchio A, et al. Differential change in left ventricular mass and regional wall thickness after cardiac resynchronization therapy for heart failure. Eur Heart J 2006;27: 1423–30.
[20] Auricchio A, Stellbrink C, Sack S, et al. Long-term clinical effect of hemodynamically optimized cardiac resynchronization therapy in patients with heart failure and ventricular conduction delay. J Am Coll Cardiol 2002;39:2026–33.
[21] Cazeau S, Leclercq C, Lavergne T, et al. Effects of multisite biventricular pacing in patients with heart failure and intraventricular conduction delay. N Engl J Med 2001;344:873–80.
[22] Abraham WT, Fisher WG, Smith AL, et al. Cardiac resynchronization in chronic heart failure. N Engl J Med 2002;346:1845–53.
[23] Lozano I, Bocchiardo M, Achtelik M, et al. Impact of biventricular pacing on mortality in a randomized crossover study of patients with heart failure and ventricular arrhythmias. Pacing Clin Electrophysiol 2000;23:1711–2.
[24] Young JB, Abraham WT, Smith AL, et al. Combined cardiac resynchronization and implantable cardioversion defibrillation in advanced chronic heart failure: the MIRACLE ICD Trial. JAMA 2003;289:2685–94.
[25] Bristow MR, Saxon LA, Boehmer J, et al. Cardiac-resynchronization therapy with or without an implantable defibrillator in advanced chronic heart failure. N Engl J Med 2004;350:2140–50.
[26] Cleland JG, Daubert JC, Erdmann E, et al. The effect of cardiac resynchronization on morbidity and mortality in heart failure. N Engl J Med 2005; 352:1539–49.
[27] Lecoq G, Leclercq C, Leray E, et al. Clinical and electrocardiographic predictors of a positive response to cardiac resynchronization therapy in advanced heart failure. Eur Heart J 2005;26:1094–100.
[28] Bax JJ, Bleeker GB, Marwick TH, et al. Left ventricular dyssynchrony predicts response and prognosis after cardiac resynchronization therapy. J Am Coll Cardiol 2004;44:1834–40.
[29] Pitzalis MV, Iacoviello M, Romito R, et al. Ventricular asynchrony predicts a better outcome in patients with chronic heart failure receiving cardiac resynchronization therapy. J Am Coll Cardiol 2005;45:65–9.
[30] Yu CM, Fung JW, Zhang Q, et al. Tissue Doppler imaging is superior to strain rate imaging and postsystolic shortening on the prediction of reverse remodeling in both ischemic and nonischemic heart failure after cardiac resynchronization therapy. Circulation 2004;110:66–73.
[31] Beshai JF, Grimm RA, Nagueh SF, et al. Cardiac-resynchronization therapy in heart failure with narrow QRS complexes. N Engl J Med 2007; 357(24):2461–71.
[32] Cleland JG, Abdellah AT, Khaleva O, et al. Clinical trials update from the European Society of cardiology congress 2007: 3CPO, ALOFT, PROSPECT

and statins for heart failure. Eur J Heart Fail 2007;9: 1070–3.

[33] De Boeck BW, Meine M, Leenders GE, et al. Practical and conceptual limitations of tissue Doppler imaging to predict reverse remodelling in cardiac resynchronisation therapy. Eur J Heart Fail 2008; 10(3):281–90.

[34] Bax JJ, Ansalone G, Breithardt OA, et al. Echocardiographic evaluation of cardiac resynchronization therapy: ready for routine clinical use? A critical appraisal. J Am Coll Cardiol 2004;44:1–9.

[35] Wyman BT, Hunter WC, Prinzen FW, et al. Mapping propagation of mechanical activation in the paced heart with MRI tagging. Am J Physiol 1999; 276:H881–91.

[36] Lardo AC, Abraham TP, Kass DA. Magnetic resonance imaging assessment of ventricular dyssynchrony: current and emerging concepts. J Am Coll Cardiol 2005;46:2223–8.

[37] Breithardt OA, Stellbrink C, Herbots L, et al. Cardiac resynchronization therapy can reverse abnormal myocardial strain distribution in patients with heart failure and left bundle branch block. J Am Coll Cardiol 2003;42:486–94.

[38] Suffoletto MS, Dohi K, Cannesson M, et al. Novel speckle-tracking radial strain from routine black-and-white echocardiographic images to quantify dyssynchrony and predict response to cardiac resynchronization therapy. Circulation 2006;113:960–8.

[39] Helm RH, Leclercq C, Faris OP, et al. Cardiac dyssynchrony analysis using circumferential versus longitudinal strain: implications for assessing cardiac resynchronization. Circulation 2005;111:2760–7.

[40] Jansen AH, Kirn B, Bracke F, et al. Abstract 2016: myocardial internal strain fraction predicts volume response in patients with cardiac resynchronization therapy. Circulation 2006;114:405.

[41] Daubert JC, Ritter P, Le Breton H, et al. Permanent left ventricular pacing with transvenous leads inserted into the coronary veins. Pacing Clin Electrophysiol 1998;21:239–45.

[42] Ansalone G, Giannantoni P, Ricci R, et al. Doppler myocardial imaging to evaluate the effectiveness of pacing sites in patients receiving biventricular pacing. J Am Coll Cardiol 2002;39:489–99.

[43] Murphy RT, Sigurdsson G, Mulamalla S, et al. Tissue synchronization imaging and optimal left ventricular pacing site in cardiac resynchronization therapy. Am J Cardiol 2006;97:1615–21.

[44] Dekker AL, Phelps B, Dijkman B, et al. Epicardial left ventricular lead placement for cardiac resynchronization therapy: optimal pace site selection with pressure-volume loops. J Thorac Cardiovasc Surg 2004;127:1641–7.

[45] Jaïs P, Takahashi A, Garrigue S, et al. Mid-term follow-up of endocardial biventricular pacing. Pacing Clin Electrophysiol 2000;23:1744–7.

[46] van Gelder BM, Scheffer MG, Meijer A, et al. Transseptal endocardial left ventricular pacing: an alternative technique for coronary sinus lead placement in cardiac resynchronization therapy. Heart Rhythm 2007;4:454–60.

[47] Joshi S, Steinberg JS, Ashton RC Jr, et al. Follow-up of robotically assisted left ventricular epicardial leads for cardiac resynchronization therapy. J Am Coll Cardiol 2005;46:2358–9.

[48] Zenati MA, Bonanomi G, Chin AK, et al. Left heart pacing lead implantation using subxiphoid videopericardioscopy. J Cardiovasc Electrophysiol 2003;14: 949–53.

[49] Sosa E, Scanavacca M, d'Avila A, et al. A new technique to perform epicardial mapping in the electrophysiology laboratory. J Cardiovasc Electrophysiol 1996;7:531–6.

[50] Maessen JG, Phelps B, Dekker AL, et al. Minimal invasive epicardial lead implantation: optimizing cardiac resynchronization with a new mapping device for epicardial lead placement. Eur J Cardiothorac Surg 2004;25:894–6.

[51] Leclercq C, Gadler F, Kranig W, et al. A randomized comparison of triple versus dual site ventricular stimulation in patients with congestive heart failure. J Am Coll Cardiol, in press.

[52] Burri H, Sunthorn H, Shah D, et al. Optimization of device programming for cardiac resynchronization therapy. Pacing Clin Electrophysiol 2006;29:1416–25.

[53] Vernooy K, Verbeek XA, Cornelussen RN, et al. Calculation of effective VV interval facilitates optimization of AV delay and VV interval in cardiac resynchronization therapy. Heart Rhythm 2007;4: 75–82.

[54] Auricchio A, Stellbrink C, Sack S, et al. The Pacing Therapies for Congestive Heart Failure (PATH-CHF) study: rationale, design, and endpoints of a prospective randomized multicenter study. Am J Cardiol 1999;83:130D–135D.

[55] Abraham WT, Young JB, Leon AR, et al. Effects of cardiac resynchronization on disease progression in patients with left ventricular systolic dysfunction, an indication for an implantable cardioverter-defibrillator, and mildly symptomatic chronic heart failure. Circulation 2004;110:2864–8.

[56] Bleeker GB, Schalij MJ, Holman ER, et al. Cardiac resynchronization therapy in patients with systolic left ventricular dysfunction and symptoms of mild heart failure secondary to ischemic or nonischemic cardiomyopathy. Am J Cardiol 2006;98:230–5.

[57] Landolina M, Lunati M, Gasparini M, et al. Comparison of the effects of cardiac resynchronization therapy in patients with class II versus class III and IV heart failure (from the InSync/InSync ICD Italian Registry). Am J Cardiol 2007;100:1007–12.

[58] Kass DA. An epidemic of dyssynchrony: but what does it mean? J Am Coll Cardiol 2008;51:12–7.

[59] Bleasdale RA, Turner MS, Mumford CE, et al. Left ventricular pacing minimizes diastolic ventricular interaction, allowing improved preload-dependent systolic performance. Circulation 2004;110:2395–400.

ELSEVIER
SAUNDERS

Heart Failure Clin 4 (2008) 347–360

HEART
FAILURE
CLINICS

A New Look at Diastole

Julien I.E. Hoffman, MD[a,*], Aman Mahajan, MD, PhD[b], Cecil Coghlan, MD[c], Saleh Saleh, MD[b], Gerald D. Buckberg, MD[b]

[a]*University of California at San Francisco, San Francisco, CA, USA*
[b]*University of California at Los Angeles, Los Angeles, CA, USA*
[c]*University of Alabama at Birmingham, Birmingham, AL, USA*

The word "diastole" comes from two Greek roots: *dia* (apart) and *stellein* (put or make); one meaning of this combination is expansion or dilatation. Its counterpart is "systole," from *sus* (together) and *stellein*, and the combination can be interpreted as contraction. As early as 1628, William Harvey [1], in his publication *De Motu Cordis*, used these terms for these meanings. Both of these terms imply a volume change. These two periods of decreased and increased ventricular volumes are separated by periods in which volume does not change. An isovolumic period precedes systolic emptying. During this period ventricular pressure rises until it exceeds aortic pressure, the aortic valve opens, and blood begins to be ejected. This isovolumic period is termed the presystolic period. When ventricular pressure begins to decrease and the aortic valve closes, another isovolumic period begins, and it lasts until ventricular pressure decreases below atrial pressure, the atrioventricular valve opens, and blood begins to enter the ventricle. By analogy to the presystolic period, this should be termed the "prediastolic period." Care is needed in using these terms, because sometimes the presystolic and emptying periods are combined and called "systole," and the prediastolic and filling periods are combined and called "diastole." There are advantages to keeping the four periods separate because different mechanisms are associated with each of them.

Initially, studies of left ventricular function were confined to examining changes in pressures and the dimensions of the long and short axes, because only these measurements could easily be made with available tools. Left ventricular volumes were derived from angiographic or echocardiographic measurements based on geometric formulas, and then much later directly by the conductance method [2]. Although torsion of the ventricle (difference in rotational twisting between the base and apex of the ventricle) had been observed centuries ago, as initially described by Borelli in 1660 [3], it was not measured in human beings until the study by Ingels and colleagues in 1975 [4]. Arts and colleagues [5] included torsion in their modeling of the left ventricle, and subsequently implanted markers on the dog heart, made detailed measurements of torsion, and concluded that torsion was important in equalizing stresses across the ventricular wall [6]. More recently, torsion has been measured in the human ventricle by noninvasive measurements with tagged magnetic resonance imaging (MRI) [7,8], Doppler tissue imaging [8–12], or speckle tracking imaging [8,13–17], and described as an angular number that quantifies the difference between clockwise and counterclockwise rotation of the base and apex of the left ventricle, respectively. These studies have confirmed the magnitude and time course of torsion in systole and untwisting in diastole, and have shown that the rate of early diastolic untwisting is decreased in cardiac hypertrophy because of aortic stenosis [7], dilated cardiomyopathy [16], and in myocardial ischemia

* Corresponding author. University of California at San Francisco, 925 Tiburon Boulevard, Tiburon, CA 94920-1525.
E-mail address: julien.hoffman@ucsf.edu (J.I.E. Hoffman)

1551-7136/08/$ - see front matter
doi:10.1016/j.hfc.2008.02.013

[18]. The normal increase in untwisting with exercise is decreased with hypertrophic cardiomyopathy [10] or aging [13]. Ischemia, too, decreases intraventricular pressure gradients and apical filling [19,20].

During systole there is not only a decrease in the dimensions of the long and short axes of the ventricle, but the entire ventricle, including the base, mid, and apex undergoes rotation and reciprocal twisting leading to creation of torsion [7,15]. The torsion aids ventricular emptying in the same way that wringing out a wet towel removes more water than merely squeezing the towel would [3]. At the end of systole, when the aortic valve closes, there is a rapid untwisting of the ventricle. This untwisting creates a negative pressure or a suction in the ventricular cavity, and this negative pressure helps to open the atrioventricular valves and draws the blood into the ventricles [21–23]. As a result, most ventricular filling (especially the rapid suction phase that accounts for 50% or more of left ventricular filling) occurs well before atrial contraction. Abnormal untwisting decreases the suction, delays ventricular filling, and can lead to diastolic dysfunction.

The time interval between closure of the aortic valve until opening of the mitral valve during deceleration of ventricular pressure is termed the "isovolumic relaxation interval," because ventricular volume does not change during this phase of developing a negative intraventricular pressure. The changes of untwisting and the creation of negative ventricular pressure have been attributed to passive elastic recoil of a ventricle below its equilibrium volume. If one stops squeezing a rubber ball, the deformed ball returns to its resting volume because of restoring elastic forces. If one stops twisting a child's swing, it untwists because of restoring forces recovering the energy of twisting. These analogies have been used for the left ventricle in early diastole. The restoring forces have been regarded as caused by a "release of energy from previously distorted extra- ... and intracellular ... elastic structures [12]." The structures referred to are titin [24] and interstitial tissue [25].

There is, however, reason to believe that other major factors also play a part in untwisting, because recent studies (see below) have shown that the subepicardial spiral muscle band that forms the right half of the ventricular septum and left ventricular outflow tract (and corresponds to the ascending segment of the ventricular helix configuration) is still contracting during prediastole (Fig. 1) [26,27]. This observation suggests that the conventional term for this phase of cardiac cycle, isovolumic relaxation (IVR), must be reexamined to explain why such evidence of muscle contraction exists, provide a mechanical explanation for the muscular apparatus that may cause this normal physiologic event, examine how this

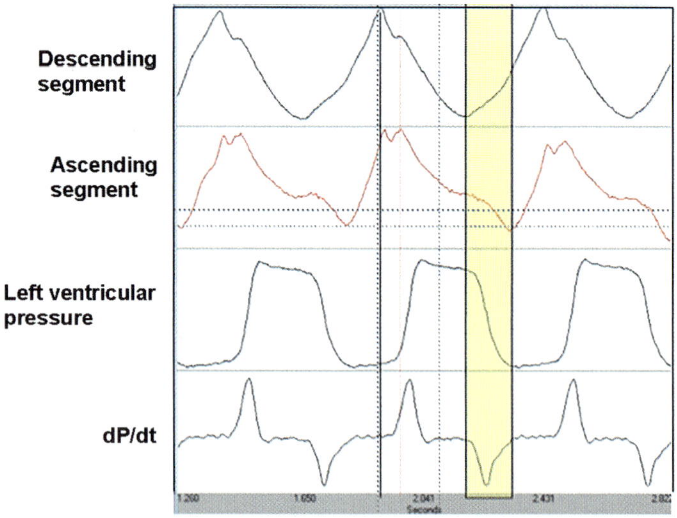

Fig. 1. Sonomicrometer tracings of the descending and ascending muscle bands. From above downward are sonomicrometer tracings of the descending and ascending muscle bands, with shortening moving down, and tracings of the left ventricular pressure and dP/dt. Note that in prediastole (*yellow rectangle*), the ascending band is still shortening while the descending band is relaxing.

phase may interact with events that interfere with diastolic untwisting, and determine if better understanding of its mechanisms can further our ability to use such knowledge to offset adverse diastolic dysfunction changes.

Structural observations

A brief description of the architecture of ventricular muscle is needed to make the involved mechanisms understandable. Although oblique fibers on the left ventricular surface had been described centuries ago, it was not until Streeter's studies that adequate details were provided [28,29]. Streeter used a T-shaped configuration, with the horizontal portion to sample the base and the vertical portion (that he called the "leg") to sample the muscle toward the apex. By making successive sections through the left ventricular free wall, he showed that the fiber angles varied with depth (Figs. 2 and 3).

At the base there were three main sets or layers of fibers. The outer (subepicardial) 20% of the left ventricular free wall has roughly parallel fibers that run at an angle of about 20 degrees to 80 degrees (mean about 50 degrees to 60 degrees) to the equatorial or short axis of the left ventricle. There is an abrupt change of direction to the fibers that occupy about 60% of the midwall and are approximately in the short axis plane at angles of 10 degrees to −10 degrees from that plane. Another abrupt change of direction leads to the 20% of deep (subendocardial) fibers that also have an angle of about 20 degrees to 80 degrees (mean about 60 degrees) to the equatorial plane, but in a direction opposite to the subepicardial fibers; the two oblique layers cross like an X. These findings have been confirmed by many later studies [30,31]. Note that because of the greater radius of subepicardial than subendocardial fibers, there is more subepicardial than subendocardial muscle. At the lower left ventricular wall toward the apex Streeter found predominantly two layers that crossed each other at about −60 degree and +60 degree angles, with "zero" at the mid ventricular position. This angulation is shown in the image of "leg" fiber angles in Fig. 3.

Streeter's studies did not include the septum, and were done on small blocks of ventricular tissue; therefore, he did not describe a spiral arrangement of fibers. His description of the base of the free wall, however, has been corroborated by recent studies with diffusion tensor MRI, a technique that has the ability to detect anisotropy because of differences in the orientation of muscle fibers [32,33]. These studies show

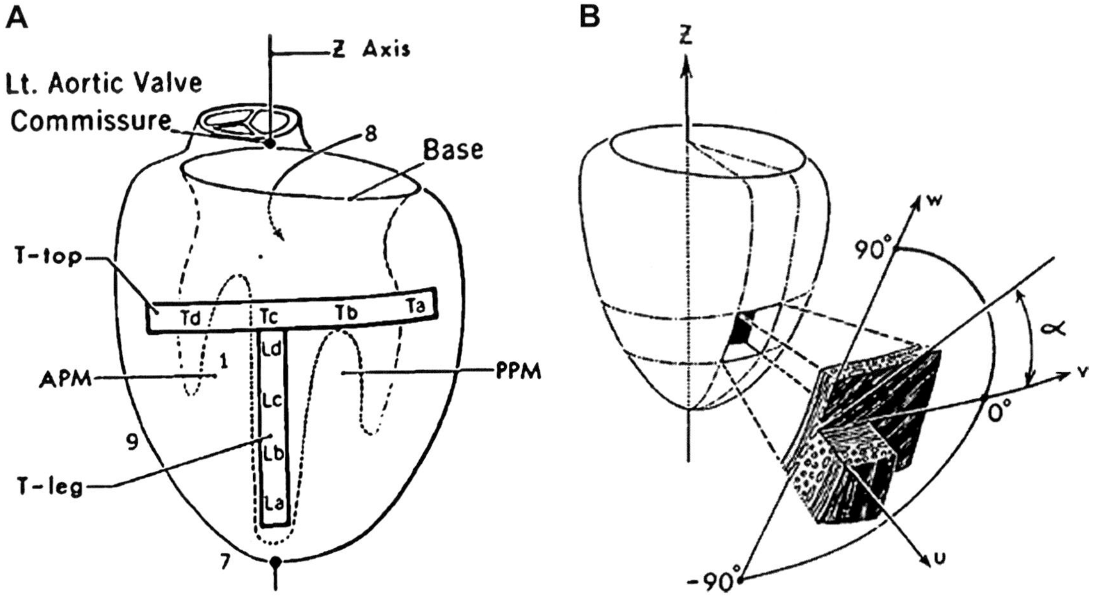

Fig. 2. Diagrams showing method of sectioning the wall and measuring the fiber angles. (*A*) Sites of sampling. (*B*) Method of measuring angles. (*From* Streeter DD, Jr., Spotnitz HM, Patel DP, et al. Fiber orientation in the canine left ventricle during diastole and systole. Circ Res 1969;24(3):339–47; with permission.)

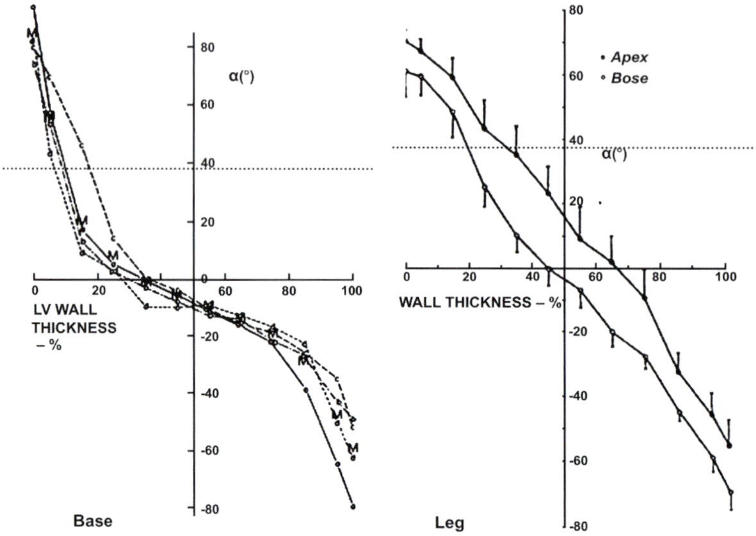

Fig. 3. Distribution of fiber angles across the left ventricular wall at the base and the leg (near the apex). Note that there is no circumferential layer near the apex. (*From* Streeter DD, Jr., Spotnitz HM, Patel DP, et al. Fiber orientation in the canine left ventricle during diastole and systole. Circ Res 1969;24(3):339–47; with permission.)

three layers of the free wall: an outer layer with a fiber angle of about 60 degrees to the equatorial plane, a horizontal (circumferential) middle layer, and an inner layer with a fiber angle of about 60 degrees in the opposite direction (see Fig. 3; Fig. 4). These transverse fibers are particularly well shown in the imaging by Zhukov and Barr [34] (Fig. 5), together with the oblique clockwise and counterclockwise fibers of the left and right handed helical arms of the subepicardium and subendocardium. The circumferential muscle does not reach the apex, which has therefore,

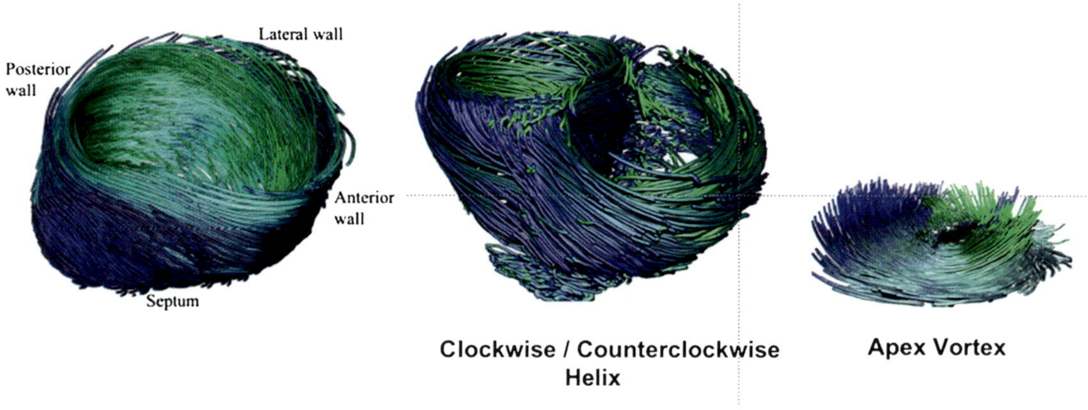

Fig. 4. View of left ventricular fibers in the human heart, with septum at bottom. Green: subendocardial spiral fibers. Light blue: circumferential fibers. Dark blue: fibers on right ventricular side of septum ("subepicardial"). (*Left panel*) Clockwise and counterclockwise helixes in the left ventricle, with circumferential fibers between them. (*Center panel*) Continuity of fibers from right to left ventricle. (*From* Rohmer D, Sitek A, Gullberg GT. Visualization of fiber structure in the left and right ventricle of a human heart. Lawrence Berkeley National Laboratory Report LBNL-61064, 2006; with permission.) (*Right panel*) Apical fibers showing descending subendocardial fibers forming vortex with ascending subepicardial fibers. The pale blue in this figure is an artifact of the rapid change of fiber angle. (*Left panel and right panel from* Rohmer D, Sitek A, Gullberg GT. Reconstruction and visualization of fiber and laminar structure in the normal human heart from ex vivo diffusion tensor magnetic resonance imaging (DTMRI) data. Invest Radiol 2007;42(11):777–89; with permission.)

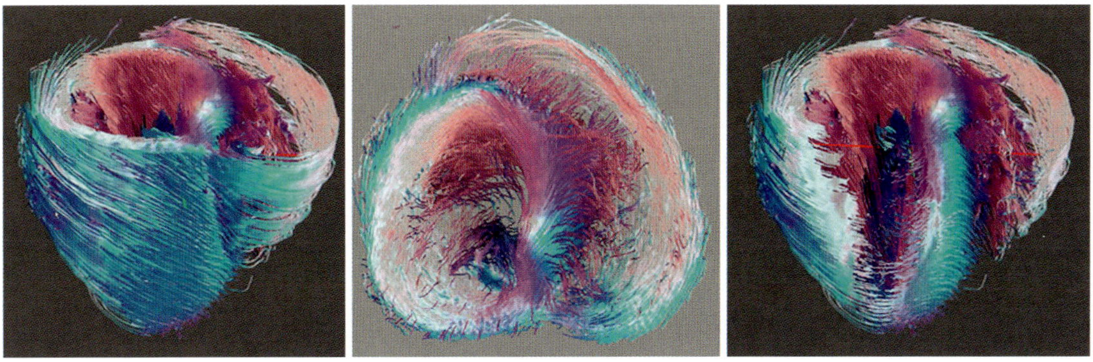

Fig. 5. Diffusion tensor MRI image of canine heart seen from behind. The clockwise subendocardial spiral fibers are in purple, the counterclockwise subepicardial fibers are shown in green-blue, and the circumferential fibers are in white. (*From* Zhukov L, Barr AH. Heart-muscle fiber reconstruction from diffusion tensor MRI. Proceedings of the 14th IEEE Visualization Conference 2003:597–602; with permission. Copyright © 2008, IEEE.)

only two layers of muscle. The circumferential muscle involving the outer ventricular wall and attached to the septum thus resembles a barrel with open upper and lower ends. The deep subendocardial fibers are arranged in a spiral that moves to the apex and forms a partial figure-8 loop, to ascend as another spiral layer on the right ventricular side of the ventricular septum (see Fig. 4). From the point of view of the left ventricle, these spiral bands are the inner and outer layers of its walls (see Figs. 4 and 5).

The embryologic development of these sets or layers of fibers is unknown, although this pattern has been seen as early as in 13 to 14 weeks of gestation in human beings [35,36]. These investigators, like Streeter, concluded that the ventricular muscle was arranged like geodesics on a set of nested twisted pretzels that resembled two doughnuts side by side. An alternative model was posited by Torrent-Guasp and colleagues [37], who regarded the ventricular muscle as a continuous band. The band starts at the base of the main pulmonary artery, passes horizontally to the left to form the basal loop that comprises the posterior walls of the right and left ventricles with predominantly horizontal fiber orientation, and continues as the circumferential muscle (middle layer) of the left ventricle. This description is common to all previously published studies of heart architecture [38]. At its left upper margin, the band turns or develops a mid-ventricular fold upon itself to produce obliquely oriented fiber bands into the left ventricle and to form the helical apical loop. This loop consists of a descending deep spiral muscle that develops a vortex at the apex and becomes the ascending spiral muscle of the left anterior free wall and left side of the septum, a muscle that is anchored to the aortic root. There are differences of detail among these models and many others that have been proposed, but they all agree on the presence of a clockwise and counterclockwise spiral and circumferential muscle bands.

The Torrent-Guasp model provides a simple and functional explanation for the spatial architectural structure of basal and apical loops. The model's principle anatomic contribution was to demonstrate that the myocardial fold changed fiber orientation and thus separated the basal and apical loop into predominantly horizontal and oblique fibers. Whatever the underlying model may be, we need to understand what roles each muscle layer or band plays during the contraction-relaxation cycle.

The presence of discrete muscle bands has been questioned, because cardiac muscle has been described as a syncytium. This is, however, only partly true, because Le Grice and colleagues [39,40] have shown that sheets of myofibers are enclosed by connective tissue to form a laminated structure that allows sliding of one sheet over another. They found, for example, that less than 50% of the wall thickening in systole could be explained by thickening of individual myofibers, the remainder being caused by slippage and rearrangement of muscle sheets.

Physiologic implications

One of the assumptions about the prediastolic period has been that because the decrease in left ventricular pressure after aortic valve closure indicates cessation of shortening and force generation of the ventricular muscle fibers, this cessation of myofiber contraction occurs synchronously throughout the ventricular muscle. For this reason, many investigators have referred to this period as the period of early diastolic relaxation or isovolumic relaxation. We now know that this is an oversimplification. For ventricular pressure to decrease, all that is needed is for some of the muscle to cease contraction. Newer knowledge about the prediastolic period shows that indeed, relaxation is not synchronous throughout the ventricular muscle (see Fig. 1). In fact, there is good evidence that relaxation in left ventricular muscle begins before aortic valve closure [41,42], and does so asynchronously [43]. We know too that contraction of the ascending (anterior wall and septal) spiral muscle continues as post systolic shortening throughout the whole prediastolic period and beyond it [26,27,44]. For this reason, the terms "diastolic relaxation" or "isovolumic ventricular relaxation" are ambiguous, and should be avoided unless qualified by specific descriptions.

An example of the effect of prolonged systolic forces during ejection was observed by Stuber, employing tagged MRI studies in patients with aortic stenosis (Fig. 6) [7]. Systolic contraction extended into the isovolumic phase (termed early diastole), and torsion was prolonged. The mechanism in aortic stenosis relates to maintenance of the descending segment's dominant role of abnormally prolonging shortening during the ejection phase and keeping the simultaneously contracting ascending segment in the shortened position. As a result, the "hiatus" during which the expected lengthening from unimpeded ascending contraction can lengthen the ventricle does not occur, and there is interference with the clockwise rotation that characterizes untwisting during the isovolumic phase. Furthermore, a similar pattern was observed following transient ischemia [45] to produce diastolic dysfunction (Fig. 7). Sonomicrometer crystal studies demonstrated that prolonged descending segment contraction limits the normal hiatus (approximately an 80-msec interval) between cessation of descending and ascending segment shortening to generate an abnormal pattern that is remedied by sodium-hydrogen exchange inhibitors. Recognition of this active process may lead to selection of new drugs that can modify a contractile mechanism for cardiac dynamics during the phase of rapid filling [45], and therefore remedy the diastolic dysfunctional component of congestive heart failure that affects approximately 50% of patients [46,47].

The change in shape of the left ventricle during prediastole and diastole has been described by Notomi and colleagues [10]. They observed that as soon as the left ventricle begins to untwist in prediastole, it widens slightly and lengthens. This creates a paradox, because prediastole is an isovolumic period and blood is incompressible. The resolution of the paradox is that the change in an irregular shape as occurs in the left ventricular cavity cannot be quantified by two linear measurements. In fact, studies of dimensional change in different regions of the left ventricle have shown that in the prediastolic period some regions nearer the apex decrease their dimensions slightly [48,49]. Lengthening of the left ventricle in the prediastolic period did not occur in one study [50]. In that study, however, there might be differences associated with cardiopulmonary bypass that was used, because this procedure may cause septal stunning. This issue was considered in regard to disruption of the normal prediastolic patterns (see Fig. 8). The physiologic untwisting action, that begins in the prediastolic period and is caused by a geometric dynamic change in shape, has been characterized by a series of hemodynamic changes that include measuring the rate of untwisting [51] as well as tau (change in time related to change in deceleration change in left ventricular pressure) [52,53], and also measuring the intraventricular pressure gradient that is maximal just after the mitral valve opens [12]. Each of these measured hemodynamic effects is caused by geometric ventricular dynamic mechanisms, and their understanding is therefore dependent upon recognizing the responsible initiating muscular structure.

Studies done to define the mechanisms of untwisting must be assessed with care. The complex anatomy of ventricular muscle mandates that markers or sonomicrometer crystal implanted in the wall must take account of fiber orientation and depth. Furthermore, because substantial shearing forces occur during twisting and untwisting, observations on the endocardial and epicardial surfaces may not coincide because the shortening output from surface crystals reflects the end result only of forces developed by the immediately underlying muscle. For example, Ashikaga and colleagues [31] used implanted markers tracked by biplane cinematography, and

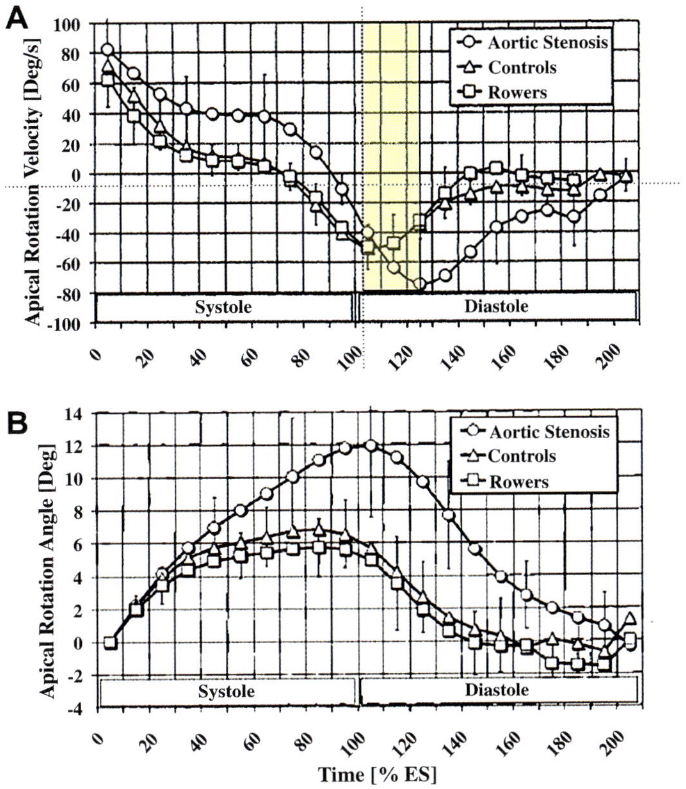

Fig. 6. Apical torsion in controls, trained athletes (rowers), and patients with aortic stenosis. In the last group, apical torsion continues beyond the end of systole. (*A*) Apical rotation velocity. (*B*) Apical rotation angle. The yellow rectangle marks the prediastolic period. (*From* Stuber M, Scheidegger MB, Fischer SE, et al. Alterations in the local myocardial motion pattern in patients suffering from pressure overload due to aortic stenosis. Circulation 1999;100(4):361–8; with permission.)

observed that in the prediastolic period the subepicardial fibers lengthened but the subendocardial fibers shortened. There are also possible differences between an open and a closed pericardium that might affect ventricular shape and thus fiber angles. Furthermore, Ingels and colleagues [54] found that shortening was most marked in the longitudinal fiber direction, as would be expected, so that a long axis measurement would not reveal the full magnitude of shortening if muscle with a different orientation on the endocardium contributed. The studies described above indicate the inability of a single global axial measurement to reflect the degree of contraction of each fiber layer.

Studies of muscle shortening and lengthening done with sonomicrometer crystals placed parallel to the long axes of the spiral muscle bands on the subepicardium and subendocardium, as well as the transversely oriented muscle at the base, have shown that early in prediastole muscle lengthening (positive strain) occurs in circumferential muscle of the base and deep descending spiral muscle fiber of the left ventricle, and 10 msec later in the lateral free wall of the left ventricle [26]. During ejection there is co-contraction of muscle in the subendocardum and subepicardium. Contraction ends nearly simultaneously in the lateral free wall and the subendocardium, but while this relaxation is occurring (reflected by absence of shortening and even crystal lengthening in these fibers), muscle of the subepicardial or ascending spiral fibers that are superficial (in terms of the left ventricular cavity) are still shortening (negative strain) and continue to do so for another 90 msec until they too relax and begin to lengthen (Fig. 8) [26,44]. These subepicardial fibers form the right side of the ventricular septum and anterior left ventricular free wall.

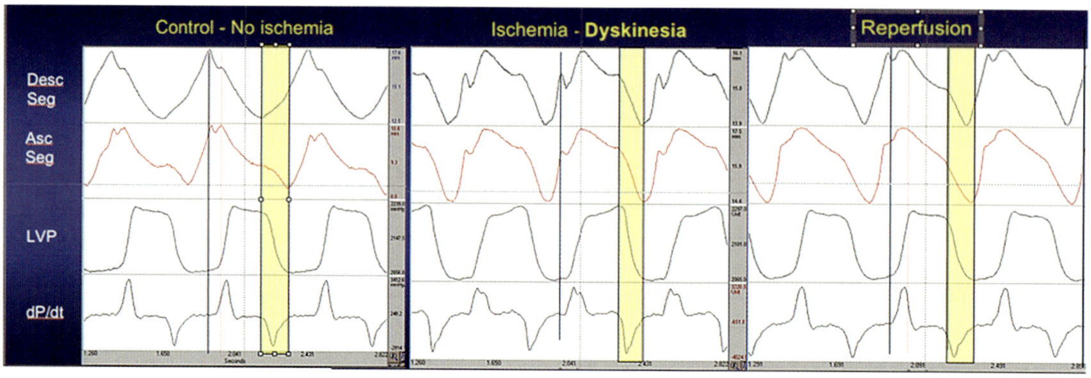

Fig. 7. Sonomicrometer tracings of length of fibers in descending and ascending bands, (shortening downward deflection) left ventricular pressure and dP/dt, shown from above down. Yellow box indicates prediastolic period. (*Left panel*) Control state to show continued shortening of ascending (epicardial) fibers in prediastole. Note that the descending (endocardial) fibers stop shortening as this interval begins, and the normal "hiatus" between end of contraction of ascending and descending fibers. (*Central panel*) Ischemia produces an abnormal lengthening pattern on both ascending and descending fibers, with lengthening continuing on both sets of fibers in prediastole. (*Right panel*) Reperfusion to show that the descending segment has prolonged contraction during the prediastole interval, thus nearly obliterating the "hiatus" between when it normally stops shortening (as in the normal sequence during control conditions) and the end of the ascending segment contraction. Asc Seg, ascending segment; Desc Seg, descending segment; LVP, left ventricular pressure. (*From* Buckberg GD, Castella M, Gharib M, et al. Structure/function interface with sequential shortening of basal and apical components of the myocardial band. Eur J Cardiothorac Surg 2006;29(Suppl 1):S75–97; with permission.)

MRI myocardial tissue tagging has confirmed the same asynchrony. These elegant MRI studies show that at the onset of prediastole, there is a reversal of the counterclockwise motion velocity of the apex, while the mid ventricular wall and base continue to show ongoing but diminished clockwise contraction as evidenced by diminishing radial velocities in these regions [55]. At this time the septum does not show any outward movement, so that the directional velocity arrows convey the lengthening motion that is described by the echo reports cited earlier. Failure to copy the reversal of tangential motion (clockwise movement) of the free wall suggests that some septal muscle is still contracting, as predicted from the sonomicrometer studies. Furthermore this differential simultaneous motion is consistent with actions of two groups of muscle fibers that consist of the basal and ascending component of the apical loop, especially since the change in directions occurs during ongoing radial velocities, as shown in Fig. 9. As prediastole continues into the interval of early rapid filling, which occurs after the mitral valve opens and when the ventricular pressure is lower than atrial pressure and the ascending septal band fibers begin to relax.

The explanation for change to clockwise apical rotation during the isovolumic phase relates to the helical fiber pattern in the apical loop. During ejection, the descending segment shortens the ventricle and causes the clockwise rotation of the base, while the torque of the ascending segment results in a counter clockwise motion at the apical region to produce torsion, thus causing counterclockwise descending segment rotation in the apical region (Fig. 10). Descending segment contraction stops at the initiation of the isovolumic phase, as does the basal segment. However, the descending segment remains a taut spring during the ongoing ascending segment contraction and lengthening (see Fig. 1). Consequently it untwists in the observed clockwise direction as similarly described when speckle tracking echo tracing recorded this motion [12]. These changes occur before end systole (see Fig. 9), but MRI demonstrates that the counterclockwise motion of the ascending segment is reduced because radial compressive velocity forces diminish during this interval. Simultaneously, prominent isovolumic clockwise apical regional tangential velocities develop, as shown in Fig. 9, which implies that unwinding of the stretched descending segment, coupled with recoil of the base, become the dominating forces that untwist the apical region to return it to its original helical starting point. Conversely, the epicardial or ascending segment

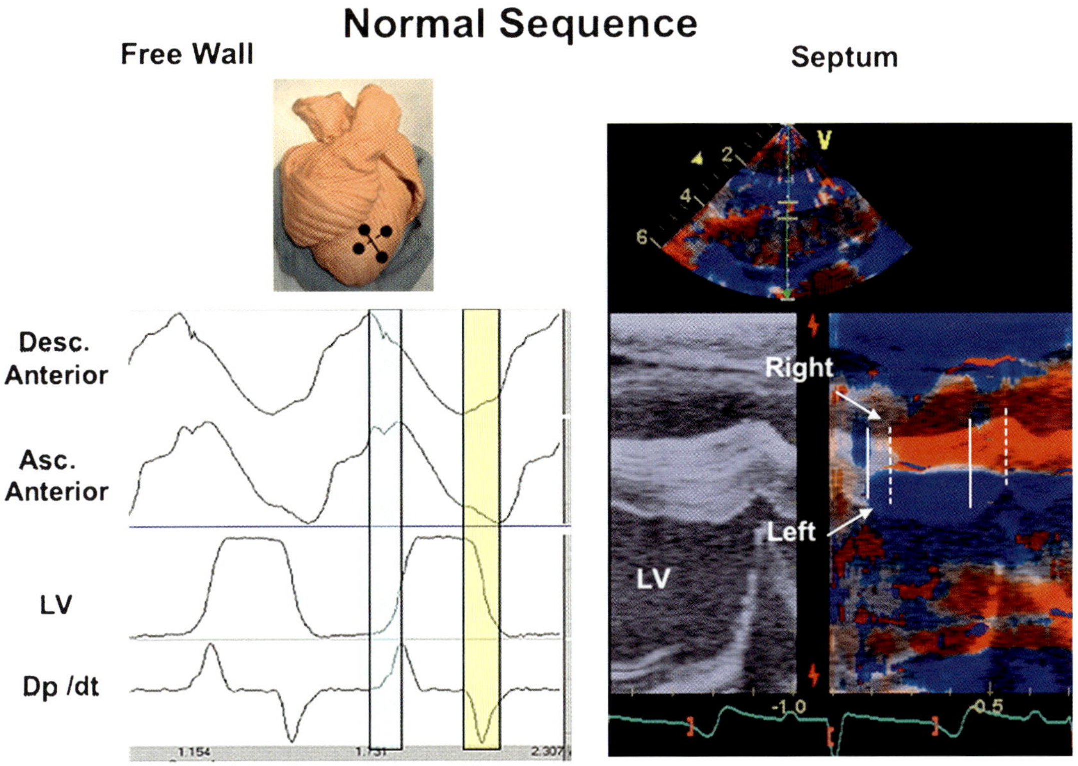

Fig. 8. Different views of sonomicrometer findings. (*Upper left panel*) Diagram to show placement of sonomicrometer crystals. (*Upper right panel*) High-resolution echocardiogram taken from porcine right ventricle (*above*) to left ventricle (*below*). (*Lower left panel*) From above down—sonomicrometer tracings in the descending anterior and ascending anterior muscle bands, left ventricular pressure tracings, and dP/dt tracings. The blue band shows the presystolic period and the yellow band the prediastolic period. (*Lower right panel*) The color coded picture of the septum shows negative strain (*red*) of the muscle on the right ventricular side of the septum (*ascending band*) while the muscle on the left ventricular side of the septum shows positive strain (*blue*). This confirms the sonomicrometer findings of contraction of the ascending band after the remaining muscle has relaxed.

fibers have ongoing contraction (see Fig. 1), and thus cannot be responsible for the clockwise apical untwisting movement, during the isovolumic interval.

What effect does the delayed relaxation of the ascending spiral muscle band have on ventricular function and how does this action relate to the untwisting that exists during rapid filling? The effect on the shape of the ventricular cavity has been mentioned above. The second effect is on the untwisting and creation of ventricular suction. As the ventricle untwists in prediastole, it lengthens and widens slightly, but the cavity volume does not change. In addition, the mitral valve itself tends to get sucked in toward the apex. The lengthening and general widening create a negative pressure. Widening might be because of recoil, but what causes the lengthening? It cannot be the result of inflow of blood because the flow of blood from atrium to ventricle has not yet started. It cannot be the result of recoil of the ascending fibers because they are still contracting. The probable explanation of the lengthening seen at this time is the continued contraction of the ascending band of antero-lateral and septal fibers, because these are the only fibers still generating force. At the end of systole the septum has a marked curvature concave to the left ventricular cavity. If the muscle of the outer ascending band is still contracting while the remaining muscle is relaxing, it will continue to thicken and straighten the septum from its curved position, thereby separating the two ends of the curved septum and lengthening the ventricular cavity. It may appear strange that muscle contraction can lengthen a structure. An analogy to help explain

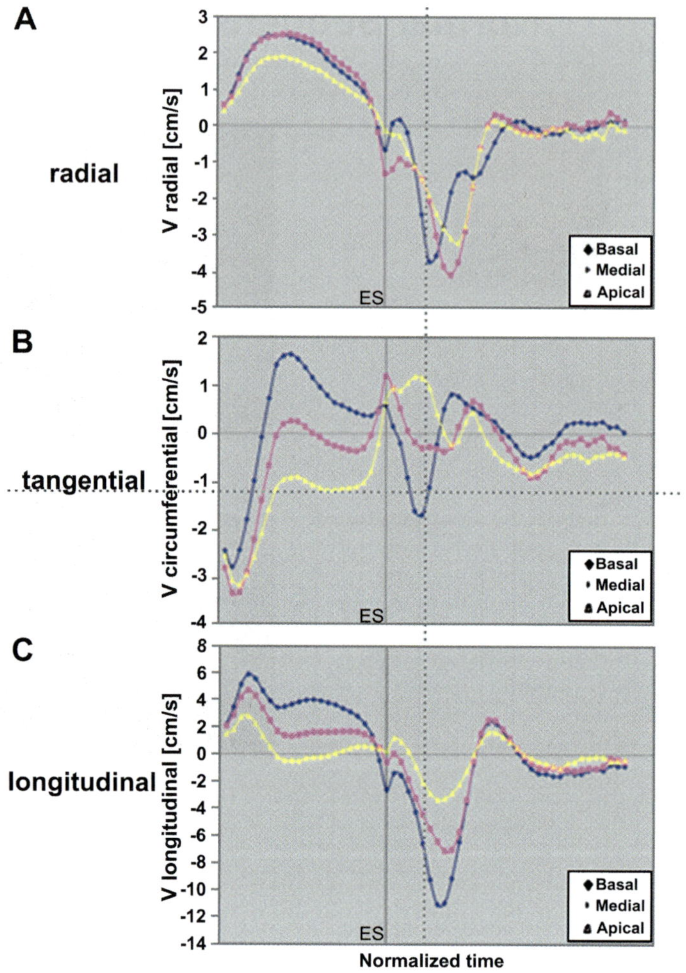

Fig. 9. Tagged MRI studies to show apical clockwise motion that exists during radial velocities that show contraction, accentuation of basal clockwise motion during this phase, and basal lengthening. Each occurs before end systole (ES), defined as absent radial compression. The tangential velocities show that positive numbers on vertical scale-clockwise, negative numbers anticlockwise. The bottom tracing shows longitudinal velocities above and below the zero line. (*From* Buckberg GD, Castella M, Mahajan A, Jung B, et al. MRI myocardial motion and fiber tracking: a confirmation of knowledge from different imaging modalities. Eur J Cardiothorac Surg 2006;29(Suppl 1):S165–77; with permission.)

this occurrence is that of a coiled cobra that rears up full length when its back muscles contract (Fig. 11).

When the mitral valve opens, the ascending band is still contracting, and does so for approximately another 40 msec. Dong and colleagues [51] have reported that 40% of untwisting occurs during the isovolumic interval, and that an additional 40% occurs during rapid filling. This continued contraction may perpetuate the suction and aid in rapid ventricular filling from the left atrium. During the prediastolic and early filling periods there is clockwise rotation at the apex, and this motion cannot be caused by the ascending loop because it is still shortening from the continuing contraction of the left-handed spiral ascending band. Simultaneously, there is accentuated clockwise motion of the base, a movement that is associated with relaxation of the basal loops. This clockwise untwisting accentuates rapid filling, as Rademakers and colleagues [48] have shown that during this time 50% of ventricular filling occurs, and filling increases to 60% with inotropic stimulation. The ascending muscle segment then stops shortening and develops recoil that accentuates untwisting during early rapid

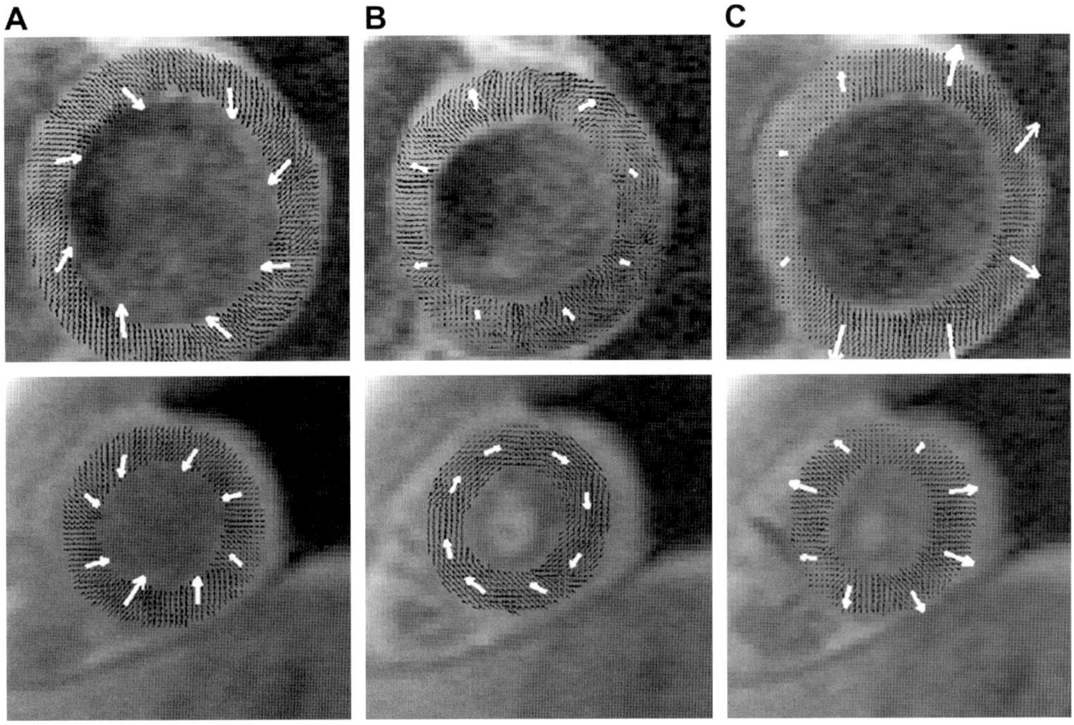

Fig. 10. Pixelwise arrow plots of the in-plane velocity component in the short axis view in a healthy volunteer. Cardiac frame during (*A*) mid-systole, (*B*) the isovolumic phase previously thought to be relaxation (IVR), and (*C*) mid-diastole. The two slice positions (basal, and apical) demonstrate the velocity twist with an inversion of rotation between IVC (presystolic contraction) and mid-systole and a counter rotation of basal and apical slices during mid-systole. The large arrows represent the absolute mean velocities in eight left ventricular angular areas of equal size for better visualization. Note reversal of apical twist during the isovolumic phase, with continuing clockwise rotation of base.

filling, as shown in Fig. 9. Following that phase, the ascending segment relaxes without such spring-like recoil, and the left ventricle fills passively with continued relaxation of all the noncontracting and thinning ventricular wall. The consolidation of these processes in the base and apex occurs when more passive ventricular filling occurs, and this filling interval becomes accentuated when the atrium contracts against a completely relaxed and thin left ventricular wall. Untwisting is the dynamic counterforce to systolic ventricular torsion, and completely reverses these rotational events toward a neutral relaxed position in the ventricle until the next heartbeat. The ascending muscle band then relaxes and the left ventricle fills passively to widen the remaining noncontracting muscle and thin the ventricular wall. More passive ventricular filling occurs after this process and then the atrium contracts against a completely relaxed and thin left ventricular wall. The systolic ventricular torsion has now been completely reversed.

In summary, during systolic ejection, the base rotates clockwise and the apex counterclockwise to give torsion that helps to empty the left ventricle. When the aortic valve closes, the upper lateral wall of the left ventricle surrounding the base of the chamber ceases contracting and begins to recoil during relaxation to accentuate the clockwise rotation of the base that is a dominant force, and thus also rotates the apex in a clockwise direction, and the lateral wall begins to get thinner and widens. Simultaneously, the ascending septal fibers that are still contracting lengthen the ventricle, and stretch the connected descending segment as they elongate. Although the ascending segment continues to impart a counterclockwise twist to the apex, the basal clockwise rotation governs the apical clockwise motion that exists during the isovolumic interval. The midwall and base show the same significant clockwise rotation and also lengthen. These changes in shape generate negative pressures in the left ventricle, and aid the opening of the mitral valve.

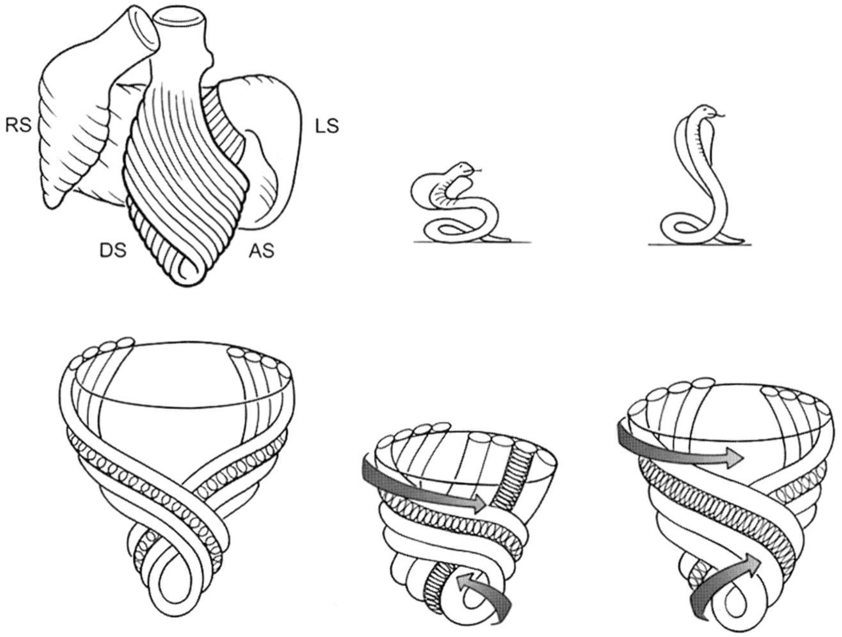

Fig. 11. Conceptual view of ventricular helix with apical and basal loops (*upper left*), with RS and LS showing the left and right segments of the basal loop and DS and AS showing the descending and ascending segments of the apical loop. There is breakdown of helical motions during diastole (*lower right*), systole (*middle*), and isovolumic phase (*lower right*). The coil springs are placed within the muscles, and define the dominant region by the tightness of coils at each stage. The correlation of lengthening during the post systolic isovolumetric phase is shown by the analogy to a cobra snake having ongoing contraction to elevate, with a change from a spiral to a lengthened height, together with a shorter but thicker muscle in upper middle and right images.

The mechanisms described above are important to consider, because if they are correct then they implicate active muscle contraction in the important untwisting period of prediastole and potentially open the door to development of novel pharmaceutic methods of adjusting calcium dynamics, to help restore more efficient means of untwisting the ventricle to aid in its capacity to efficiently suction blood for efficient venous return. Delayed untwisting is an early sign of diastolic dysfunction. If the delayed untwisting opposes the continued contraction of the ascending fibers, then the approximately 90-msec "hiatus" between the expected ends of descending and ascending contraction becomes narrowed or lost. Consequently, recoil to produce untwisting and lengthening from ascending spiral segment contraction is impeded, ongoing systolic torsion persists, limited lengthening occurs, and suction will be impaired when the mitral valve opens. Sonomicrometer crystal studies have demonstrated that extended descending segment contraction limits the normal hiatus (approximately 80-msec interval) between cessation of descending and ascending segment shortening to generate an abnormal pattern that is remedied by sodium hydrogen exchange inhibitors [45]. Recognition of this active process may lead to selection of new drugs that can modify a contractile mechanism for cardiac dynamics during the phase of rapid filling, and therefore remedy the diastolic dysfunctional component of congestive heart failure that affects approximately 50% of patients [46,47].

References

[1] Harvey W. An anatomical disposition on the motion of the heart and blood in animals, 1628. In: Willis FA, Keys TE, editors. Cardiac classics. London: Henry Kimpton; 1941. p. 19–79.

[2] Baan J, van der Velde ET, de Bruin HG, et al. Continuous measurement of left ventricular volume in animals and humans by conductance catheter. Circulation 1984;70(5):812–23.

[3] Borelli GA. In: Bishop LF, Neilson J Jr, editors. History of cardiology. New York: Medical Life Press; 1927.

[4] Ingels NB Jr, Daughters GT 2nd, Stinson EB, et al. Measurement of midwall myocardial dynamics in intact man by radiography of surgically implanted markers. Circulation 1975;52(5):859–67.
[5] Arts T, Reneman RS, Veenstra PC. A model of the mechanics of the left ventricle. Ann Biomed Eng 1979;7(3–4):299–318.
[6] Arts T, Veenstra PC, Reneman RS. Epicardial deformation and left ventricular wall mechanisms during ejection in the dog. Am J Physiol 1982; 243(3):H379–90.
[7] Stuber M, Scheidegger MB, Fischer SE, et al. Alterations in the local myocardial motion pattern in patients suffering from pressure overload due to aortic stenosis. Circulation 1999;100(4):361–8.
[8] Notomi Y, Lysyansky P, Setser RM, et al. Measurement of ventricular torsion by two-dimensional ultrasound speckle tracking imaging. J Am Coll Cardiol 2005;45(12):2034–41.
[9] Notomi Y, Setser RM, Shiota T, et al. Assessment of left ventricular torsional deformation by Doppler tissue imaging: validation study with tagged magnetic resonance imaging. Circulation 2005; 111(9):1141–7.
[10] Notomi Y, Martin-Miklovic MG, Oryszak SJ, et al. Enhanced ventricular untwisting during exercise: a mechanistic manifestation of elastic recoil described by Doppler tissue imaging. Circulation 2006;113(21):2524–33.
[11] Notomi Y, Srinath G, Shiota T, et al. Maturational and adaptive modulation of left ventricular torsional biomechanics: Doppler tissue imaging observation from infancy to adulthood. Circulation 2006; 113(21):2534–41.
[12] Notomi Y, Popovic ZB, Yamada H, et al. Ventricular untwisting: a temporal link between left ventricular relaxation and suction. Am J Physiol Heart Circ Physiol 2008;294(1):H505–13.
[13] Burns AT, La Gerche A, Macisaac AI, et al. Augmentation of left ventricular torsion with exercise is attenuated with age. J Am Soc Echocardiogr 2008;21(4):315–20.
[14] Cirillo M, Arpesella G. Rewind the heart: a novel technique to reset heart fibers' orientation in surgery for ischemic cardiomyopathy. Med Hypotheses 2008;70(4):848–54.
[15] Hui L, Pemberton J, Hickey E, et al. The contribution of left ventricular muscle bands to left ventricular rotation: assessment by a 2-dimensional speckle tracking method. J Am Soc Echocardiogr 2007; 20(5):486–91.
[16] Jin SM, Noh CI, Bae EJ, et al. Decreased left ventricular torsion and untwisting in children with dilated cardiomyopathy. J Korean Med Sci 2007;22(4): 633–40.
[17] Kim HK, Sohn DW, Lee SE, et al. Assessment of left ventricular rotation and torsion with two-dimensional speckle tracking echocardiography. J Am Soc Echocardiogr 2007;20(1):45–53.
[18] Buchalter MB, Rademakers FE, Weiss JL, et al. Rotational deformation of the canine left ventricle measured by magnetic resonance tagging: effects of catecholamines, ischaemia, and pacing. Cardiovasc Res 1994;28(5):629–35.
[19] Courtois M, Kovacs SJ, Ludbrook PA. Physiological early diastolic intraventricular pressure gradient is lost during acute myocardial ischemia. Circulation 1990;81(5):1688–96.
[20] Steine K, Stugaard M, Smiseth OA. Mechanisms of retarded apical filling in acute ischemic left ventricular failure. Circulation 1999;99(15):2048–54.
[21] Yellin EL, Hori M, Yoran C, et al. Left ventricular relaxation in the filling and nonfilling intact canine heart. Am J Physiol 1986;250(4 Pt 2):H620–9.
[22] Nikolic S, Yellin EL, Tamura K, et al. Passive properties of canine left ventricle: diastolic stiffness and restoring forces. Circ Res 1988;62(6):1210–22.
[23] Nikolic SD, Feneley MP, Pajaro OE, et al. Origin of regional pressure gradients in the left ventricle during early diastole. Am J Physiol 1995;268(2 Pt 2): H550–7.
[24] Helmes M, Trombitas K, Granzier H. Titin develops restoring force in rat cardiac myocytes. Circ Res 1996;79(3):619–26.
[25] Waldman LK, Nosan D, Villarreal F, et al. Relation between transmural deformation and local myofiber direction in canine left ventricle. Circ Res 1988;63(3): 550–62.
[26] Buckberg GD, Castella M, Gharib M, et al. Structure/function interface with sequential shortening of basal and apical components of the myocardial band. Eur J Cardiothorac Surg 2006;29(Suppl 1): S75–97.
[27] Sengupta PP, Krishnamoorthy VK, Korinek J, et al. Left ventricular form and function revisited: applied translational science to cardiovascular ultrasound imaging. J Am Soc Echocardiogr 2007;20(5):539–51.
[28] Streeter DD Jr, Spotnitz HM, Patel DP, et al. Fiber orientation in the canine left ventricle during diastole and systole. Circ Res 1969;24(3):339–47.
[29] Streeter DD Jr. Gross morphology and fiber geometry of the heart. In: Berne RM, Sperelakis N, editors. Handbook of physiology, section 2: the cardiovascular system, volume 1: the heart. Bethesda (MD): American Physiological Society; 1979. p. 61–112.
[30] Rademakers FE, Rogers WJ, Guier WH, et al. Relation of regional cross-fiber shortening to wall thickening in the intact heart. Three-dimensional strain analysis by NMR tagging. Circulation 1994; 89(3):1174–82.
[31] Ashikaga H, Criscione JC, Omens JH, et al. Transmural left ventricular mechanics underlying torsional recoil during relaxation. Am J Physiol Heart Circ Physiol 2004;286(2):H640–7.
[32] Wu MT, Tseng WY, Su MY, et al. Diffusion tensor magnetic resonance imaging mapping the fiber

architecture remodeling in human myocardium after infarction: correlation with viability and wall motion. Circulation 2006;114(10):1036–45.

[33] Rohmer D, Sitek A, Gullberg GT. Reconstruction and visualization of fiber and laminar structure in the normal human heart from ex vivo diffusion tensor magnetic resonance imaging (DTMRI) data. Invest Radiol 2007;42(11):777–89.

[34] Zhukov L, Barr AH. Heart-muscle fiber reconstruction from diffusion tensor MRI. In: Proceedings of the 14th IEEE Visualization Conference; 2003. p. 597–602.

[35] Sanchez-Quintana D, Garcia-Martinez V, Climent V, et al. Morphological changes in the normal pattern of ventricular myoarchitecture in the developing human heart. Anat Rec 1995;243(4):483–95.

[36] Jouk PS, Usson Y, Michalowicz G, et al. Three-dimensional cartography of the pattern of the myofibres in the second trimester fetal human heart. Anat Embryol (Berl) 2000;202(2):103–18.

[37] Torrent-Guasp F, Ballester M, Buckberg GD, et al. Spatial orientation of the ventricular muscle band: physiologic contribution and surgical implications. J Thorac Cardiovasc Surg 2001;122(2):389–92.

[38] Robb J, Robb R. The normal heart: anatomy and physiology of the structural units. Am Heart J 1942;23:455–67.

[39] LeGrice IJ, Smaill BH, Chai LZ, et al. Laminar structure of the heart: ventricular myocyte arrangement and connective tissue architecture in the dog. Am J Physiol 1995;269(2 Pt 2):H571–82.

[40] LeGrice IJ, Takayama Y, Covell JW. Transverse shear along myocardial cleavage planes provides a mechanism for normal systolic wall thickening. Circ Res 1995;77(1):182–93.

[41] Noble MI. The contribution of blood momentum to left ventricular ejection in the dog. Circ Res 1968; 23(5):663–70.

[42] Solomon SB, Nikolic SD, Frater RW, et al. Contraction-relaxation coupling: determination of the onset of diastole. Am J Physiol 1999;277(1 Pt 2): H23–7.

[43] Rosen BD, Gerber BL, Edvardsen T, et al. Late systolic onset of regional LV relaxation demonstrated in three-dimensional space by MRI tissue tagging. Am J Physiol Heart Circ Physiol 2004;287(4):H1740–6.

[44] Buckberg GD, Clemente C, Cox JL, et al. The structure and function of the helical heart and its buttress wrapping. IV. Concepts of dynamic function from the normal macroscopic helical structure. Semin Thorac Cardiovasc Surg 2001;13(4):342–57.

[45] Castella M, Buckberg GD, Saleh S. Diastolic dysfunction in stunned myocardium: a state of abnormal excitation-contraction coupling that is limited by Na(+)-H(+) exchange inhibition. Eur J Cardiothorac Surg 2006;29(Suppl 1):S107–14.

[46] Mosterd A, Hoes AW, de Bruyne MC, et al. Prevalence of heart failure and left ventricular dysfunction in the general population; The Rotterdam Study. Eur Heart J 1999;20(6):447–55.

[47] Bursi F, Weston SA, Redfield MM, et al. Systolic and diastolic heart failure in the community. JAMA 2006;296(18):2209–16.

[48] Rademakers FE, Buchalter MB, Rogers WJ, et al. Dissociation between left ventricular untwisting and filling. Accentuation by catecholamines. Circulation 1992;85(4):1572–81.

[49] Sengupta PP, Khandheria BK, Korinek J, et al. Apex-to-base dispersion in regional timing of left ventricular shortening and lengthening. J Am Coll Cardiol 2006;47(1):163–72.

[50] Goetz WA, Lansac E, Lim HS, et al. Left ventricular endocardial longitudinal and transverse changes during isovolumic contraction and relaxation: a challenge. Am J Physiol Heart Circ Physiol 2005;289(1): H196–201.

[51] Dong SJ, Hees PS, Siu CO, et al. MRI assessment of LV relaxation by untwisting rate: a new isovolumic phase measure of tau. Am J Physiol Heart Circ Physiol 2001;281(5):H2002–9.

[52] Simari RD, Bell MR, Schwartz RS, et al. Ventricular relaxation and myocardial ischemia: a comparison of different models of tau during coronary angioplasty. Cathet Cardiovasc Diagn 1992;25(4):278–84.

[53] Davis KL, Mehlhorn U, Schertel ER, et al. Variation in tau, the time constant for isovolumic relaxation, along the left ventricular base-to-apex axis. Basic Res Cardiol 1999;94(1):41–8.

[54] Ingels NB Jr, Hansen DE, Daughters GT 2nd, et al. Relation between longitudinal, circumferential, and oblique shortening and torsional deformation in the left ventricle of the transplanted human heart. Circ Res 1989;64(5):915–27.

[55] Jung B, Markl M, Foll D, et al. Investigating myocardial motion by MRI using tissue phase mapping. Eur J Cardiothorac Surg 2006;29(Suppl 1):S150–7.

ELSEVIER
SAUNDERS

Heart Failure Clin 4 (2008) 361–370

HEART
FAILURE
CLINICS

Surgical Restoration of the Postinfarction Dilated Ventricle

Constantine L. Athanasuleas, MD[a], Gerald D. Buckberg, MD[b,*]

[a]*University of Alabama Birmingham, Birmingham, AL, USA*
[b]*David Geffen School of Medicine at UCLA, Los Angeles, CA, USA*

Heart failure consumes an increasing proportion of the total health care cost [1,2]. Coronary artery disease accounts for at least two thirds of cases and the majority of patients with CHF have sustained prior infarctions and ventricular dilation [3]. Ventricular dilation changes the size and shape of the normal conical or elliptic ventricular form into a sphere configuration. In 2000, $56 billion was spent on CHF: $36 billion on decompensated CHF, $18 billion or maintenance therapy, and only $2 billion on surgical treatment [2]. The surgical options included ventricular assist devices and transplantation. This article introduces an alternate approach that restores the postinfarction spherical ventricular geometry into a conical form. The article also shows how this geometric change returns more normal form/function relationships and improves the adverse mechanical and rhythm consequences that follow ventricular dilation.

Ventricular remodeling postinfarction

Early revascularization has been advocated and implemented in the treatment of acute myocardial infarction (MI). Left ventricular dilation, however, occurs in about 20% of patients undergoing successful early revascularization of the infarct-related artery [4,5]. The process of progressive ventricular dilation that ultimately impairs cardiac function is called "remodeling," a term that is absent from the dictionary, but its antonym is "unhealthy or away from normal." Conversely, the term "restore" means "to bring things back to normal." During the course of ventricular remodeling, the remote noninfarcted myocardium undergoes changes in volume and shape. The normal elliptic shape becomes spherical. Global systolic function deteriorates resulting in CHF and ventricular arrhythmias [6,7]. The prognosis of patients with ischemic cardiomyopathy is more closely related to left ventricle (LV) volume rather than to ejection fraction (Fig. 1A and B) [8].

Surgical approaches in the treatment of CHF post infarction are based on an understanding of normal cardiac structure and function. Morphologic changes in the diseased ventricle explain reduced global myocardial performance, functional mitral regurgitation, and ventricular arrhythmias. Operative techniques must be directed toward normalizing the altered spherical shape of the heart toward a more conical one while simultaneously reducing ventricular volume.

Shape

The conical heart shape has been well-known since Hippocrates and Galen, and it was further described by the forefathers of anatomy [9]. A helical spiral at the cardiac apex was demonstrated by Lower in the seventeenth century and an internal helix was postulated by Senec in the eighteenth century. In 1891 Krehl [10] described circular fibers that encircled the left ventricle (the "Triebwerkzeug") and were thought to be responsible for the force of ventricular ejection. How the helical form relates to function has long been a mystery called the "Gordian Knot," by cardiac

* Corresponding author. David Geffen School of Medicine at UCLA, 10833 Le Conte Avenue, 62-258 CHS, Los Angeles, CA 90095.
E-mail address: gbuckberg@mednet.ucla.edu (G.D. Buckberg).

doi:10.1016/j.hfc.2008.02.004

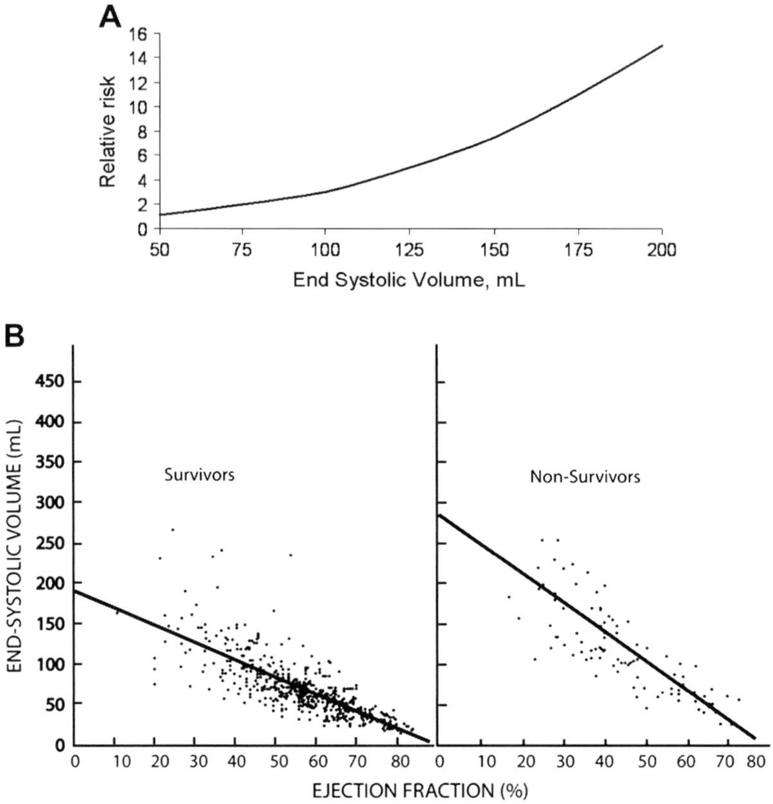

Fig. 1. (*A*) Relative death risk post MI. Relationship between LV end systolic volume index (LVESVI) and mortality. (*B*) Post MI. LV volume versus ejection fraction (EF). Among patients with the same EF after infarction, survival is better among those with smaller LV volume. (*From* White HD, Norris RM, Brown MA, et al. Left ventricular end-systolic volume as the major determinant of survival after recovery from myocardial infarction. Circulation 1987;76:44–51; with permission.)

anatomists. Torrent-Guasp's [11] studies of the relationship between cardiac form and function date back to 1950. He spatially unfolded the intact heart by macroscopic dissection to demonstrate that a muscular band begins at the pulmonary artery and ends at the aorta. This band contains a myocardial fold that separates the heart into two simple loops called the "basal" and "apical" loops. The structural components include: a horizontal or transverse fiber orientation for the basal loop that surrounds the right and left ventricles; and a change in fiber direction through a spiral fold in the ventricular band to form a ventricular helix that now contains obliquely oriented fibers. These form descending and ascending segments of the apical loop with an apical vortex. These components are shown in an earlier article in this issue. The helical architecture of the normal heart has been confirmed by strain relationships using MRI, corrosion casts showing spiral architecture, and by sonomicrometry [12–15]. Each pattern reflects the normal oblique fiber orientation that conveys maximum force during ejection and suction [16].

Myocardial shape determines systolic ejection. The normally oriented oblique myocardial fibers produce an ejection fraction of approximately 60%. The infarcted, dilated ventricle becomes spherical and the myocardial fibers become transversely oriented (Fig. 2). When this occurs, the ejection fraction falls to about 30%, even when the intrinsic fiber shortening of the myocytes remain unchanged [17,18]. This architectural disadvantage limits deformation (ie, twisting) that is visible at operation or by MRI and speckle echocardiography, negatively impacting the natural increment of strain development from mid-wall to apex [19]. This further impairs sequential contraction efficiency and reduces ventricular function by producing mechanical dyssynchrony [20].

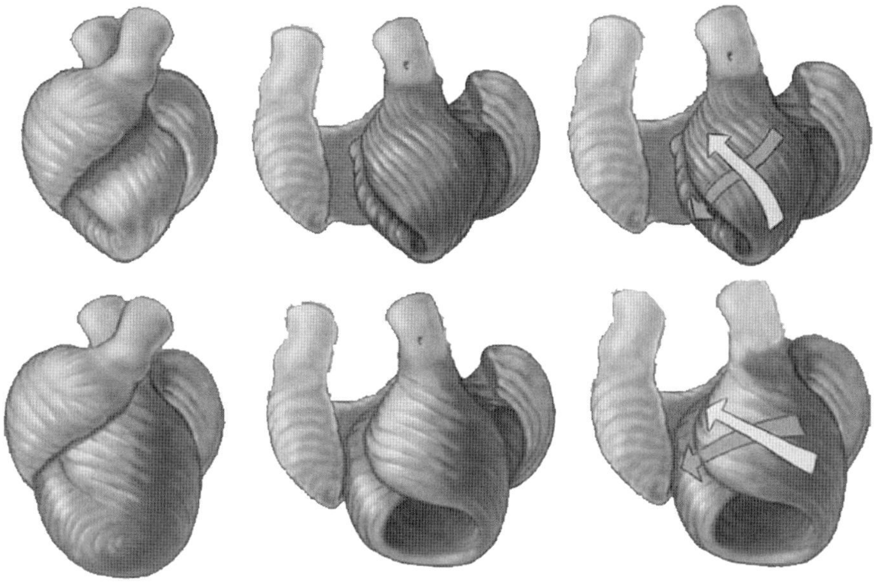

Fig. 2. The normal heart is shown above and the dilated heart below. Note the transverse orientation of fibers in the dilated heart, which decrease the force of suction and ejection. (*From* Coghlan C, Hoffman J. Leonardo da Vinci's flights of the mind must continue: cardiac architecture and the fundamental relation of form and function revisited. Eur J Cardiothorac Surg 2006;29(Suppl 1):S4–17; with permission.)

The morphologic characteristics in ischemic and nonischemic heart disease are directly related to clinical outcome. Increasing the left ventricle's spherical shape in both ischemic and nonischemic cardiomyopathy portends a poor prognosis [21–23]. The surgeon must identify scarred regions that can be excluded at operation in cases of ischemic cardiomyopathy. This preservation of spherical shape is also important in nonischemic cardiomyopathy where there are no homogenous changes in the myocardium, contrary to prior opinion. It has been recently shown that myocardial scarring is site-specific within the ventricle. The surgeon can identify these changes and tailor intraventricular repair based on intraoperative echocardiographic findings during cardiopulmonary bypass by varying ventricular filling and noting its effects on regional wall motion [24]. Localizing major segments of intrinsic disease is essential because surgery must reshape the ventricle into a more conical structure and exclude regions of damaged myocardium.

Size

Left ventricular enlargement and increased spherical shape are characteristic findings in dilated cardiomyopathy. Several pathologic processes are involved. In ischemic disease, extensive focal scar or multiple patchy areas of smaller scar can lead to dilation of the remote noninfarcted segment. In nonischemic cardiomyopathy, some segments show more extensive scarring than others. This also leads to global ventricular dilation.

Urgent reperfusion of an infarcted ventricular segment shrinks ventricular size by converting the acutely dyskinetic segment into a smaller akinetic one. An important measurement after infarction, rarely obtained in clinical practice, is the left ventricular end systolic volume index (LVESVI). The Global Utilization of Streptokinase and Tissue Plasminogen Activator for Occluded Coronary Arteries (GUSTO)–1 trial recorded LVESVI within 90 minutes of acute infarction and showed that in spite of successful reperfusion of the infarct-related artery, 17% of patients had LVESVI > 40 mL/m^2 (normal 25 mL/m^2). Progressive CHF and death rates were correlated with increasing ventricular volumes above this value [5]. These findings were confirmed in another study that documented early LVESVI > 50 mL/m^2 in 20% of patients in whom ventricular dilation over 3 years led to CHF by progressive dysfunction of the remote noninfarcted myocardium [4].

Left ventricular dilation often has other pathologic consequences such as functional mitral regurgitation. Leaflet coaptation is reduced and, when the papillary muscles widen, there is tethering of the mitral apparatus. This process results in mitral regurgitation. The hemodynamic burden placed by adding mitral regurgitation further raises ventricular volume, reducing forward cardiac output and worsening heart failure. Increased ventricular volume also accentuates ventricular dysrhythmia and can cause dyssynchronous mechanical contraction [7,20]. This change may be a contributing factor in sudden death [7,25].

Surgical options

The concept that "form defines function" is the principle behind surgical ventricular restoration (SVR). SVR is designed to treat patients with CHF who sustained postinfarction ventricular dilation, by exclusion of the infarcted segment. This approach dates back to the classic left ventricular aneurysmectomy procedure. Transmural necrosis after infarction is rare, given the success of early coronary intervention after infarction. Dor [26,27] first described intraventricular infarct exclusion in the more common setting of the akinetic ventricle recognizing the adverse consequences of ventricular dilation in the presence of akinesia as well as dyskinesia. During SVR, the infarcted segment of the left ventricle is excluded, usually with an intraventricular patch, thereby creating a smaller and more elliptic chamber ventricular chamber (Fig. 3).

SVR addresses the scarred ventricular segment and thus is quite different from partial left ventriculectomy (the Batista procedure), which was not site-specific and involved resection of the functional lateral wall in both ischemic and nonischemic disease. Partial left ventriculectomy has largely been abandoned due to poor outcomes [28,29].

The full surgical treatment of dilated ischemic cardiomyopathy must address the coronary vessels, ventricle, and the valve (the three "V's" of CHF). Coronary bypass alone, in the treatment of ischemic CHF, may not be enough if the ventricle has significantly enlarged. Similarly, attempts to treat ischemic mitral valve regurgitation at the annular level (ring annuloplasty) are not as predictable or durable as previously thought because the mechanism of functional mitral regurgitation is related to the ventriculo-mitral interaction. SVR is usually performed as an adjunct to coronary bypass and mitral valve repair.

Surgical ventricular restoration outcomes

Dor's contributions inspired a multinational study of ventricular restoration. A collaborative

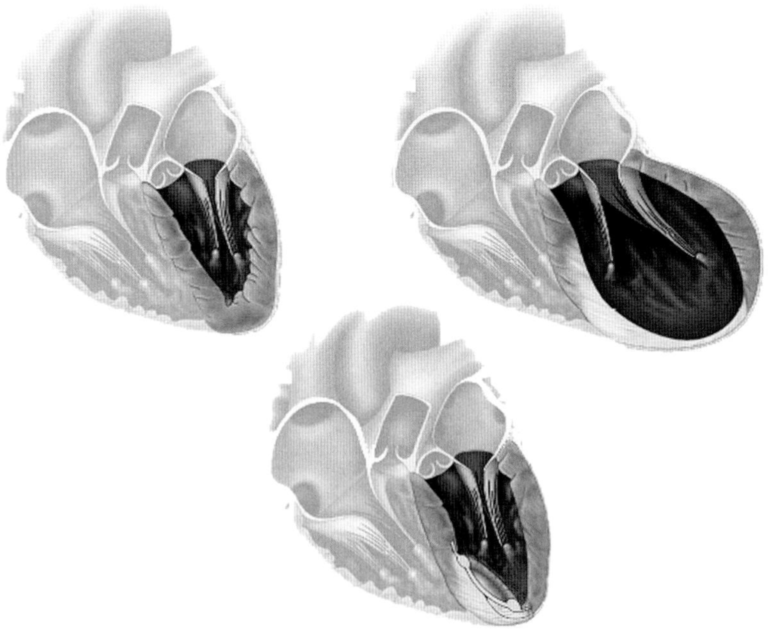

Fig. 3. SVR excludes the infarcted segment with an intraventricular patch and restores shape toward a more conical form. (*From* Coghlan C, Hoffman J. Leonardo da Vinci's flights of the mind must continue: cardiac architecture and the fundamental relation of form and function revisited. Eur J Cardiothorac Surg 2006;29(Suppl 1):S4–17; with permission.)

group of cardiologists and cardiac surgeons (the RESTORE Group) from four continents (North America, Europe, Asia, and South America) applied SVR in 1198 patients between 1998 and 2003 [30]. Patients were included in the registry if SVR was performed with the following criteria: prior anterior MI; significant ventricular dilation (LVESVI $\geq$ 60 mL/m^2); and a regional asynergic (noncontractile) area of $\geq$35%. SVR was most often done as a concomitant procedure: 90% received coronary bypass grafting and mitral valve repair was required in about 20%.

In the RESTORE registry, 86% of patients had New York Heart Association (NYHA) class III/IV symptoms of CHF preoperatively. Such patients have a high mortality with medical therapy, or with surgical revascularization without left ventricular restoration, where late deaths are attributable to CHF [31,32]. Echocardiography, ventriculography, or magnetic resonance angiography (MRA) was used to confirm the asynergic area and calculate the ejection fraction (EF). LVESVI was determined by ventriculography or MRA.

Hospital mortality after SVR was 5.3% and it increased as preoperative ventricular volume rose: 2.3% if LVESVI was <60 mL/m^2; 5.7% if LVESVI was 60–90 mL/m^2; 8.1% if LVESVI was 90–120 mL/m^2; and 8.4% if LVESVI was >120 mL/m^2. These findings are comparable to recently reported mortality rates (5.5%–11%) in ischemic patients with left ventricular dysfunction (EF < 35%) undergoing coronary artery bypass grafting alone. The addition of mitral valve repair influenced early outcome. Hospital mortality was 8.7% with mitral repair versus 4.0% without repair ($P<.001$). Perioperative mechanical support with intra-aortic balloon pumping was uncommon (<9%). Global systolic function improved postoperatively as EF increased from 29.6 $\pm$ 11.0% preoperatively to 39.5 $\pm$ 12.3% postoperatively ($P<.001$). LVESVI decreased from 80.4 $\pm$ 51.4 mL/m^2 preoperatively to 56.6 $\pm$ 34.3 mL/m^2 postoperatively ($P<.001$). The geometric changes in size and shape after SVR are shown in Figs. 3 and 4.

The overall 5-year probability of survival after SVR was 68.6 $\pm$ 2.8 %. This rate confirms Dor's [26] extensive experience and is unprecedented in the treatment of advanced ischemic cardiomyopathy. A detailed analysis of these findings has been reported that breaks down the data for each volume subset [30]. The multivariate analysis of SVR demonstrated that major risk factors were age, preoperative EF, LVESVI, and NYHA functional class.

The RESTORE data further emphasized the importance of measuring LVEVI as a surrogate marker of left ventricular function. EF and LVESVI are not directly related, as there is a wide variation in volume for a given EF [33].

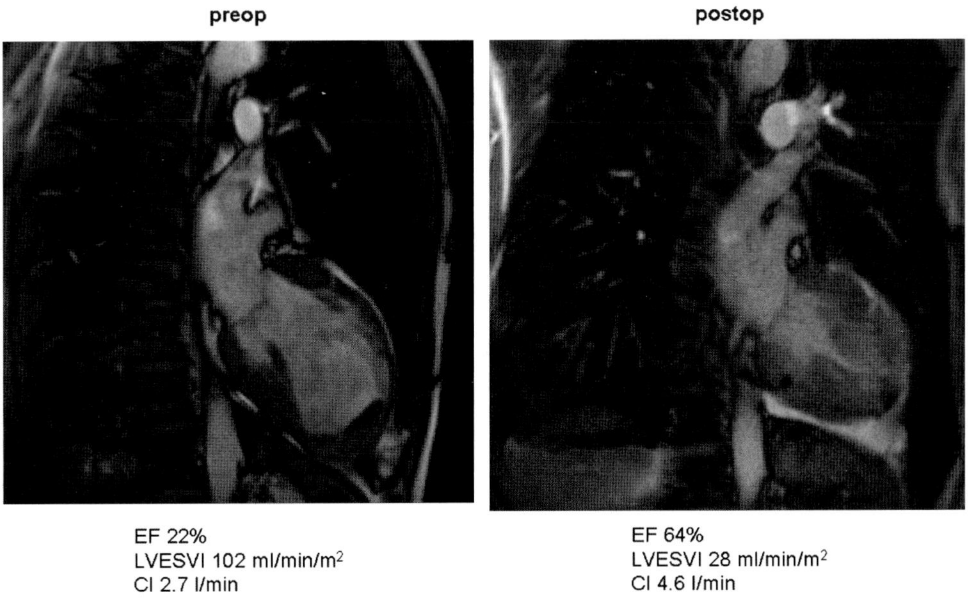

Fig. 4. Pre- and postoperative changes in left ventricular end systolic size after SVR. (*Courtesy of* Vincent Dor, MD, Monte Carlo, Monaco.)

Patients with preoperative LVESVI $\leq$ 80 mL/m^2 had long-term survival of 79.4 $\pm$ 3.3% as compared with 67.2 $\pm$ 3.2% for those with larger hearts. Preoperative NYHA functional class was also predictive of outcome with decreased 5-year survival in patients with preoperative class IV symptoms (49.7 $\pm$ 5.8% versus 69.9 $\pm$ 4.7% in class III). These predictors of long-term outcome after SVR are similar to those previously reported [34]. A small number of patients (9%) in functional class I underwent SVR as an adjunct to coronary artery bypass grafting (CABG) because ventricular dilation (LVESVI > 60 mL/m^2) has been shown to be a precursor of late development of CHF and early death [5,8].

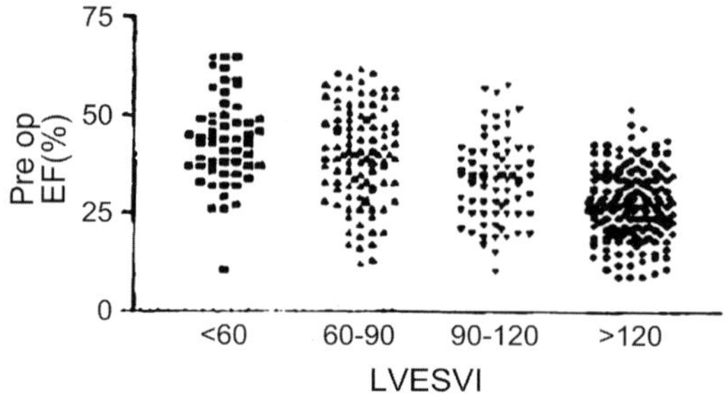

Fig. 5. Preoperative EF and ESVI (mL/m^2). Left ventricular volumes can widely vary for a given ejection raction. (*Courtesy of* Vincent Dor, MD, Monte Carlo, Monaco, and Marisa DiDonato, MD, Milano, Italy.)

Ventricular scar: the "culprit muscle"

Coronary artery plaque is often referred to as the "culprit lesion." In discussing heart failure, perhaps one should think of the ventricular scar as the "culprit muscle" since this is the catalyst for secondary changes in the remote ventricle that lead to the clinical manifestations of CHF.

Urgent thrombolysis or angioplasty of the infarct-related artery salvages myocardium, but its effectiveness is time-related. Even early successful reperfusion is associated with some myocardial necrosis. The epicardium may be spared, but the endocardium is often injured. This situation results in akinesia of a left ventricular segment rather than dyskinesia, which follows transmural necrosis. The latter is seen less often due to increasingly successful intervention for MI.

Diagnostic guidelines when considering surgical ventricular restoration

The workup of the patients following MI who are candidates for SVR must include consideration of the extent of myocardial injury and its effect on the remote muscle. Measurements should include: (1) left ventricular size; (2) asynergic area; and (3) viability of remote (noninfarcted) myocardium. These are rarely reported in routine clinical practice, but they are easily obtainable. Ejection fraction alone is misleading, as there is often great variability in ventricular volume for a given ejection fraction (Fig. 5).

Left ventricular volume can be obtained by echocardiography, multiple gated acquisition scan, MRA, or contrast ventriculography. Transthoracic or transesophageal echocardiography is easily obtained, but may provide the least reliable data regarding volume because the apex is not well seen and it is very technician dependent. Nuclear studies such as the multiple gated acquisition scans have a variability of $\pm$ 15%. Biplane ventriculography based on Simpson's rule for approximation of volume is the most accurate method for measuring volume in the catheterization laboratory, but it is not often done because most labs obtain single plane images. Right anterior oblique (RAO) ventriculography actually underestimates volume and must be considered in clinical decisions [35]. MRA is the most accurate, but cannot be done in patients with pacemakers or defibrillators and is often not available.

Clinicians often report left ventricular end diastolic dimension (LVEDD). This dimension is often misleading because it measures the distance between the bases of the papillary muscles. Anterior infarction often causes nonhomogeneous structural changes and damage may exist beyond this point. Consequently, LVEDD can be normal in the presence of a large akinetic or dyskinetic anteroseptal wall as a result of anterior MI. LVEDD is more useful during the later stages of ventricular remodeling in ischemic cardiomyopathy after global dilation occurs and in nonischemic cardiomyopathy with global dilation.

Asynergy is most accurately measured by the centerline method, which calculates how much scar occupies the LV perimeter [36]. A reasonable estimate can be obtained from the RAO ventriculogram or from the echocardiogram.

Myocardial viability can be obtained by nuclear studies, dobutamine stress testing, or gadolinium enhanced magnetic resonance imaging (MRI). Improvement in contractility of infarcted segments after revascularization is rare when the transmural extent of delayed enhancement is greater than 50% (Fig. 6) [37]. Progressive left

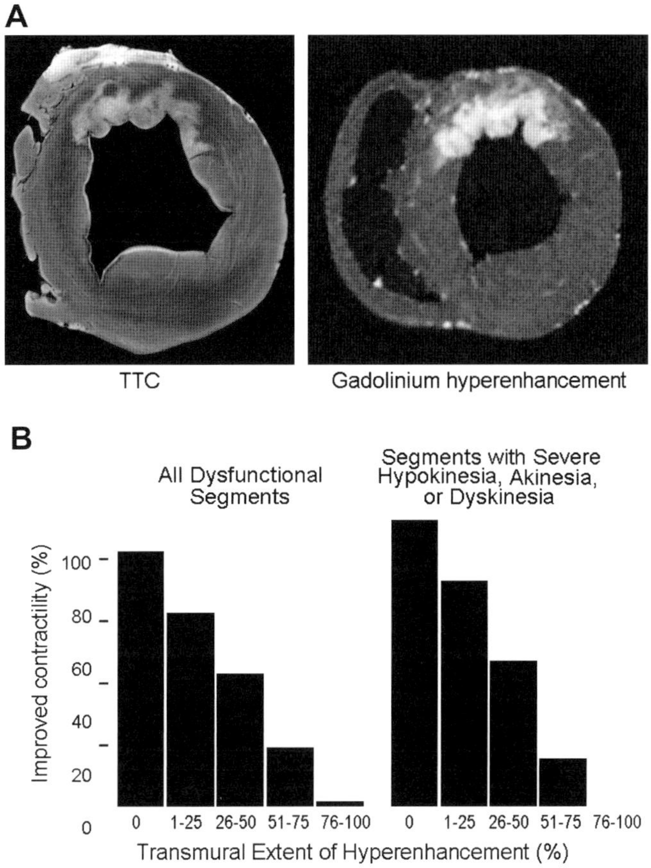

Fig. 6. (*A*) Myocardial Infarction. Postinfarction myocardial necrosis, determined by TTC (tetrazolium chloride) on left and MRI gadolinium hyperenhancement on right. (*Courtesy of* Robert M. Judd, PhD, Chicago, IL.) (*B*) CMR and Ventricular Recovery Post-CABG. Recovery of contractile function after revascularization is related to degree of wall thickness gadolinium hyperenhancement. (*From* Kim RJ, Wu E, Rafael A, et al. The use of contrast-enhanced magnetic resonance imaging to identify reversible myocardial dysfunction. N Engl J Med 2000;343:1445–53; with permission.)

ventricular dilation occurs if greater than 20% of the muscle mass was scarred by infarction [38]. In patients followed 1 year after infarction, progressive dilation occurs if greater than 30% of left ventricular circumference is asynergic [39]. These observations lend credibility to the concept of the culprit muscle that is the persistent activator of changes in the remote muscle, perhaps mediated by neurohumoral components. Retention of the scarred segment may be related to the relative inefficacy of increasing doses of carvedilol in improving the ejection fraction in patients with ischemic versus nonischemic cardiomyopathy [40].

Assessment of the remote noninfarcted muscle post infarction is a crucial component in the evaluation of patients who may undergo SVR. Often there are significant coronary obstructions in vessels supplying the remote muscle and possible prior subendocardial infarctions. Echocardiography or biplane ventriculography are useful tools in evaluating remote regional wall motion. In the presence of marked thinning (<5 mm) and severe hypokinesia on echocardiography, revascularization is unlikely to improve contractility. In questionable cases, gadolinium MRA is very useful in determining viability. The presence of even severe hypokinesia of the remote segment does not exclude patients from SVR because the remote myocardial function is greatly enhanced by reduction of left ventricular volume and reshaping of the ventricular chamber [41]. Even high septal akinesia reverts to normal function as the wall stress is reduced after operation.

Ventricular arrhythmia and surgical ventricular restoration

Increased ventricular size and shape increase ventricular arrhythmias as shown in the Survival and Ventricular Enlargement Trial (SAVE) [42]. In a subset of patients studied in the RESTORE group, investigators examined 382 patients with electrophysiologic testing. They found a clear relationship between ventricular volume and arrhythmia. Spontaneous ventricular arrhythmias were more common in the most dilated hearts (LVESVI $>$ 120/ml/m^2); inducible events more frequent if LVESVI was 100–120 mL/m^2; and no arrhythmias were induced if LVESVI was $<$100 mL/m^2 [43]. SVR reduced inducible ventricular tachycardia from 41% preoperatively (144/352) to 8% (26/307) at early study, and 8% (14/177) 1 year later. Cardiac mortality was low at 5 years and not different between groups with and without evidence of spontaneous or inducible preoperative arrhythmias. If SVR had not been performed, many of these patients whose ejection fractions were below 35% might have otherwise undergone defibrillator placement as the Multicenter Automatic Defibrillator Implantation Trial (MADIT) criteria suggest [44]. A few patients (26 of 382) had postoperative induced arrhythmia by paired ventricular stimulation. Amiodarone was successful in treating such patients after SVR. This finding is consistent with the observation that amiodarone is most effective in the treatment of atrial fibrillation when the atrium is not massively enlarged [25].

Surgical ventricular restoration and global ventricular function

A recent analysis of 30 consecutive patients undergoing SVR showed that preoperative LV contraction was highly asynchronous, because pressure/volume (P/V) loops displayed abnormal isometric phases with a right shifting [20]. Moreover, endocardial time motion was either early or delayed at the end-systolic phase as demonstrated by the pressure/length (P/L) loops, which were markedly abnormal in size, shape, and orientation. SVR shifted the P/V loops leftwards toward normal and the P/L loops almost normalized demonstrating cardiac resynchronization. Hemodynamic measurements after SVR indicated improved systolic function (EF 30 $\pm$ 13% to 45 $\pm$ 12%; P = .001). Diastolic function also improved as evidenced by a more rapid peak-filling rate.

Surgical ventricular restoration and remote muscle function

Impaired function of the noninfarcted remote myocardium after MI worsens CHF. Recovery of remote muscle function has been demonstrated after SVR by MRA tagging; circumferential shortening and deformation improved [45]. This is linked to clinical recovery as data shows improved NYHA status and 6-minute walking tests after SVR in addition to improvement in quality of life. These findings are sustainable up to 2 years after operation [46].

The morphologic change in shape of the remote muscle after SVR has physiologic implications as well. Myocardial oxygen consumption (MVO_2) is closely related to wall tension, which in turn is related to the radius of the ventricle. If the ventricle is spherical, then the ventricular volume (V) is related to radius (r) as follows: $V = 4/3\pi \cdot r^3$. Substituting this relationship into the LaPlace relationship, tension (T) is related to $P \cdot \sqrt[3]{V}$. However, if the ventricle is cylindric, then tension is reduced by its relation to the square of the radius: $P \cdot \sqrt[2]{V}$. Deformation increases and efficiency improves as the ventricle anisotropically thickens and the chamber dimension narrows toward the apex.

SVR has also been shown to favorably alter the neurohumoral components that aggravate heart failure. Norepinepherine, angiotensin II, and plasma renin activity all fall after operation as a consequence of the reduced ventricular stretch [47]. The full extent of this recovery may be delayed for over 4 months because of the turnover of collagen [48].

Surgical ventricular restoration and helical fiber orientation

The helical architecture of the normal heart has been confirmed by strain relationships using MRI, by corrosion casts showing spiral architecture, and by sonomicrometry crystals [12–15]. Each pattern reflects the normal oblique fiber orientation that conveys maximum force during ejection and suction. The fiber orientation changes when dilation occurs because of flattening of the double helical arms of the apical loop. The principle underlying SVR is the reversal of abnormal cardiac architecture back to normal, thereby improving function.

Ventricular assist or replacement

Other surgical approaches in the treatment of ischemic cardiomyopathy include ventricular assist devices (LVAD) and transplantation. The recent Randomized Evaluation of Mechanical Assistance for the Treatment of Congestive Heart Failure (REMATCH) trial was designed to evaluate the suitability of LVAD as long-term myocardial replacement therapy in patients who were ineligible for cardiac transplantation. Patients were randomized to LVAD or optimal medical therapy. Although LVAD showed a 48% reduction in death compared with medical therapy, less than 10% of patients survived to 3 years in the LVAD treated group, compared with no survivors among patients treated medically [49]. Cardiac transplantation is another alternative in the management of these difficult patients and 5-year survival is 70% [50]. Lack of donors, however, remains a significant problem.

In summary, dilated cardiomyopathy is associated with morphologic changes in the ventricle; volume increases and there is a change in the shape of the heart from the normal conical structure into a spherical one. These changes directly affect global systolic function, mechanical efficiency, and arrhythmogenesis. The spherical shape may arise from ischemia, valve insufficiency, or myocyte disease. Surgical ventricular restoration supplements correction of vascular or valvular pathology by simultaneously addressing ventricular pathology to reshape the heart and improve functional ventricular performance.

References

[1] Hunt SA, Baker DW, Chin MH, et al. ACC/AHA Guidelines for the evaluation and management of chronic heart failure in the adult: executive summary a report of the American College of Cardiology/American Heart Association Task Force on Practice Guidelines (Committee to Revise the 1995 Guidelines for the evaluation and management of heart failure): developed in collaboration with the International Society for Heart and Lung Transplantation; endorsed by the Heart Failure Society of America. Circulation 2001;104:2996–3007.
[2] O'Connell JB. The economic burden of heart failure. Clin Cardiol 2000;23:III6–10.
[3] Gheorghiade M, Bonow RO. Chronic heart failure in the United States: a manifestation of coronary artery disease. Circulation 1998;97:282–9.
[4] Gaudron P, Eilles C, Kugler I, et al. Progressive left ventricular dysfunction and remodelling after myocardial infarction. Potential mechanisms and early predictors. Circulation 1993;87:755–62.
[5] Migrino RQ, Young JB, Ellis SG, et al. End-systolic volume index at 90 to 180 minutes into reperfusion therapy for acute myocardial infarction is a strong predictor of earlyl and late mortality. Circulation 1997;96:116–21.
[6] Mann DL. Left ventricular size and shape: determinants of mechanical signal transduction pathways. Heart Fail Rev 2005;10:95–100.
[7] Babuty D, Lab MJ. Mechanoelectric contributions to sudden cardiac death. Cardiovasc Res 2001;50:270–9.
[8] White HD, Norris RM, Brown MA, et al. Left ventricular end-systolic volume as the major determinant of survival after recovery from myocardial infarction. Circulation 1987;76:44–51.
[9] Robb JS, Robb RC. The normal heart: anatomy and physiology of the structural units. Am Heart J 1942;23:455–67.
[10] Krehl L. Kenntniss der fallung entleerung des herzens. Abhandl Math Phys 1891;29:341–62.
[11] Torrent-Guasp F, Ballester M, Buckberg GD, et al. Spatial orientation of the ventricular muscle band: physiologic contribution and surgical implications. J Thorac Cardiovasc Surg 2001;122:389–92.
[12] Gorodkov A, Dobrova NB, Dubernaud J, et al. Anatomic structures determining blood flow in the heart left ventricle. J Mater Sci Mater Med 1996;7:153–60.
[13] Jung B, Schneider B, Markl M, et al. Measurement of left ventricular velocities: phase contrast MRI velocity mapping versus tissue-doppler-ultrasound in healthy volunteers. J Cardiovasc Magn Reson 2004;6:777–83.
[14] Buckberg GD, Castella M, Gharib M, et al. Structure/function interface with sequential shortening of basal and apical components of the myocardial band. Eur J Cardiothorac Surg 2006;29(Suppl 1):S75–97.
[15] Jung BA, Kreher BW, Markl M, et al. Visualization of tissue velocity data from cardiac wall motion measurements with myocardial fiber tracking: principles and implications for cardiac fiber structures. Eur J Cardiothorac Surg 2006;29(Suppl 1):S158–64.
[16] Buckberg GD, Weisfeldt ML, Ballester M, et al. Left ventricular form and function: scientific priorities and strategic planning for development of new views of disease. Circulation 2004;110:e333–6.
[17] Ingels NB Jr. Myocardial fiber architecture and left ventricular function. Technol Health Care 1997;5:45–52.
[18] Sallin EA. Fiber orientation and ejection fraction in the human ventricle. Biophys J 1969;9:954–64.

[19] Bogaert J, Rademakers FE. Regional nonuniformity of normal adult human left ventricle. Am J Physiol Heart Circ Physiol 2001;280:H610–20.

[20] Di Donato M, Toso A, Dor V, et al. Surgical ventricular restoration improves mechanical intraventricular dyssynchrony in ischemic cardiomyopathy. Circulation 2004;109:2536–43.

[21] Douglas PS, Morrow R, Ioli A, et al. Left ventricular shape, afterload and survival in idiopathic dilated cardiomyopathy. J Am Coll Cardiol 1989;13:311–5.

[22] Brzezinska B, Loboz-Grudzien K, Sokalski L. Patterns of post-MI left ventricular volume changes–clinical implications. Kardiol Pol 2007;65:1190–8.

[23] Yokusoglu M, Uzun M, Baysan O, et al. Elongation index as a new index determining the severity of left ventricular systolic dysfunction and mitral regurgitation in patients with congestive heart failure. Echocardiography 2005;22:555–60.

[24] Suma H, Isomura T, Horii T, et al, the RESTORE Group. Role of site selection for left ventriculoplasty to treat idiopathic dilated cardiomyopathy. Heart Fail Rev 2005;9:329–36.

[25] Buckberg GD. Sudden cardiac death after heart failure; symptomatic versus disease treatment? An editorial comment. Heart Fail Rev 2004;9:347–51.

[26] Dor V, Sabatier M, Montiglio F, et al. Endoventricular patch reconstruction of ischemic failing ventricle. A single center with 20 years experience. Advantages of magnetic resonance imaging assessment. Heart Fail Rev 2004;9:269–86.

[27] Di Donato M, Sabatier M, Dor V, et al. Effects of Dor procedure on left ventricular dimension and shape and geometric correlates of mitral regurgitation one year after surgery. J Thorac Cardiovasc Surg 2001;121:91–6.

[28] Ascione R, Lim KH, Chamberlain M, et al. Early and late results of partial left ventriculectomy: single center experience and review of the literature. J Cardiovasc Surg 2003;18:190–6.

[29] Buckberg GD. Form versus disease: optimizing geometry during ventricular restoration. Eur J Cardiothorac Surg 2006;29(Suppl 1):S238–44.

[30] Athanasuleas CL, Buckberg GD, Stanley AW, et al. Surgical ventricular restoration in the treatment of congestive heart failure due to post-infarction ventricular dilation. J Am Coll Cardiol 2004;44:1439–45.

[31] Levy D, Kenchaiah S, Larson MG, et al. Long-term trends in the incidence of and survival with heart failure. N Engl J Med 2002;347:1397–402.

[32] Shah PJ, Hare DL, Raman JS, et al. Survival after myocardial revascularization for ischemic cardiomyopathy: a prospective ten-year follow-up study. J Thorac Cardiovasc Surg 2003;126:1320–7.

[33] Buckberg GD. Ventricular structure and surgical history. Heart Fail Rev 2004;9:255–68.

[34] Di Donato M, Toso A, Maioli M, et al. Intermediate survival and predictors of death after surgical ventricular restoration. Semin Thorac Cardiovasc Surg 2001;13:468–75.

[35] Sheehan FH, Schofer J, Mathey DG, et al. Measurement of regional wall motion from biplane contrast ventriculograms: a comparison of the 30 degree right anterior oblique and 60 degree left anterior oblique projections in patients with acute myocardial infarction. Circulation 1986;74:796–804.

[36] Mahrholdt H, Wagner A, Parker M, et al. Relationship of contractile function to transmural extent of infarction in patients with chronic coronary artery disease. J Am Coll Cardiol 2003;42:505–12.

[37] Klein MD, Herman MV, Gorlin R. A hemodynamic study of LV aneurysm. Circulation 1967;35:614–30.

[38] Pfeffer MA, Lamas GA, Vaughan DE, et al. Effect of captopril on progressive ventricular dilatation after anterior myocardial. N Engl J Med 1988;319:80–6.

[39] Bristow MR, Gilbert EM, Abraham WT, et al. Carvedilol produces dose-related improvements in left ventricular function and survival in subjects with chronic heart failure. MOCHA Investigators. Circulation 1996;94:2807–16.

[40] Di Donato M, Sabatier M, Toso A, et al. Regional myocardial performance of non-ischaemic zones remote from anterior wall left ventricular aneurysm. Eur Heart J 1995;16:1285–92.

[41] St John SM, Lee D, Rouleau JL, et al. Left ventricular remodeling and ventricular arrhythmias after myocardial infarction. Circulation 2003;107: 2577–82.

[42] DiDonato M, Sabatier M, Dor V, et al, RESTORE Group. Ventricular arrhythmias after LV remodeling: surgical ventricular restoration or ICD? Heart Fail Rev 2005;9:299–306.

[43] Moss AJ, Greenberg H, Case RB, et al. Long-term clinical course of patients after termination of ventricular tachyarrhythmia by an implanted defibrillator. Circulation 2004;110:3760–5.

[44] Kramer CM, Magovern JA, Rogers WJ, et al. Reverse remodeling and improved regional function after repair of left ventricular aneurysm. J Thorac Cardiovasc Surg 2002;123:700–6.

[45] Sartipy U, Anders ALD. Improved health-related quality of life and functional status after surgical ventricular restoration. Ann Thorac Surg 2007;83: 1381–7.

[46] Schenk S, McCarthy PM, Starling RC, et al. Neurohormonal response to left ventricular reconstruction surgery in ischemic cardiomyopathy 1021. J Thorac Cardiovasc Surg 2004;128:38–43.

[47] Caulfield JB, Janicki JS. Structure and function of myocardial fibrillar collagen. Technol Health Care 1997;5:95–113.

[48] Rose EA, Gelijns AC, Moskowitz AJ, et al. Long-term mechanical left ventricular assistance for end-stage heart failure. N Engl J Med 2001;345:1435–43.

[49] Keck BM, Bennett LE, Rosendale J, et al. World-wide thoracic organ transplantation: a report from the UNOS/ISHLT International Registry for Thoracic Organ Transplantation. Clin Transplant 1999;35–49.

ELSEVIER
SAUNDERS

Heart Failure Clin 4 (2008) 371–378

HEART FAILURE CLINICS

Computational Modeling for Bedside Application

Roy C.P. Kerckhoffs, PhD[a,*], Sanjiv M. Narayan, MD, FACC[b], Jeffrey H. Omens, PhD[a], Lawrence J. Mulligan, PhD[c], Andrew D. McCulloch, PhD[a]

[a]*University of California San Diego, La Jolla, CA, USA*
[b]*VA Medical Center, San Diego, CA, USA*
[c]*Medtronic Inc., Mounds View, MN, USA*

In the Physiome Project, integrative physiological function is described by computational modeling [1]. The project was motivated by the current wealth of biological data, especially by data from the molecular and cellular levels that are based, in part, on improved instrumentation such as nuclear magnetic resonsance and confocal microscopy. Improved imaging modalites such as MRI and CT, along with other types of instrumentation, are also producing data at higher levels of biology.

Various workshops and panel recommendations have recognized and addressed the importance in interpreting experimental multiscale results. The Multiscale Modeling Consortium, in conjunction with the Interagency Modeling and Analysis Group (comprised of members of several federal agencies), aim to promote the development and exchange of tools, models, data and standards for the multi-scale modeling community [2]. These goals also represent a major part of the mission of the Physiome Project [1]. Recently, the NSF blue ribbon panel recognized that simulation-based engineering science, [3] applied to the multiscale study of simulation based medicine, may lead further toward the realization of predictive, preventative, personalized, and participatory medicine [2].

During the last few decades, tremendous progress has been made in computer power, diagnostic and therapeutic medical technologies, and the knowledge of pathophysiology from gene to organ systems. When these advances are combined with efforts to create online databases and tools to share this knowledge, it is increasingly feasible to apply multiscale patient-specific modeling based on proven disease mechanisms to guide and predict the response to therapy in many aspects of medicine. This is an exciting and relatively new approach. These models will provide a better understanding of human physiology and, most importantly, will allow for predictive capabilities of surgery and therapy.

This work was supported by Medtronic Inc., UC Discovery Grant ITL06-10159 (to A.D.M.), a grant from the UCSD von Liebig Center for Entrepreneurship and Technology Advancement (to A.D.M.), the National Biomedical Computation Resource (NIH grant P41 RR08605) (to A.D.M), the National Science Foundation (BES-0506252) (to A.D.M), NIH grant HL83359 and a grant from the Doris Duke Clinical Foundation (to S.M.N), NIH grant HL32583 (to J.H.O.). This investigation was conducted in part using a facility constructed with support from Research Facilities Improvement Program Grant Number C06 RR-017588-01 from the National Center for Research Resources, National Institutes of Health.

Andrew McCulloch and Jeffrey Omens are cofounders of and consultants to Insilicomed Inc., a licensee of UCSD-owned software used in this research. Insilicomed was not involved in this research. Lawrence Mulligan is an employee of Medtronic.

* Corresponding author. Department of Bioengineering, The Whitaker Institute for Biomedical Engineering, University of California, San Diego, 9500 Gilman Drive, La Jolla, CA 92093-0412.

E-mail address: rkerckhoffs@ucsd.edu (R.C.P. Kerckhoffs).

1551-7136/08/$ - see front matter
doi:10.1016/j.hfc.2008.02.009

This article provides a brief overview of recent accomplishments. The requirements for accurate predictive patient-specific models are outlined. A patient-specific heart model for cardiac resynchronization therapy is described, briefly.

Computational modeling

A mathematical model is a description of a system in mathematical form; models are used extensively in physics and biophysics. For many such models, it is impossible to find an analytical mathematical solution. Computers can be used to obtain approximate solutions, numerically, and they are therefore usually referred to as computational models.

Many computational models of physiology are written in terms of (coupled) ordinary and/or partial differential equations (ODEs and/or PDEs). An ordinary differential equation is an equation of an unknown function (ie, the dependent variable) of an independent variable that relates the values of the function itself and of its derivatives of various orders. Differential equations are coupled when they share a common dependent variable. An example of a set of coupled ODEs is the description of the circulatory system, where changes in volumes and/or pressures in compartments of the circulatory system are described as a function of time [4]. A partial differential equation is an equation where a function depends on more than one variable. An example of a set of coupled PDEs in solid mechanics is the equation of motion, where stress (ie, the force per unit area) depends on three spatial dimensions and time. An example of a set of coupled PDEs in electrophysiology is the bidomain model, where intracellular and extracellular voltages are "solved for" as a function of space and time. The equation of motion and the bidomain model are examples of so-called "deterministic continuum models," where it is assumed that stochastic and discrete events are negligible [5].

Typically, it takes more computational effort to solve a PDE than it does to solve for an ODE, because of the diversity in possible solutions. Probably one of the best-known computational tools for solving PDEs is the finite element method. This method was mainly developed in the 1950s, to address the needs for methods in designing complex structures in civil engineering. The method is suitable for solving PDEs on complex domains, like the blood flow in the aorta, or a deformation in the heart. In the finite element method, a continuous domain is discretized into elements and nodes; the solution is approximated on the domain by linear or higher order functions, which are defined in the elements. For a basic explanation of the finite element method and its application in surgery, see Hashim and Richens (2006) [6]. For an in-depth explanation of the finite element method, see for example Bathe (1996) [7].

Because computational models quantify physiology mathematically, they also define working hypotheses that are testable, reproducible, and have already been used to improve our understanding of physiologic systems and disease [8]. In the cardiovascular system, computational models have been used to develop subsequently validated hypotheses on the role of repolarization dynamics in initiating life-threatening [9] as well as benign [9] rhythm disturbances. Furthermore, models have provided important insights into the electrophysiologic effects of defibrillation [10–12] and information about the electrical and mechanical impact of pacing normal [13–15] and failing [16–18] hearts (Fig. 1). Because detailed information on the ion channel kinetics of individual myocytes is now available [19], computational models can also suggest the cellular mechanisms underlying these disease states [20].

In the clinical arena, computational modeling has provided diagnostic indices [21,22], virtual surgery training platforms [23–26], and assessments of the effects of surgery [27–30].

Multiscale modeling

The need to model at multiple levels, both spatially and temporally, becomes clear by simply considering physiology: organisms consist of organs, which are made of different tissues; these tissues are made up of specialized connected cells; and within these cells complex biochemical processes take place, which can only take place because of the underlying protein kinetics and gene expressions. This is, of course, a simplified view on scalar organization because many more levels can be identified, ranging in size from nanometers at the molecule level to 1 m at the whole body level [1]. A strong interconnection exists between all levels: normal function at a given level depends on the underlying synergy of sublevels, but also on higher levels, when feedback mechanisms are considered. A significant disturbance at any level will affect normal function on a higher level, demonstrating the need for multiscale patient-specific models.

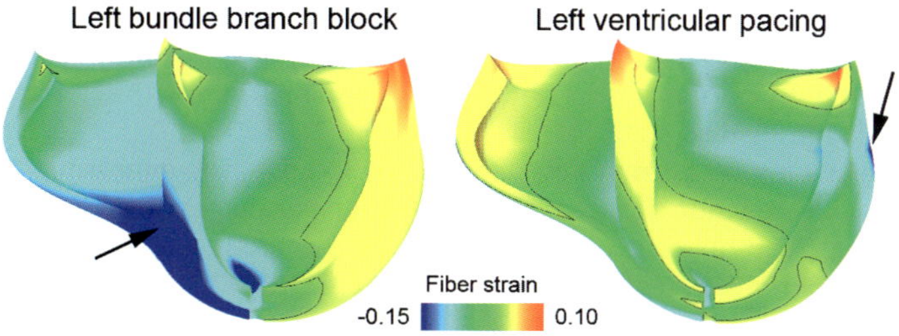

Fig. 1. Simulated isovolumic fiber strain (strain at opening of aortic valve with reference at end-diastole) in the ventricles for a failing canine heart, for left bundle branch block and pacing at the left ventricular free wall. Pacing sites are indicated by arrows. The black line in the ventricles indicates zero strain.

However, designing a multiscale model that encompasses all biophysical detail on all levels is an impossible task because of the enormous human effort and computer power required. Nonetheless, such a model would not be very useful because a model is a representation of reality designed to help people better understand that reality; a model should be focused on solving a specific problem. For a patient-specific model, efforts should be directed at the pathology in question.

A highly detailed physiologic model demands high computational effort. To reduce computational load, Crampin and colleagues [31], as well as Bassingthwaighte and colleagues [8], have acknowledged and addressed the need for simplified models at particular physiologic levels. Taking into account the tradeoff between physiologic—and thus, computational—complexity of the model and accuracy of the results, Bassingthwaighte and colleagues [8] proposed a strategy for the design of a multiscale model of physiologic systems. This strategy involves a six-step approach to design and validation of an initial high-resolution multiscale model. Specific components will be simplified in order to gain computational speed, but these simplified components will be kept within a specific valid range. If it is necessary, then inadequate components will be replaced by more detailed ones. The resultant multiscale model will then be validated again.

Mechanistic patient-specific modeling

Significance

The results of randomized clinical trials might not apply directly to individual patients, not even to those who participated in the trial [32]. Important differences exist between individuals in respective treatment groups; these differences can dramatically impact the likelihood of an individual benefiting from a specific therapy. Averaging the effects across different patients can give misleading results about the prospective treatment of an individual whose characteristics likely differ from the mean of a population. This problem is especially highlighted in children, where variability in dimensions is much greater than in adults [33,34].

Patient-specific regression models have been successful in identifying patients that would most likely benefit from a certain therapy [35,36]. However, one drawback of these types of models is that they may not provide much insight into pathophysiologic mechanisms in any specific individual. Modeling mechanistically from a biophysical base would not only provide predictions of certain therapies or surgical interventions, but also the modeling would also provide insight into the success (or failure) of these therapies and interventions.

Many important biophysical properties cannot be measured directly in patients although they can be quantitatively modeled. For example, stress (ie, force per unit area) cannot be measured accurately without damaging tissue. Assuming that stress is a key factor for a specific pathology, information on the dynamics and distribution of biophysical stress may shed light on: (1) cardiac mechanics because stress is closely related to cardiac oxygen consumption [37]; (2) the mechanics and likelihood of tissue rupture in vascular aneurysms [38–40], if stress exceeds a certain threshold; and (3) potential stimuli for growth and remodeling in soft tissues [41–43] and bone [44].

Requirements

Initial considerations for modeling should be focused on clinically relevant parameters. There could be more than one parameter used; for example, in the heart, cardiac output is an important measured parameter, yet cardiac output may remain normal due to compensatory mechanisms that mask the disease state [45]. In this way, cardiac output may be normal despite altered cardiac contractile function (ie, reduced ejection fraction) with high end-diastolic pressures in heart failure; dyssynchronous regional wall function, that independently predicts remodeling [46,47]; or valvular abnormalities. Computational modeling has the unique strength of being based on parameters that are not typically measurable (eg, stress), yet that are clinically important. An example is using a model to have prior knowledge of the distribution of stress in a residual limb that will be fitted with a prosthetic socket. With use of a model, stress distributions, which can cause pressure ulcers, can be prevented by optimizing the prosthesis [48].

Operationally, the patient-specific model should generate parameter output that will aid clinicians in their decision-making. The model should contain most key factors (ie, submodels at lower scales) that will influence the output parameter, but to maintain decent computability, the model should not become overly intricate. For example, an important parameter in predicting the outcome of cardiac resynchronization therapy (CRT) in patients with heart failure and wide QRS is mechanical synchrony of contraction in the ventricular walls. A patient-specific model of cardiac electromechanics for this disease and the related therapy may include ventricular geometry, fiber architecture, an impulse conduction model, passive and dynamic active mechanical properties, and a blood circulation model.

A patient-specific model needs input from the patient. As tomographic imaging (eg, CT, MRI) and image segmentation are important for obtaining information on geometric structures, obtaining material properties is equally important, preferably non-invasively. For patient-specific bone models, methods have been proposed and tested for obtaining a linear stress-strain relation of bone (ie, the Young's modulus) by converting Hounsfield units (a quantitative scale of radiodensity) by CT imaging [49,50]. For patient-specific cardiac models, methods have been proposed to estimate passive and contractile properties from tagged MR images [30,40,51,52] and cavity pressure measurements. With regard to the latter, methods aimed at deriving end-diastolic and end-systolic pressure-volume relations from single beats [53,54] can also be helpful in estimating material properties from these relations [30,40], but these methods should always be used in combination with data on regional shortening [55].

Because it is impossible to obtain all possible input parameters for each patient, existing data can be used for completion. For the patient-specific heart model previously described, cardiac fiber architecture will be obtained from the Johns Hopkins University's online datasets (http://www.ccbm.jhu.edu/research/dSets.php) and morphed into the patient-specific cardiac geometries, using the original data on a "host-mesh" [56]. Efforts to create more online databases and tools on biological organization, which is one of the goals of the Physiome Project [57], will help in this matter. Another possibility is to estimate parameter values with adaptation algorithms, for example, for bone density [44], cardiac fiber architecture [58], or circulation resistance [59]. A potential problem with these algorithms is that biological adaptation, on which the algorithms are based, might be part of the pathology: for example, in the case of cardiac fiber architecture, genetic defects can lead to fiber disarray [60]. Such a fiber-related pathology may render the adaptation algorithm to fall outside the range of validity.

Prediction

The next logical step in using a patient-specific model is to predict, and if necessary, optimize, outcomes from therapy or surgical interventions by applying appropriate interventions. These model interventions can be exactly the same as the intervention to be performed in reality, or to apply the effects, if known, of a particular intervention in a model. In cardiac surgery, an example of the former is to remove tissue in a cardiac ventricular model, exactly as performed in ventricular reduction surgery (ie, the Batista procedure) [28]. To study prostate thermal therapy, one may model acoustic signals to assess pelvic bone heating in the thermal ablation of the prostate [61]. An example of modeling intervention effects indirectly is constraining the motion of myocardium at two opposite regions in the left ventricle to investigate the influence of a myosplint on cardiac function and wall stress, without the need of having to model the physical contact between the myosplint and myocardium [29].

Predictions of the patient-specific models should be validated by comparison against clinical follow-up whenever possible. If model predictions and clinical follow-up are not congruent, several possibilities must be considered. First, components of the patient-specific model may be oversimplified. If so, these inadequate components should be replaced with more detailed models [8] that may require additional measurements. Second, the model may be based on an incomplete pathophysiologic understanding of the disease; additional theoretical or experimental studies may be needed to adequately revise the model.

For example, a model prediction may fail due to biological adaptation, especially in the long-term. Most existing models of interventions to patient-specific models are used to study acute output parameters, and they do not consider longer-term physiologic adaptation. Although acute parameters may accurately predict long-term outcome, the implementation of adaptation algorithms may enhance the predictive capabilities of patient-specific models after an intervention [41,43,44,59,62,63].

Examples of patient-specific modeling

Investigators have been working on the design of patient-specific models in almost all areas of human physiology, at many spatial levels including that of bone structures [56,63–66], skeletal muscle [67], brain [68,69], eye [70], tongue [71], teeth [72], lungs [73], heart [33,51,74], large arteries [38,39,75,76], and digestive system [77,78]. Modeled physics include electrophysiology, solid mechanics, fluid dynamics (gas and fluid), chemistry, thermal dynamics, and combinations of these. Efforts are also being made to model specific pathologies like cancer on the subcellular [79,80] and tissue levels [68,81].

Patient-specific modeling of dilated cardiomyopathy and CRT

The most significant recent advance in management of heart failure (HF) with a conduction block has come from CRT [82,83] and defibrillator [84] therapy. However, as many as 30% of currently eligible patients fail to respond to CRT. Notably, exact estimation of the percentage of non-responders and enumeration of factors predicting non-response are difficult because of the varying criteria used to define "response." These criteria include: improvements in the distance walked in 6 minutes in the peak oxygen utilization (VO_2 max) during exercise; and a decrease in left ventricular end-systolic volume (indicating that cardiac dilatation is reversing). Although these factors make it difficult to select optimal patients for CRT, optimal selection remains of paramount importance to reduce unnecessary implants, procedural risks, and health care expenses.

Because computational models of cardiac electromechanics are currently able to predict the effects of ventricular pacing on regional wall mechanics and global function [18,85,86], the authors of this article propose to develop new computational tools for optimally selecting patients for CRT and for optimizing CRT to each individual patient. Having acquired Institutional Review Board approval, two to five patients with New York Heart Association (NYHA) class III or IV will be recruited at the San Diego VA Medical Center. Implementing the strategy outlined above, investigators will develop patient-specific computational models of the human heart from detailed mapping and test the models' ability to predict observed short-term functional improvements after CRT. The clinical procedures that will be performed include: cardiac contrast CT to obtain ventricular geometry; electroanatomic mapping of both ventricles to obtain ventricular activation patterns during native (dyssynchronous) ventricular activation and during CRT; cardiac ultrasound to obtain dynamic ventricular (ie, pseudo-) volumes; and invasive dynamic pressure measurements during cardiac catheterization. Pressure-volume loops will be obtained during maneuvers to alter pre-load and afterload. Three and six month follow-ups will be performed to assess the long-term outcomes, to determine the predictive accuracy of our models, and also, to provide an opportunity for the patient-specific models to optimize CRT in a patient-tailored fashion.

In summary, efforts are being put in place to develop efficient methods and computational tools for the design of mechanistic multiscale patient-specific models on many levels of physiology. Combined with the abundance of physiological data, these models will be useful on a large scale in the clinic to predict outcomes of surgeries and therapies.

References

[1] Hunter PJ, Borg TK. Integration from proteins to organs: the Physiome Project. Nat Rev Mol Cell Biol 2003;4:237–43.

[2] Liao J-C, Reinbolt J, Kerckhoffs R, et al. Multiscale modeling and simulation session: from molecules to

cells to organisms. Pac Symp Biocomput 2008;13: 327–31.
[3] Oden JT, Belytschko T, Fish J, et al. Revolutionizing Engineering Science through Simulation, in National Science Foundation Blue Ribbon Panel on Simulation-Based Engineering Science: National Science Foundation, 2006.
[4] Lu K, Clark JW, Ghorbel FH, et al. A human cardiopulmonary system model applied to the analysis of the Valsalva maneuver. Am J Physiol Heart Circ Physiol 2001;281:H2661–79.
[5] Crampin EJ, Smith NP, Hunter PJ. Multi-scale modelling and the IUPS physiome project. J Mol Histol 2004;35:707–14.
[6] Hashim S, Richens D. Finite element method in cardiac surgery. Interact CardioVasc Thorac Surg 2006;5:5–8.
[7] Bathe K-J. Finite element procedures. Upper Saddle River (NJ): Prentice Hall, Inc.; 1996.
[8] Bassingthwaighte JB, Chizeck HJ, Atlas LE. Strategies and tactics in multiscale modeling of cell-to-organ systems. Proceedings of the IEEE 2006;94: 819–31.
[9] Weiss JN, Karma A, Shiferaw Y, et al. From pulsus to pulseless: the saga of cardiac alternans. Circ Res 2006;98:1244–53.
[10] Aguel F, Eason J, Trayanova N. Advances in modeling cardiac defibrillation. Int J Bifurcat Chaos 2003;13:3791–803.
[11] Rodriguez B, Tice BM, Eason JC, et al. Cardiac vulnerability to electric shocks during phase 1A of acute global ischemia. Heart Rhythm 2004;1: 695–703.
[12] Sambelashvili A, Efimov IR. Dynamics of virtual electrode-induced scroll-wave reentry in a 3D bidomain model. Am J Physiol Heart Circ Physiol 2004;287:H1570–81.
[13] Kerckhoffs RCP, Bovendeerd PHM, Prinzen FW, et al. Intra- and interventricular asynchrony of electromechanics in the ventricularly paced heart. J Eng Math 2003;47:201–16.
[14] Kerckhoffs RCP, Faris O, Bovendeerd PHM, et al. Electromechanics of paced left ventricle simulated by straightforward mathematical model: comparison with experiments. Am J Physiol Heart Circ Physiol 2005;289:H1889–97.
[15] Usyk TP, McCulloch AD. Relationship between regional shortening and asynchronous electrical activation in a three-dimensional model of ventricular electromechanics. J Cardiovasc Electrophysiol 2003;14:S196–202.
[16] Kerckhoffs RCP, Healy SN, Usyk TP, et al. Computational modeling of cardiac electromechanics. Proceedings of the IEEE 2006;94:769–83.
[17] Kerckhoffs RCP, McCulloch AD, Omens JH, et al. Effect of pacing site and infarct location on regional mechanics and global hemodynamics in a model based study of heart failure. Lect Notes Comput Sci 2007;4466:350–60.
[18] Usyk TP, McCulloch AD. Electromechanical model of cardiac resynchronization in the dilated failing heart with left bundle branch block. J Electrocardiol 2003;36:57–61.
[19] ten Tusscher KHWJ, Panfilov AV. Alternans and spiral breakup in a human ventricular tissue model. Am J Physiol Heart Circ Physiol 2006;291: H1088–100.
[20] Livshitz LM, Rudy Y. Regulation of Ca2+ and electrical alternans in cardiac myocytes: role of CAMKII and repolarizing currents. Am J Physiol Heart Circ Physiol 2007;292:H2854–66.
[21] Herz SL, Ingrassia CM, Homma S, et al. Parameterization of left ventricular wall motion for detection of regional ischemia. Ann Biomed Eng 2005;33: 912–9.
[22] Ingrassia CM, Usyk TP, Kerckhoffs RCP, et al. Model-based development of four-dimensional wall motion measures. Computer Methods in Applied Mechanics and Engineering 2007;196: 3061–9.
[23] Chiu AM, Dey D, Drangova M, et al. 3-D image guidance for minimally invasive robotic coronary artery bypass. Heart Surg Forum 2000;3:224–31.
[24] Coste-Maniere E, Adhami L, Mourgues F, et al. Planning, simulation, and augmented reality for robotic cardiac procedures: the STARS system of the ChIR team. Semin Thorac Cardiovasc Surg 2003;15:141–56.
[25] Friedl R, Preisack MB, Klas W, et al. Virtual reality and 3D visualizations in heart surgery education. Heart Surg Forum 2005;5:E17–21.
[26] Wierzbicki M, Drangova M, Guiraudon G, et al. Validation of dynamic heart models obtained using non-linear registration for virtual reality training, planning, and guidance of minimally invasive cardiac surgeries. Med Image Anal 2004;8:387–401.
[27] Dang ABC, Guccione JM, Zhang P, et al. Effect of ventricular size and patch stiffness in surgical anterior ventricular restoration: a finite element model study. Ann Thorac Surg 2005;79:185–93.
[28] Guccione JM, Moonly SM, Wallace AW, et al. Residual stress produced by ventricular volume reduction surgery has little effect on ventricular function and mechanics: a finite element model study. J Thorac Cardiovasc Surg 2001;122:592–9.
[29] Guccione JM, Salahieh A, Moonly SM, et al. Myosplint decreases wall stress without depressing function in the failing heart: a finite element model study. Ann Thorac Surg 2003;76:1171–80.
[30] Wall ST, Walker JC, Healy KE, et al. Theoretical impact of the injection of material into the myocardium: a finite element model simulation. Circulation 2006;114:2627–35.
[31] Crampin EJ, Halstead M, Hunter P, et al. Computational physiology and the physiome project. Exp Physiol 2004;89:1–26.
[32] Kent DM, Hayward RA. Limitations of applying summary results of clinical trials to individual

patients: the need for risk stratification. JAMA 2007; 298:1209–12.

[33] Jolley M, Triedman J, Westin C-F, et al. Image based modeling of defibrillation in children. In: Triedman J, editor. Engineering in Medicine and Biology Society, 2006. 28th Annual International Conference of the IEEE. p. 2564–7.

[34] Pekkan K, Frakes D, de Zelicourt D, et al. Coupling pediatric ventricle assist devices to the fontan circulation: simulations with a lumped-parameter model [Miscellaneous Article]. ASAIO J 2005;51:618–28.

[35] Selker HP, Griffith JL, Beshansky JR, et al. Patient-specific predictions of outcomes in myocardial infarction for real-time emergency use: a thrombolytic predictive instrument. Ann Intern Med 1997; 127:538–56.

[36] Visweswaran S, Cooper GF. Patient-Specific Models for Predicting the Outcomes of Patients with Community Acquired Pneumonia. AMIA Annu Symp Proc 2005;759–63.

[37] Hisano R, Cooper G. Correlation of force-length area with oxygen consumption in ferret papillary muscle. Circ Res 1987;61:318–28.

[38] Berguer R, Bull JL, Khanafer K. Refinements in mathematical models to predict aneurysm growth and rupture. Ann NY Acad Sci 2006;1085:110–6.

[39] Speelman L, Bohra A, Bosboom EMH, et al. Effects of wall calcifications in patient-specific wall stress analyses of abdominal aortic aneurysms. J Biomech Eng 2007;29:105–9.

[40] Walker JC, Ratcliffe MB, Zhang P, et al. MRI-based finite-element analysis of left ventricular aneurysm. Am J Physiol Heart Circ Physiol 2005;289: H692–700.

[41] Gleason RL, Humphrey JD. A mixture model of arterial growth and remodeling in hypertension: altered muscle tone and tissue turnover. J Vasc Res 2004;41:352–63.

[42] Kuhl E, Maas R, Himpel G, et al. Computational modeling of arterial wall growth. Biomech Model Mechanobiol 2007;6:321–31.

[43] Rodriguez EK, Hoger A, McCulloch AD. Stress-dependent finite growth in soft elastic tissues. J Biomech 1994;27:455–67.

[44] Huiskes R, Weinans H, Grootenboer HJ, et al. Adaptive bone-remodeling theory applied to prosthetic-design analysis. J Biomech 1987;20:1135–50.

[45] Starfinger C, Hann CE, Chase JG, et al. Model-based cardiac diagnosis of pulmonary embolism. Comput Methods Programs Biomed 2007;87:46–60.

[46] Jansen AHM, Bracke F, van Dantzig JM, et al. The influence of myocardial scar and dyssynchrony on reverse remodeling in cardiac resynchronization therapy. Eur J Echocardiogr 2007, in press.

[47] Yu C-M, Fung W-H, Lin H, et al. Predictors of left ventricular reverse remodeling after cardiac resynchronization therapy for heart failure secondary to idiopathic dilated or ischemic cardiomyopathy. Am J Cardiol 2002;91:684.

[48] Portnoy S, Yarnitzky G, Yizhar Z, et al. Real-time patient-specific finite element analysis of internal stresses in the soft tissues of a residual limb: a new tool for prosthetic fitting. Ann Biomed Eng 2007; 35:120–35.

[49] Cattaneo PM, Dalstra M, Frich LH. A three-dimensional finite element model from computed tomography data: a semi-automated method. Proc Inst Mech Eng [H] 2001;215:203–13.

[50] Diamant I, Shahar R, Masharawi Y, et al. A method for patient-specific evaluation of vertebral cancellous bone strength: in vitro validation. Clin Biomech 2007;22:282–91.

[51] Linte CA, Wierzbicki M, Aladl U, et al. Towards a Biomechanical-Based Method for Assessing Myocardial Tissue Viability. In: Engineering in Medicine and Biology Society, 2006. Annual International Conference of the IEEE. p. 2884–7.

[52] Sermesant M, Moireau P, Camara O, et al. Cardiac function estimation from MRI using a heart model and data assimilation: advances and difficulties. Med Image Anal 2006;10:642–56.

[53] Chen C-H, Fetics B, Nevo E, et al. Noninvasive single-beat determination of left ventricular end-systolic elastance in humans. J Am Coll Cardiol 2001;38:2028–34.

[54] Klotz S, Hay I, Dickstein ML, et al. Single beat estimation of the end-diastolic pressure-volume relationship: a novel method with the potential for noninvasive application. Am J Physiol Heart Circ Physiol 2006;291:H403–12.

[55] Kjorstad KE, Korvald C, Myrmel T. Pressure-volume-based single-beat estimations cannot predict left ventricular contractility in vivo. Am J Physiol Heart Circ Physiol 2002;282:H1739–50.

[56] Fernandez J, Hunter P. An anatomically based patient-specific finite element model of patella articulation: towards a diagnostic tool. Biomech Model Mechanobiol 2005;4:20–38.

[57] Hunter P, Robbins P, Noble D. The IUPS human physiome project. Pflügers Arch 2002;445:1–9.

[58] Arts T, Rijcken JM, Bovendeerd PHM, et al. Predicting myofiber direction in the cardiac wall by mathematical modeling. Faseb Journal 1999;13: A1076.

[59] Arts T, Delhaas T, Bovendeerd P, et al. Adaptation to mechanical load determines shape and properties of heart and circulation: the CircAdapt model. Am J Physiol Heart Circ Physiol 2005;288:H1943–54.

[60] Karlon WJ, McCulloch AD, Covell JW, et al. Regional dysfunction correlates with myofiber disarray in transgenic mice with ventricular expression of ras. Am J Physiol Heart Circ Physiol 2000;278: H898–906.

[61] Wootton JH, Ross AB, Diederich CJ. Prostate thermal therapy with high intensity transurethral ultrasound: the impact of pelvic bone heating on treatment delivery. Int J Hyperthermia 2007; 23:609–22.

[62] Kroon W, Delhaas T, Arts T, et al. Constitutive modeling of cardiac tissue growth. Lect Notes Comput Sci 2007;4466:340–9.
[63] Lengsfeld M, Burchard R, Günther D, et al. Femoral strain changes after total hip arthroplasty—patient-specific finite element analyses 12 years after operation. Med Eng Phys 2005;27:649–54.
[64] Anderson DD, Goldsworthy JK, Li W, et al. Physical validation of a patient-specific contact finite element model of the ankle. J Biomech 2007;40:1662–9.
[65] Matthews F, Messmer P, Raikov V, et al. Patient-specific three-dimensional composite bone models for teaching and operation planning. J Digit Imaging; [Epub ahead of print].
[66] Kessler O, Stefan W, Mayr E, et al. D'Lima, Bony impingement affects range of motion after total hip arthroplasty: a subject-specific approach. J Orthop Res 2008;26:443–52.
[67] Reinbolt JA, Haftka RT, Chmielewski TL, et al. A computational framework to predict post-treatment outcome for gait-related disorders. Med Eng Phys 2007, in press.
[68] Hogea C, Davatzikos C, Biros G. An image-driven parameter estimation problem for a reaction-diffusion glioma growth model with mass effects. J Math Biol 2007;56:793–825.
[69] Wittek A, Miller K, Kikinis R, et al. Patient-specific model of brain deformation: Application to medical image registration. Journal of biomechanics 2007; 40:919–29.
[70] Sakamoto JA, Barrett HH, Goncharov AV. Inverse optical design of the human eye using likelihood methods and wavefront sensing. Opt. Express 2008;16:304–14.
[71] Buchaillard S, Brix M, Perrier P, et al. Simulations of the consequences of tongue surgery on tongue mobility: implications for speech production in post-surgery conditions. Int J Med Robot 2007;3: 252–61.
[72] Magne P. Efficient 3D finite element analysis of dental restorative procedures using micro-CT data [official publication of the Academy of Dental Materials]. Dent Mater 2007;23:539–48.
[73] De Backer JW, Vos WG, Gorle CD. Flow analyses in the lower airways: patient-specific model and boundary conditions. Med Eng Phys 2008, in press.
[74] Saber NR, Wood NB, Gosman AD, et al. Progress towards patient-specific computational flow modeling of the left heart via combination of magnetic resonance imaging with computational fluid dynamics. Ann Biomed Eng 2003;31:42–52.
[75] Hunter KS, Lanning CJ, Chen S-YJ, et al. Simulations of congenital septal defect closure and reactivity testing in patient-specific models of the pediatric pulmonary vasculature: a 3D numerical study with fluid-structure interaction. J Biomech Eng 2006; 128:564–72.
[76] Wolters BJBM, Rutten MCM, Schurink GWH, et al. A patient-specific computational model of fluid-structure interaction in abdominal aortic aneurysms. Med Eng Phys 2005;27:871–83.
[77] Buist ML, Cheng LK, Yassi R, et al. An anatomical model of the gastric system for producing bioelectric and biomagnetic fields. Physiol Meas 2004;25: 849–61.
[78] Schöber W, Kopp A, Scherf C, et al. Clinical evaluation of a computer simulated prediction model of contrast enhancement of the liver in spiral CT. Eur J Radiol 2004;51:19–26.
[79] de Pillis LG, Radunskaya AE, Wiseman CL. A validated mathematical model of cell-mediated immune response to tumor growth. Cancer Res 2005;65: 7950–8.
[80] Ruths DA, Nakleh L, Iyengar MS, et al. Hypothesis generation in signaling networks. J Comput Biol 2006;13:1546–57.
[81] Cristini V, Lowengrub J, Nie Q. Nonlinear simulation of tumor growth. J Math Biol 2003;46:191–224.
[82] Bristow MR, Saxon LA, Boehmer J, et al. Cardiac-resynchronization therapy with or without an implantable defibrillator in advanced chronic heart failure. N Engl J Med 2004;350:2140–50.
[83] Cleland JGF, Daubert J, Erdmann E, et al. The effect of cardiac resynchronization on morbidity and mortality in heart failure. N Engl J Med 2005; 352:1539–49.
[84] Josephson M, Wellens HJJ. Implantable defibrillators and sudden cardiac death. Circulation 2004; 109:2685–91.
[85] Kerckhoffs RCP, Lumens J, Vernooy K, et al. Cardiac Resynchronization: insight from experimental and computational models. Prog Biophys Mol Biol 2008;[epub ahead of print].
[86] Nickerson D, Nash M, Nielsen P, et al. Computational multiscale modeling in the UPS physiome project: modeling cardiac electromechanics. IBM Journal of Research and Development 2006;50: 617–30.

ELSEVIER
SAUNDERS

Heart Failure Clin 4 (2008) 379–382

HEART
FAILURE
CLINICS

Reclassifying Heart Failure: Predominantly Subendocardial, Subepicardial, and Transmural

Partho P. Sengupta, MD[a], Jagat Narula, MD, PhD[b,*]

[a]*Mayo Clinic, Scottsdale, AZ, USA*
[b]*University of California Irvine, Irvine, CA, USA*

"Everything should be made as simple as possible, but not more so."

—Albert Einstein

Heart failure remains a major public health burden in the United States. Approximately 5 million people sustain chronic heart failure, and 500,000 new patients are diagnosed with heart failure every year [1,2]. Timely recognition, classification, and grading of heart failure require a robust and practical algorithm. Whereas the classification by the World Health Organization has focused primarily on the etiologic and pathogenetic factors [3], the recent American College of Cardiology/American Heart Association (ACC/AHA) guidelines for chronic heart failure [4] emphasize the development and progression of disease (Table 1). The classification based on the clinical manifestations has customarily described heart failure by the left ventricular ejection fraction (LVEF) in two distinct forms: (1) diastolic heart failure or (2) heart failure with preserved LV function and systolic heart failure. Such classification is somewhat reminiscent of the distinction between backward and forward cardiac failure emphasized in the mid-twentieth century. A broader look at the heart failure population suggests that such demarcation is artificial because heart failure consists of a continuous spectrum wherein systolic and diastolic abnormalities are inseparable [6–9].

This review proposes a framework for describing heart failure using a combination of symptoms and patterns of aberrant myocardial mechanics that are discerned through noninvasive cardiac imaging techniques. We believe this approach can identify cohorts of patients with similar presentations, prognosis, and response to therapeutic interventions. One can classify the pathophysiology of heart failure into three broad subgroups: (1) heart failure with predominant subendocardial dysfunction, (2) heart failure with predominant subepicardial dysfunction, and (3) heart failure with transmural dysfunction (Table 2). This classification scheme corresponds to the structural and functional subunits of the left ventricle that govern the normal ejection and suction performance of a beating heart. The counterdirectional right- and left-handed helical myofiber geometry of the subendocardial and subepicardial regions support two fundamental forms of muscle action that work in close rhythmic balance [10–13]. To better describe this continuum of action, we use the structural analogy of natural vortex patterns [10]. The inside core of vortex swirls inwards and downwards, gathering implosive suction energy by centripetal action. The outer core expels and disburses energy upwards and outwards simultaneously by centrifugal action. For example, stirring cream in a cup of coffee leaves an inward swirl with aggregation and dissolution in the center while an outward expansion and separation occurs in an opposite direction. The suction and expulsion processes of a vortex motion occur in different regions yet are interlinked. The diastolic and systolic performance of the LV depends on the functional integrity of the subendocardial and subepicardial regions but is coupled

* Corresponding author. Division of Cardiology, University of California Irvine School of Medicine, 101 The City Drive, Building 53, Mail Route 81, Orange, CA 92705.

E-mail address: narula@uci.edu (J. Narula).

1551-7136/08/$ - see front matter
doi:10.1016/j.hfc.2008.03.013

Table 1
Progression of cardiomyopathy

At risk for cardiomyopathy or heart failure (no structural disease)	Asymptomatic cardiomyopathy (structural heart disease)	Symptomatic cardiomyopathy
Stage A[a]	Stage B[a]	Stage C and stage D[a]
Stage 1[b]	Stage 2[b]	Stage 3[b]
Normal subendocardial and subepicardial function	Subendocardial, subepicardial, or transmural dysfunction	Subendocardial, subepicardial, or transmural dysfunction

[a] American College of Cardiology/American Heart Association diagnosis and management of chronic heart failure in the adult [4].

[b] Heart Failure Society of America definition, classification, and staging of adult cardiomyopathies: proposal for revision [5].

synergistically. If the subendocardial region is affected, the outcome predominantly affects the suction performance, although ejection is still maintained with compensation offered from the outer subepicardial region. If compensation is not possible due to concomitant dysfunction of the subepicardial region, expulsion dynamics are reduced and the LV dilates.

Noninvasive techniques such as MRI and echocardiography are useful for understanding LV longitudinal and circumferential dynamics in clinical settings. Observational data regarding the utility of characterizing transmural mechanics in clinical settings are rapidly accumulating.

Heart failure with predominant subendocardial dysfunction

Most progressive myocardial diseases, including coronary ischemia, have been shown to cause subendocardial dysfunction. This dysfunction results in an early preferential involvement of longitudinal LV mechanics [14]. The timing of contraction-relaxation crossover is the most vulnerable period of myofiber mechanics [15,16]. In early stages, ventricular relaxation either regionally or globally becomes abnormally slow and impaired with a progressive delay in the timing of onset of relaxation. The epicardial function which governs the circumferential strain and twist mechanics of the LV remains either normal or shows an exaggerated compensation. Compensatory features such as myocardial hypertrophy of the subepicardial region attempt to reduce subendocardial stress, thereby preserving the global LVEF [17]. Interestingly, hearts undergoing regression of cardiac hypertrophy show marked apoptosis within the subepicardial region, which supports the hypothesis that changes within the subepicardial region in hypertrophied heart may, indeed, reflect a compensatory mechanism [18].

Progressive remodeling of the subepicardium and loss of cardiac muscle resilience by fibrosis result in gradual loss of early diastolic longitudinal relaxation and a delay in LV untwisting. These changes are accompanied by elevation of LV filling pressures and the appearance of varying grades of diastolic dysfunction. This stage manifests clinically as heart failure with preserved systolic function.

Heart failure with predominant subepicardial dysfunction

Predominant subepicardial myofiber dysfunction has been shown to manifest with loss of

Table 2
Classification of cardiac mechanics in heart failure

Functional impairment	Longitudinal mechanics	Circumferential mechanics	Torsional mechanics	Global EF	Diastolic filling pressures	Clinical syndrome
Predominant subendocardial dysfunction	Impaired	Preserved	Preserved	Preserved	Elevated	Diastolic HF/ HENEF
Predominant subepicardial dysfunction	Preserved	Impaired	Impaired	Preserved	Elevated	Diastolic HF, HENEF
Transmural dysfunction	Impaired	Impaired	Impaired	Impaired	Elevated	Systolic HF

Abbreviations: EF, ejection fraction; HF, heart failure; HFNEF, heart failure and normal ejection fraction.

cardiac circumferential strain and LV twist. For example, pericardial diseases cause subepicardial tethering and predominant loss of circumferential strain and LV twist mechanics while relatively sparing subendocardial function [19]. Normal twist results in storage of potential energy. This energy is used for LV diastolic recoil and contributes to ventricular suction and early diastolic filling [20]. Loss of early diastolic untwisting mechanics leads to reduced LV suction and progressive elevation in diastolic filling pressures. The subendocardial region remains unaffected and attempts to compensate, maintaining the overall LVEF.

Heart failure with transmural dysfunction

Progressive myocardial diseases with marked transmural involvement result in concomitant subendocardial and subepicardial dysfunction. This dysfunction results in attenuation of the longitudinal and circumferential mechanics of the LV [21,22]. Circumferential shortening of the LV has a key role in LV ejection performance [12]. Progressive loss of LV circumferential shortening impairs LV ejection performance, resulting in LV dilatation and systolic heart failure. An acute transmural infarction also has been shown to result in simultaneous impairment of LV longitudinal and circumferential mechanics, resulting in LV systolic dysfunction.

Correlates of myocardial mechanics at the subcellular level

The proposal that transmural mechanics may better define the spectrum of myocardial dysfunction in heart failure is supported by experimental observations that show the existence of marked subcellular and receptor differences in the subendocardial and subepicardial regions. For example, norepinephrine uptake is significantly diminished in the subendocardium compared with subepicardial myocyte regions due to a significant reduction of beta receptors in the subendocardium but not subepicardium [23]. Likewise, cAMP and phosphodiesterase activities are significantly decreased in endocardial but not epicardial layers [24]. A marked transmural gradient in sarcoplasmic reticulum Ca ATPase (SERCA2a) is also seen, with levels significantly reduced in the subendocardial region. On the contrary, the Na-Ca exchanger gradient that is normally higher in the epicardium and lower in the endocardium is reversed [25]. Rat models of cardiac hypertrophy have also shown shifts in the V-myosin isoform that occur most evidently in subendocardium [25]. Overall, these findings indicate that the subendocardium is affected most by structural and functional alterations. This observation would be consistent with studies that have reported an early onset of diastolic dysfunction due to loss of subendocardial long axis function while the subepicardial function and global LVEF remain relatively unchanged [26]. Long-term metoprolol therapy is associated with an increase in myocardial beta receptor density in the subendocardium. This increase results in a significant improvement in LV long axis function, even before changes in global LVEF have appeared [27]. Furthermore, it has been shown that decreased tissue Doppler velocity is significantly related to decreased beta receptor density [28].

In summary, technologic innovations in cardiac imaging have provided new mechanistic insights for understanding the phenotypic diversity of heart failure syndromes. The application of new algorithms for classifying the transmural extent of myocardial dysfunction based on longitudinal and circumferential myocardial mechanics may provide a useful clinical measure for early recognition of a subclinical state that is likely to progress to either systolic or diastolic heart failure. New techniques for the characterization of LV transmural mechanics hold great promise for improving the quality of care for the growing population of patients who have heart failure.

References

[1] Rosamond W, Flegal K, Furie K, et al. Heart disease and stroke statistics–2008 update: a report from the American Heart Association Statistics Committee and Stroke Statistics Subcommittee. Circulation 2008;117:e25–146.
[2] Redfield MM, Jacobsen SJ, Burnett JC Jr, et al. Burden of systolic and diastolic ventricular dysfunction in the community: appreciating the scope of the heart failure epidemic. J Am Med Assoc 2003;289:194–202.
[3] Richardson P, McKenna W, Bristow M, et al. Report of the 1995 World Health Organization/International Society and Federation of Cardiology task force on the definition and classification of cardiomyopathies. Circulation 1996;93:841–2.
[4] Hunt SA. ACC/AHA 2005 guideline update for the diagnosis and management of chronic heart failure in the adult: a report of the American College of Cardiology/American Heart Association Task Force on

practice guidelines (writing committee to update the 2001 guidelines for the evaluation and management of heart failure). J Am Coll Cardiol 2005;46:e1–82.
[5] Giles TD, Chatterjee K, Cohn JN, et al. Definition, classification, and staging of the adult cardiomyopathies: a proposal for revision. J Card Fail 2004;10: 6–8.
[6] De Keulenaer GW, Brutsaert DL. Diastolic heart failure: a separate disease or selection bias? Prog Cardiovasc Dis 2007;49:275–83.
[7] Brutsaert DL. Cardiac dysfunction in heart failure: the cardiologist's love affair with time. Prog Cardiovasc Dis 2006;49:157–81.
[8] Maurer MS, Spevack D, Burkhoff D, et al. Diastolic dysfunction: can it be diagnosed by Doppler echocardiography? J Am Coll Cardiol 2004;44: 1543–9.
[9] Geske JB, Sorajja P, Nishimura RA, et al. Evaluation of left ventricular filling pressures by Doppler echocardiography in patients with hypertrophic cardiomyopathy: correlation with direct left atrial pressure measurement at cardiac catheterization. Circulation 2007;116:2702–8.
[10] Sengupta PP, Korinek J, Belohlavek M, et al. Left ventricular structure and function: basic science for cardiac imaging. J Am Coll Cardiol 2006;48: 1988–2001.
[11] Sengupta PP, Khandheria BK, Korinek J, et al. Apex-to-base dispersion in regional timing of left ventricular shortening and lengthening. J Am Coll Cardiol 2006;47:163–72.
[12] Sengupta PP, Krishnamoorthy VK, Korinek J, et al. Left ventricular form and function revisited: applied translational science to cardiovascular ultrasound imaging. J Am Soc Echocardiogr 2007;20:539–51.
[13] Sengupta PP, Khandheria BK, Korinek J, et al. Left ventricular isovolumic flow sequence during sinus and paced rhythms: new insights from use of high-resolution Doppler and ultrasonic digital particle imaging velocimetry. J Am Coll Cardiol 2007;49: 899–908.
[14] Vinereanu D, Nicolaides E, Tweddel AC, et al. "Pure" diastolic dysfunction is associated with long-axis systolic dysfunction: implications for the diagnosis and classification of heart failure. Eur J Heart Fail 2005;7:820–8.
[15] Pouleur H. Diastolic dysfunction and myocardial energetics. Eur Heart J 1990;11(Suppl C):30–4.
[16] Abe T, Ohga Y, Tabayashi N, et al. Left ventricular diastolic dysfunction in type 2 diabetes mellitus model rats. Am J Physiol Heart Circ Physiol 2002; 282:H138–48.
[17] Zhang J. Myocardial energetics in cardiac hypertrophy. Clin Exp Pharmacol Physiol 2002;29:351–9.
[18] Tea BS, Dam TV, Moreau P, et al. Apoptosis during regression of cardiac hypertrophy in spontaneously hypertensive rats: temporal regulation and spatial heterogeneity. Hypertension 1999;34:229–35.
[19] Sengupta PP, Krishnamoorthy VK, Abhayaratna W, et al. Disparate patterns of left ventricular mechanics differentiate constrictive pericarditis from restrictive cardiomyopathy. J Am Coll Cardiol Img 2008;1:29–38.
[20] Narula J, Vannan MA, DeMaria AN. Of that waltz in my heart. J Am Coll Cardiol 2007;49:917–20.
[21] Tibayan FA, Lai DT, Timek TA, et al. Alterations in left ventricular curvature and principal strains in dilated cardiomyopathy with functional mitral regurgitation. J Heart Valve Dis 2003;12:292–9.
[22] Takeuchi M, Nishikage T, Nakai H, et al. The assessment of left ventricular twist in anterior wall myocardial infarction using two-dimensional speckle tracking imaging. J Am Soc Echocardiogr 2007;20:36–44.
[23] Beau SL, Tolley TK, Saffitz JE. Heterogeneous transmural distribution of beta-adrenergic receptor subtypes in failing human hearts. Circulation 1993; 88:2501–9.
[24] Sato N, Asai K, Okumura S, et al. Mechanisms of desensitization to a PDE inhibitor (milrinone) in conscious dogs with heart failure. Am J Physiol Heart Circ Physiol 1999;276:H1699–705.
[25] Prestle J, Dieterich S, Preuss M, et al. Heterogeneous transmural gene expression of calcium-handling proteins and natriuretic peptides in the failing human heart. Cardiovasc Res 1999;43:323–31.
[26] Lumens J, Delhaas T, Arts T, et al. Impaired subendocardial contractile myofiber function in asymptomatic aged humans, as detected using MRI. Am J Physiol Heart Circ Physiol 2006;291: H1573–9.
[27] Gruner Svealv B, Tang MS, Waagstein F, et al. Pronounced improvement in systolic and diastolic ventricular long axis function after treatment with metoprolol. Eur J Heart Fail 2007;9:678–83.
[28] Shan K, Bick RJ, Poindexter BJ, et al. Relation of tissue Doppler derived myocardial velocities to myocardial structure and beta-adrenergic receptor density in humans. J Am Coll Cardiol 2000;36: 891–6.

ELSEVIER
SAUNDERS

Heart Failure Clin 4 (2008) 383–386

HEART
FAILURE
CLINICS

Index

Note: Page numbers of article titles are in **boldface** type.

1551-7136/08/$ - see front matter
doi:10.1016/S1551-7136(08)00084-6

N

P

Q

R

S

T

V

X